The English physician enlarged with three hundred and sixty-nine medicines, made [of] English herbs, that were not in any impression until this. Being an astrologo-physical discourse of the vulgar herbs of this nation, ... By Nich. Culpepper. ...

Nicholas Culpeper

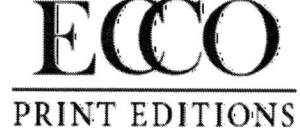

The English physician enlarged with three hundred and sixty-nine medicines, made [of] English herbs, that were not in any impression until this. Being an astrologo-physical discourse of the vulgar herbs of this nation, ... By Nich. Culpepper. ...
Culpeper, Nicholas
ESTCID: T136624
Reproduction from British Library

London : printed for the booksellers, 1785.
[12],345,[3]p. ; 12°

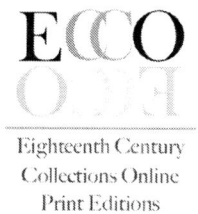

Eighteenth Century
Collections Online
Print Editions

Gale ECCO Print Editions

Relive history with *Eighteenth Century Collections Online*, now available in print for the independent historian and collector. This series includes the most significant English-language and foreign-language works printed in Great Britain during the eighteenth century, and is organized in seven different subject areas including literature and language; medicine, science, and technology; and religion and philosophy. The collection also includes thousands of important works from the Americas.

The eighteenth century has been called "The Age of Enlightenment." It was a period of rapid advance in print culture and publishing, in world exploration, and in the rapid growth of science and technology – all of which had a profound impact on the political and cultural landscape. At the end of the century the American Revolution, French Revolution and Industrial Revolution, perhaps three of the most significant events in modern history, set in motion developments that eventually dominated world political, economic, and social life.

In a groundbreaking effort, Gale initiated a revolution of its own: digitization of epic proportions to preserve these invaluable works in the largest online archive of its kind. Contributions from major world libraries constitute over 175,000 original printed works. Scanned images of the actual pages, rather than transcriptions, recreate the works *as they first appeared.*

Now for the first time, these high-quality digital scans of original works are available via print-on-demand, making them readily accessible to libraries, students, independent scholars, and readers of all ages.

For our initial release we have created seven robust collections to form one the world's most comprehensive catalogs of 18th century works.

Initial Gale ECCO Print Editions collections include:

History and Geography
Rich in titles on English life and social history, this collection spans the world as it was known to eighteenth-century historians and explorers. Titles include a wealth of travel accounts and diaries, histories of nations from throughout the world, and maps and charts of a world that was still being discovered. Students of the War of American Independence will find fascinating accounts from the British side of conflict.

Social Science
Delve into what it was like to live during the eighteenth century by reading the first-hand accounts of everyday people, including city dwellers and farmers, businessmen and bankers, artisans and merchants, artists and their patrons, politicians and their constituents. Original texts make the American, French, and Industrial revolutions vividly contemporary.

Medicine, Science and Technology
Medical theory and practice of the 1700s developed rapidly, as is evidenced by the extensive collection, which includes descriptions of diseases, their conditions, and treatments. Books on science and technology, agriculture, military technology, natural philosophy, even cookbooks, are all contained here.

Literature and Language
Western literary study flows out of eighteenth-century works by Alexander Pope, Daniel Defoe, Henry Fielding, Frances Burney, Denis Diderot, Johann Gottfried Herder, Johann Wolfgang von Goethe, and others. Experience the birth of the modern novel, or compare the development of language using dictionaries and grammar discourses.

Religion and Philosophy
The Age of Enlightenment profoundly enriched religious and philosophical understanding and continues to influence present-day thinking. Works collected here include masterpieces by David Hume, Immanuel Kant, and Jean-Jacques Rousseau, as well as religious sermons and moral debates on the issues of the day, such as the slave trade. The Age of Reason saw conflict between Protestantism and Catholicism transformed into one between faith and logic -- a debate that continues in the twenty-first century.

Law and Reference
This collection reveals the history of English common law and Empire law in a vastly changing world of British expansion. Dominating the legal field is the *Commentaries of the Law of England* by Sir William Blackstone, which first appeared in 1765. Reference works such as almanacs and catalogues continue to educate us by revealing the day-to-day workings of society.

Fine Arts
The eighteenth-century fascination with Greek and Roman antiquity followed the systematic excavation of the ruins at Pompeii and Herculaneum in southern Italy; and after 1750 a neoclassical style dominated all artistic fields. The titles here trace developments in mostly English-language works on painting, sculpture, architecture, music, theater, and other disciplines. Instructional works on musical instruments, catalogs of art objects, comic operas, and more are also included.

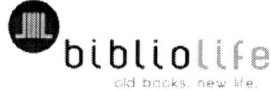

The BiblioLife Network

This project was made possible in part by the BiblioLife Network (BLN), a project aimed at addressing some of the huge challenges facing book preservationists around the world. The BLN includes libraries, library networks, archives, subject matter experts, online communities and library service providers. We believe every book ever published should be available as a high-quality print reproduction; printed on-demand anywhere in the world. This insures the ongoing accessibility of the content and helps generate sustainable revenue for the libraries and organizations that work to preserve these important materials.

The following book is in the "public domain" and represents an authentic reproduction of the text as printed by the original publisher. While we have attempted to accurately maintain the integrity of the original work, there are sometimes problems with the original work or the micro-film from which the books were digitized. This can result in minor errors in reproduction. Possible imperfections include missing and blurred pages, poor pictures, markings and other reproduction issues beyond our control. Because this work is culturally important, we have made it available as part of our commitment to protecting, preserving, and promoting the world's literature.

GUIDE TO FOLD-OUTS MAPS and OVERSIZED IMAGES

The book you are reading was digitized from microfilm captured over the past thirty to forty years. Years after the creation of the original microfilm, the book was converted to digital files and made available in an online database.

In an online database, page images do not need to conform to the size restrictions found in a printed book. When converting these images back into a printed bound book, the page sizes are standardized in ways that maintain the detail of the original. For large images, such as fold-out maps, the original page image is split into two or more pages

Guidelines used to determine how to split the page image follows:

- Some images are split vertically; large images require vertical and horizontal splits.
- For horizontal splits, the content is split left to right.
- For vertical splits, the content is split from top to bottom.
- For both vertical and horizontal splits, the image is processed from top left to bottom right.

THE
English Physician
ENLARGED

With Three Hundred and Sixty Nine

MEDICINES,

MADE of

English Herbs,

That were not in any Impression until This.

BEING

An *Astrologo-Physical* Discourse of the Vulgar Herbs of this Nation, containing a complete Method of Physic, whereby a Man may preserve his Body in Health, or cure himself, being Sick, for Three pence Charge, with such Things only as grow in England, they being most fit for English Bodies.

Herein is also shewed,

1. The Way of making Plasters, Ointments, Oils, Poultices, Syrups, Decoctions, Juleps, or Waters of all Sorts of Physical Herbs, that you may have them ready for your Use at all Times of the Year — 2. What Planet governeth every Herb or Tree (used in *Physic*) that groweth in England 3. The Time of gathering all Herbs, both Vulgarly and Astrologically — 4. The Way of drying and keeping the Herbs all the Year — 5. The Way of keeping their Juice ready for Use at all Times — 6. The Way of making and keeping all Kinds of Useful Compounds made of Herbs — 7. The Way of mixing Medicines according to the Cause and Mixture of the Disease and Part of the Body afflicted.

By NICH. CULPEPPER Gent.

STUDENT in Physic and Astrology.

LONDON

Printed for the Booksellers

An Alphabetical TABLE of all the HERBS and PLANTS in this BOOK; also what PLANET governeth every one of them.

AMARA dulcis, it is under Mercury Page 1
All Heal, it is under the dominion of Mars 2
Alkanet, it is under the dominion of Venus 3
Adders Tongue, it is under the Moon in Cancer 4
Agrimony, it is under Jupiter, and the sign Cancer 5
Water Agrimony, it is under Jupiter, and the sign Cancer 7
Alehoof, it is under Venus 8
Alexander, or Alisander, it is under Jupiter 9
Black Alder Tree, it is under Venus 10
Common Alder Tree, it is under Venus 11
Angelica, it is under the Sun in Leo 12
Amaranthus, it is under the dominion of Saturn 14
Anemone, it is under Mars 15
Garden Arrach, it is under the Moon 17
Arrach, wild and stinking, it is under the dominion of Venus and the sign Scorpio 16
Archangel, red, white yellow, they are under Venus 17
Arsmart, and Dead Arsmart, it is under Saturn and the other sorts under Mars 19
Asarabacca, it is under Mars 20
Asparagus and prickly Sparagus, are under Jupiter 22
Artichokes, are under Venus 144

Ash Tree, it is governed by the Sun 23
Avens, is under Jupiter 24
Arum, see Cuckow-pint
Alecoft, see Costmary
Aparine, see Clever
Acanthus, see Brank Ursine
Ammi and Ammios, see Bishop's weed

B

Balm is an herb of Jupiter 25
Barbary, it is under Mars 26
Barley, it is a notable plant of Saturn 27
Garden Basil, or Sweet Basil, is an herb of Mars and under the sign Scorpio 27
The Bay Tree is a tree of the Sun under the sign Leo 28
Beans are under Venus 30
French beans belong to V. 31
Ladies Bedstraw, it is under Venus 32
Beets, the red under Saturn, and the white under Jupiter 33
Water Betony, called also Brown Wort, and Bishop's Leaves, it is an herb of Jupiter 34
Wood Betony is appropriated to Jupiter and the sign Aries 35
Beech Tree, it is under Sat. 37
Bilberries is under Jupiter 38
Bifoyl is a plant of Saturn 38
Birch Tree is under Venus ib.
Birds-foot belongs to Saturn 40
Bishop's Weed, or Bulwort, is under Venus ib.
Bistort, it is under Saturn 41

A TABLE of the HERBS;

One Black, an herb of the S. 43
Bramble or Blackberry bush, a plant of Venus in Aries 43
Blites are under the dominion of Venus 44
Borage and Bugloss are under Jupiter 45
Blue bottle and Blue blow, is under Saturn 46
Brankursine and Bear's breech, are under the Moon 47
Briony is under Mars 48
Brookline is under Mars 50
Butcher's broom and Bruscus is under Mars 51
Broom and Broom rape, are under Mars 52
Bucks horn Plantane is under Saturn 53
Bucks horn is under Sat. 54
Bugles, or Brown Bugles, is under Venus 55
Burnet, an herb of the Sun 56
Butter-bur, and herb of the Sun 58
Burdock, an herb of Ven. 59
Bitter Sweet, see Amara dulcis
Spanish Bugloss, see Alkanet
Bruisewort, see Sopewort
Bear's foot, see Black Hellebore
Bishopswort, see Bentain
Brimstone wort, see Fennel
Buggiaron see Cuckow point
Balm herb, see Costmary
Bull's foot, see Colt's-foot
Blessed Thistle, see Carduus Benedictus
Bipennula, see Burnot
Bastard Agrimony, see Water Agrimony

C

Cabbages and Coleworts, are herbs of the Moon 60
The Sea Colewort, the Moon owns it 61
Calomint, or Mountain Mint, is an herb of Mercury 62
Camomile is under the Sun 63
Water Caltrops, or Caltrops, are under the government of the Moon 64
Compions Wild, are under the Sun 65
Carduus Benedictus is an herb of Mars 66
Carrots are under Mer. 67
Carraway is under Mer. 68
Celandine, is an herb of the Sun 69
The lesser Celandine is under Mars 71
The ordinary small Centuary is an herb of the Sun 72
The Cherry-tree is a tree of Venus 73
Winter Cherry, a plant of Venus 74
Chervil Cærefolium is under Jupiter 75
Sweet Chervil and Sweet Cicely are under Jupiter 76
Chesnut Tree is under Jup. 77
Earth Chesnuts and Ciper Nuts are under Venus ib
Chickweed under the Moon ib.
Chick Pease, or Cicer, is under Venus 78
Cinquefoil an herb of Jup. 79
Cives, Chives, and Chivet, is under Mars 81
Clary, or Clear Eyes, is under the Moon ib
Wild Clary, or Christ's Eye, is under the Moon 82

Clevers

As also what PLANET governeth them.

Clevers and Clavers, are under the Moon — 83
Clown's Woundwort is under Saturn — 84
Cock's Head is under Ven. 85
Columbines is under Ven. 86
Colt foot, or Coughwort, is under Venus ib.
Comfrey is an herb of Sat. 87
Coralwort, under the Moon 89
Costmary is under Jup. 90
Crowfoot is under Mars 96
Cudweed, or Cotton Wood, is an herb of Venus 90
Cowslips are under Ven. 91
Crabs Claw is under Ven. 92
Black Cresses, under Mars 93
Sciatica Cresses, under Sat. ib.
Water Cresses, is under the Moon — 94
Crosswort is under Saturn 95
Crowfoot, an herb of Mars 96
Cuckowpint, or Pintle, or Calvesfoot, is under M. 97
Cucumbers, or Cowcumbers, is under the Moon 99
Caterach, see Spleenwort
Carpenters herb, see Self heal
Cammock, see Rest harrow
Corn Role, see Poppy
Champetys, see Ground Pine
Callians, see Orchis
Catmint, see Nep
Cuckow Flowers, see Ladies Smock
Christmas herb, see Black Hellebore
Call me to you, see Hearts Ease
Cranes Bill, see Dove's foot
Crop, see Darnel
Middle Consound, Comfrey, or herb Carpenter, see Bugle

Corn Flowers, see Blue Bottle
Cummin Royal, and Ethiopian Cummin seed, for both, see Bishop's Wood
Clovewort, see Avens
Catsfoot, see Alehoof

D

Daisies are governed by Ven. and under the sign Can. 100
Dandelion is under Jupiter ib.
Daffodil is under Saturn 102
Dill is under Mercury ib.
Devil's Bit is under Ven. 103
Docks are under Jupiter 104
Dodder of Thyme, and other Dodders, are under Sat. 105
Dog's Grass is under Ju. 106
Dove's Foot is a Martial plant 107
Duck's Meat, Cancer claims the herb, and the Moon will be Lady of it 108
Down, or Cotton Thistle, is under Mars ib.
Dragons, a plant of Mars 109
Great round leaves Dock, or Bastard Rhubarb ib.
Dyer's Weed, see Wold and Weld
Dittander, see Pepper Wort
Dog's Stone, see Orchis
Dewberry Bush, see Gooseberry Bush
Drop Wort, see Filipendula
Dentaria, see Coral Wort
Dragon Wort, see Bistort
Dog's and Goat's Arrach, see Arrach wild and stinking

E

Elder Tree is under Ven. 110

A TABLE of the HERBS;

Dwarf Elder is under V. 110
Elm Tree is under Sat. 111
Endive is under Venus 112
Elecampane is under Mer. 113
Eringo is a venereal plant 114
Eye Bright, the Sun claims dominion over it, and is under the Lion — 115
Epithimum, see Dodder of Thyme Earth Nuts, see Earth Chesnuts
English Serpentary, see Adstort
Eupatorium, see Water Agrimony

F
Fern is under Mercury 116
Water Fern is under Sat. 117
Featherfew is under Ven. 118
Fennel is an herb of Mercury, and under Virgo 119
Sow Fennel and Hog's Fennel are herbs of Mercury 120
Figwort is under Venus 121
Filipendula is under Ven. 122
Fig-Tree is under Jup. 123
The yellow Water Flag, or Flower-de-luce, is under the Moon — 124
Flax weed is under Mars 125
Flea Wort is under Sat. 126
Flower-de-luce — 126
Fix-weed is under Sat. 127
Fluellin, or Luellin, is a Lunar herb — 129
Foxglove is under Venus 130
Fumitory is under Sat. 131
Furz Bush, is under Mars 133
Felwort, see Gentian
Frogs foot, see Crows foot
Fresh Water Soldier, see Crabs Claws
Foal foot, see Colts Foot

Five finger, or five leaved grass, see Cinquefoil
Fig-wort, see the lesser Celandine
Flower gentle, Floramen, and Velvet Flower, see Amaranthus

G
Gentian is under Mars 134
Clove Gilliflowers are under the dominion of Jupiter 135
Germander is under Mer. 136
Stinking Gladwin is under Saturn 137
Goldenrod, Ven. claims it 138
Gout wort or herb Gerard, Saturn rules it 139
Gromwell, three sorts, are under Venus ib.
Gooseberry bush, under Ven 140
Winter green is under Sat 141
Grounsel is under Venus 142
Garden patience, see Monks Rhubarb
Garstones, see Orchis
Gosts see Furz Bush
Quick grass, or Couch grass, see Dog's grass
Gold knobs, Gold cups, see Cowfoot
Goose grass, or Goose share, see Clevers
Ground-nuts, see Earth Chesnuts
Gill-go-by Ground, and Gillcreep-by, Ground, see Alehoof

H
Hercules All heal, see Allheal
Hercules Wound wort, see Allheal

Hearts-

As also what PLANET governeth them.

Hearts-ease is Saturn 143
Hart's-tongue is under J. 144
Hazel-nut is under Mer. 145
Hawk-weed is under Sat. 146
Hawthorn is under Mars 147
Hemlock is under Saturn ib.
Hemp is under Saturn 149
Henbane is under Saturn ib.
Hedge-hyssop, under Mars 151
Black-Hellebore is an herb of Saturn 152
Herb Robert is under V. 153
Herb Truelove, it is under Venus 154
Hyssop is under Jupiter 155
Hops are under Mars 156
Horehound is under Mer. 157
Horse-tail is under Sat. 158
Houseleek is under Jupiter 159
Hounds-tongue is under Mercury 160
Holly Holm, or Hulver-bush, is under Saturn 161
Honey-suckles, see Meadow-trefoil
Honey-suckle, see Wood-bine
Small Houseleek, see Stone-crop
Heliotropium, see Turnsole
Hook-heal, see Self-heal
Horse-rhadish, see Rhadish
Herb Two-pence, see Money-wort
Horse-strange, and Horse-strong see Hogs Fennel
Horse-hoof, see Colts-foot
Holy Thistle, see Carduus Benedictus
Harts-horn, Herba-stella, Herba-stellaria, Herb-eye, and Herb-ivy, see Buckthorn
Heart-sickle, see Blue-bottle

Herb William, see B.shop-weed
Herb Bennet, see Avens
Horse-parsley, see Alexander
Haymaids, see Alehoof
Hepatorium, see Water Agrimony

J
St John's-wort is under the Sun, and the sign Leo 161
Ivy is under Saturn 162
Juniper-bush is a Solar herb 163
St James's-wort, see Rag-wort
Juray, see Darnel
Jarus, see Cuckow-point
Ground-ivy, see Alehoof

K
Kidney-wort is under Venus 165
Knapweed is under Sat. 165
Knot-grass is under Sat. 166
King's clever, see Melilot
Knight's Pound wort, see Crab-claws
Knee-holm, Knee-holly, Knee-hulver, see Butcher's broom

L
Ladies mantle is governed by Venus 168
Lavender, Mer. owns it 169
Lavender-cotton, Mercury governs it ib.
Ladies smock, the Moon governs it 170
Lettuce, the Moon owns it ib.
Water Lilly, white and yellow, are under the Moon 171
Lilly of the Valley, Conval Lilly, May Lilly, and Lilly Contancy, are under Mercury 172

A TABLE of the Herbs;

White Lillies are governed by the Moon 173
Liquorice, Mercury governs it ib.
Liver-wort is under Jup. 174
Loose strife, under the Moon 175
Loose strife with spiked heads of flowers, is an herb of the Moon ib
Lovage, an herb of the S. 177
Lung-wort is an herb of Jupiter 178
Love in Idleness, see Heart-Ease
Locker's Goulons, see Crowfoot
Loppa Major, see Burdock
Ladies Seal, see Briony
Langue de Bœuf, see Borage and Bugloss

M

Moral, see Amora Dulcis
Madder, an herb of Mars 178
Maiden hair, or Wall-rue, is under Mercury 179
Golden Maiden-hair is an herb of Mercury 180
Mallows and Marshmallow are under Venus 181
Maple-tree is under Jup 184
Wild, Bastard, and Grove Marjoram, are under Mercury ib.
Sweet Marjoram is an herb of Mercury ib.
Marigolds are herbs of the Sun 186
Mother-wort is an herb of Mercury ib
Sweet Maudlin, an herb of Jupiter 187

Medlar is under Saturn 187
Melilot, or King's Clover, is under Mercury 188
French and Dogs Mercury, are under Venus 189
Mint is an herb of Ven. 190
Misselto is under the Sun 194
Money-wort, under Ven 195
Moon-wort, the Moon owns it 196
Mosses, Saturn owns them 197
Mother-wort, under Ven 198
Mouse-ear, under Moon 199
Mugwort is under Venus 200
Mulberry-tree, Mercury owns it 201
Mullein, Saturn owns it 202
Mustard is under Mars 203
Hedge Mustard, Mars owns it 205
Medic-fetch, see Cock's-head
Myrrhs, see Chervil
Macedonian parsley seed, see Alexander

N

Nailwort 206
Nep Calmint, under Venus ib.
Nettles are under Mars 207
Nightshade, under Saturn 209
Dead Nettles, see Archangel

O

Oak, Jupiter owns it 210
Oats 211
One Blade, Sun owns it ib.
Orchis is under Venus ib.
Onions are under Mars 212
Orpine, the Moon owns it 213
One-berry, herb True-love, is under Venus 154
Organs, Origanum, see wild Marjoram

Osmon

As also what PLANET governeth them.

Osmond Royal, see Water Fern
Ox tongue, see Bugloss
Oyster-loit, see Bistort
Orach and Oragi, see Garden Arrach
Opoponax wort, see All heal
Orchanet, see Alkanet

P
Parsley is under Mer. 214
Parsley piert, or Parsley Break stone —— 215
Parsnip is under Ven. 216
Cow Parsnip is under Mercury —— —— 217
Peach tree belongs to V. ib
Pear-tree —— 219
Pellitory of Spain is under Mercury —— 220
Pellitory of the Wall, Mercury owns it —— 221
Penny royal, Venus owns it 223
Peony, masculine and feminine the Sun owns them 224
Pepper wort is a Martial herb 225
Periwinkle, Venus owns it 226
St Peter's wort, under the Sun 227
Pimpernel is a Solar herb 229
Ground Pine, Mars owns it ib
Plantain is under Ven. 230
Plums are under Ven. 232
Pollypody of the Oak is an herb of Saturn 233
Poplar-tree, under Sat. 234
Poppy, white and black, and the wild Poppy or Corn rose the Moon rules 236

Purslain, under the Moon 238
Primroses are under Ven. 239
Privet, the Moon rules, 204
Park-leaves, see Tutsan
Prick madam, see Stonecrop
Prunel, see Self heal
Pansy, see Heart's ease
Piss a bed, see Dandelion
Priest pintle, see Cuckowpint
Poults, see Crowfoot
Peagles, see Cowslips
Pig nut, see Earth Chesnuts
Pile wort, see the lesser Celandine
Petesitis, see Butter bur
Pimpinella, see Burnet
Petitgree, see Butcher's broom
Passions, see Bistort
Porticaria, or Peach wort, or Plumbago see Arsmart,
Black potherb, see Alexander
Wild parsley, see Alexander
Panacea, see All heal

Q
Queen of the Meadows, Meadow sweet, or Mead sweet, Venus claims them 240
Quince tree, Sat owns it 241

R
Rhadish and Horse Rhadish are under Mars 243
Ragwort is under Ven 244
Rose grass, red and yellow, both are under the Moon 245
Rest harrow, or Cammock, are under Mars 235
Rocket is under Mars 247
Winter rocket, or Winter cross is under Venus 248
Red roses are under Jupiter, Damask

A TABLE of the HERBS.

Damask Roses are under Ven.
White roses are under the Moon — 249
Rasa solis, or Sun-dew, the Sun rules it 253
Rosemary, under the Sun 254
Rhubarb, or Rhapontick, Mars claims it 256
Garden Patience, or Monk Rhubarb, or Bastard Rhubarb, Mars governs them 257
Meadow Rue — 259
Garden Rue is an herb of the Sun, and under Leo 260
Rupture wort is Saturnine 262
Rushes are under Saturn 263
Rye — ib
Ramp and Wake Robin, see Cuckow pint
Red Fathering, see Cockhead
Rush Leeks, see Cives
Rulcus, see Butcher's Broom

S
Saffron is an herb of the Sun 264
Sage is an herb of Jup. ib.
Wood Sage is under Ven. 266
Solomon's Seal, Saturn owns the plant — 267
Samphire is an herb of Jup 268
Sanicle is an herb of Ven. 269
Saracens confound, or Saracen Wound wort, Sat. governs — 270
Sauce alone, or Jack by the hedge, is an herb of Mer. 271
Winter and Summer Savory Mer. governs them 272
Savine, Mars owns it ib.
The common white Saxifrage, the Moon governs 273
Burnet Saxifrage, the Moon governs it 274
Scabious, three sorts, Mercury owns them — 275
Scurvy grass is under Jup. 277
Self-heal, and Sickle wort, are under Venus 277
Service tree is under the dominion of Saturn 279
Shepherd's purse is under Sat. ib.
Smallage is an herb of Mer. 280
Sope wort is under Ven. 281
Sorrel is under Venus ib.
Wood Sorrel is under Ven. 282
Sow Thistle is under Ven. 283
Southernwood is a Mercurial plant — 284
Spignel is under Venus 285
Spleen wort is under Sat. ib.
Star-thistle is under Mars 286
Strawberries is under Ven. 287
Succory is under Jupiter 288
Stone-crop, small Houfleek, is under the Moon 289
Septfoil, see Tormentil
Silverwood, see Wild Tansy
Staggerwood, and Stammerwort and Segrum, see Ragwort
Satyrion, see Orchis
Sengreen, see Houfleek
Setter-wort, and Setter grass, see Black Hellebore
Sulphur-wort, see Sow Fennel
Sea holly, see Eringe
Starch-wort, see Cuckow pint
Sweth, see Cives
Saligot, see Caltrops
Sickle-wort, see Bugloss

Sanguinare;

As also what PLANET governeth them.

Sanguinare, and Swine-cresses, see Buckthorn
Syamus, see Blue bottle
Snakeweed, see Bistort
Sparagus, or Sparage, see Asparagus
Serpents Tongue, see Adders Tongue
Spanish Bugloss, see Alkanet

T

English Tobacco is a Martial plant — 290
Tamarisk-tree is governed by Saturn — 291
Garden Tansy is under Ven. 292
Wild Tansy, Ven. rules it 293
Thistles, mars rules them 294
Melancholy Thistle is under Capricorn, and therefore under Saturn and Mars ib
Our Lady's Thistle, is under Jupiter — 295
Welsy, or Cotton Thistle, is a plant of Mars 296
Fuller's Thistle, or Teasle, is an herb of Venus 267
Treacle and Mithridate Mustard, are herbs of Mars 298
Black Thorn, or Sloe Bush 298
Thorough-wax, or Thorough-leaf — 299
Thyme — 300
Thyme (Mother of) is under Venus — ib.
Termentil, or Septfoil, is an herb of the Sun 301
Turnsole, or Heliotropium, is an herb of the Sun 303
Meadow Trefoil, or Honey-suckles, under Mercury ib.

Heart Trefoil is under the dominion of the Sun 304
Pearl Trefoil is under the dominion of the Moon ib.
Tut-san, or Park-leaves, is an herb of the Sun 305
Three Faces in one Hood, see Heart's Ease
Throat wort, see Fig wort
Cotton Thistle, see Down
Tooth wort, toothed and Dog-teeth Violet. see Coral wort
Tribus Aquaticus, and Tribus merinus, see Water Caltrops
Tamas, see Briony
Twa-blade, see Bifoyl
Turnhoof, see Alehoof

V.

Garden Valerian is under the government of merc. 305
Vervain is under Venus 307
The Vine is under Venus 308
Violets are under Venus ib.
Vipers Bugloss is an herb of the Sun 309
Black and white Vine, Wild or Wood Vine, see Briony

W

Wall Flowers, or Winter Gilliflowers, the moon rules them — 311
Walnut, a plant of the Sun ib.
Wold, Weld, or Dyers Weed, is under mars 313
Wheat is under Venus 314
The Willow-tree is governed by the moon 315
Wood is under Saturn 316
Woodbine, or Honey suckle, is a plant of mercury 317
Wormwood, an herb of mars 318

A TABLE of the HERBS;

Whitlow grass 206
Wall-penny-royal, or Wall pennywort, see Kidney-wort
Wine berry bush, see Gooseberry-bush
Whins, see the Furz bush
Water-flag, see yellow flower de luce
Wall wort, see Elder-tree
Wray, see Darnel
Wading Pond weed, see Crabs claws, and Water Sea-green
Water nuts, and Water-chesnuts, see Caltrops
Water pimpernel, see Brooklime
Worts, and Wortle berries, see Bil-berries
Wine flower, see Anemone
Woody Night shade, see Amara Dulcis
Hercules Wound wort, see All heal

Y
Yarrow, called Nose bleed, milfoil, and Thousand-leaf, is under the influence of Venus — 325

The CONTENTS of the DIRECTIONS for making *Syrups, Conserves, Oils, Ointments, Plaisters, &c.* of *Herbs, Roots, Flowers, &c.* whereby you may have them ready for Use all the Year long.

SECT. I
The way of gathering, drying and preserving Simples, and their Juices.

Chap. 1 Of Leaves of Herbs or Trees 326
2. Of Flowers 328
3. Of Seeds ib.
4. Of Roots ib.
5. Of Barks 329
6. Of Juices 330

SECT. II.
The way of making and keeping all necessary compounds.

Chap. 1. Of distilled Waters 331
Chap. 2. Of Syrups 331
3. Of Juleps 333
4. Of Decoctions 334
5. Of Oils 335
6. Of Electuaries ib.
7. Of Conserves 336
8. Of Preserves 337
9. Of Lohochs 339
10. Of Ointments ib.
11. Of Plaisters 340
12. Of Poultices ib.
13. Of Troches 341
14. Of Pills ib.
15. The way of mixing medicines according to the cause of the Disease, and parts of the body afflicted 342

The

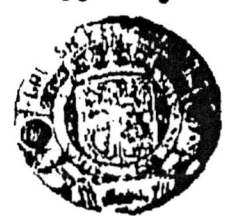

THE English Physician ENLARGED.

Amara Dulcis.

CONSIDERING divers shires in this nation give divers names to one and the same herb, and that the common name which it bears in one country is not known in another, I shall take the pains to set down all the names that I know of each herb: pardon me for setting that name first which is most common to myself. Besides Amara dulcis, some call it Mortal, others Bitter sweet, some Woody Night-shade, and others Felen-wort.

Descript.] It grows up with woody stalks even to a man's height, and sometimes higher. The leaves fall off at the approach of Winter, and spring out of the same stalks at Springtime. The branch is compassed about with a whitish bark, and hath a pith in the middle of it: The main branch brancheth itself into many small ones, with claspers, laying hold on what is next to them, as vines do: It bears many leaves, they grow in no order at all, at least in no regular order: The leaves are longish, though somewhat broad, and pointed at the ends: many of them have two little leaves growing at the end of their foot stalk; some have but one, and some none. The leaves are of a pale green colour, the flowers are of a purple colour, or of a perfect blue like to violets, and they stand many of them together in knots, the berries are green at first, but when they are ripe they are very red; if you taste them, you shall find them just as the crabs which we in Sussex call bitter sweets, *viz.* sweet at first, and bitter afterwards.

Place] They grow commonly almost throughout England, especially in moist and shady places.

Time] The leaves shoot out about the latter end of March, if the temperature of the air be ordinary; it flowereth in July, and the seeds are ripe soon after, usually in the next month.

Government

Government and Virtues.] It is under the planet Mercury, and a notable herb of his also, if it be rightly gathered under his influence. It is excellent good to remove witchcraft both in men and beasts, as also all sudden diseases whatsoever. Being tied round about the neck, is one of the admirablest remedies for the vertigo or dizziness in the head that is; and that is the reason (as Tragus saith) the people in Germany commonly hang it about their cattles necks, when they fear any such evil hath betided them. Country people commonly use to take the berries of it, and having bruised them, they apply them to felons, and thereby soon rid their fingers of such troublesome guests.

We have now shewed you the external use of the herb: we shall speak a word or two of the internal, and so conclude. Take notice, it is a Mercurial herb, and therefore of very subtle parts, as indeed all mercurial plants are; therefore take a pound of the wood and leaves together, bruise the wood (which you may easily do, for it is not so hard as oak) then put it in a pot, and put to it three pints of white wine, put on the pot-lid and shut it close; and let it infuse hot over a gentle fire twelve hours, then strain it out, so you have a most excellent drink to open obstructions of the liver and spleen, to help difficulty of breath, bruises and falls, and congealed blood in any part of the body, it helps the yellow jaundice, the dropsy and black jaundice, and to cleanse women newly brought to bed. You may drink a quarter of a pint of the infusion every morning. It purgeth the body very gently, and not churlishly, as some hold. And when you find good by this, remember me.

They that think the use of these medicines is too brief, it is only for the cheapness of the book; let them read those books of mine of the last edition, viz. *Riverius, Veslingus, Riolanus, Johnson, Sennertus,* and *Physic for the Poor.*

All-heal.

IT is called All-heal, Hercules's All heal, and Hercules's Wound wort, because it is supposed that Hercules learned the herb and its virtues from Chiron, when he learned physic of him. Some call it Panay, and others Opopane wort.

Descript.] Its root is long, thick, and exceeding full of juice, of a hot and biting taste, the leaves are great and large, and winged almost like ash-tree leaves, but that they are

something

something hairy, each leaf consisting of five or six pair of such wings set one against the other upon foot-stalks, broad below, but narrow towards the end; one of the leaves is a little deeper at the bottom than the other, of a fair, yellowish, fresh green colour; they are of a bitterish taste, when chewed in the mouth. From among these ariseth up a stalk, green in colour, round in form, great and strong in magnitude, five or six feet high in altitude, with many joints, and some leaves thereat: Towards the top come forth umbels of small yellow flowers, after which are passed away, you may find whitish, yellow, short, flat seeds, bitter also in taste.

Place.] Having given you the description of the herb from the bottom to the top, give me leave to tell you, that there are other herbs called by this name; but because they are strangers in England, I give only the description of this, which is easily to be had in the gardens of divers places.

Time.] Although Gerard saith, That they flower from the beginning of May to the end of December, experience teacheth them that keep it in their gardens, that it flowers not till the latter end of the Summer, and sheds its seed presently after.

Government and Virtues.] It is under the dominion of mars, hot biting, and choleric; and remedies what evils mars afflicts the body of man with, by sympathy, as vipers flesh attracts poison, and the loadstone iron. It kills the worms, helps the gout, cramp, and convulsions, provokes urine, and helps all joint aches. It helps all cold griefs of the head, the vertigo, falling sickness, the lethargy, the wind colic, obstructions of the liver and spleen, stone in the kidneys and bladder. It provokes the terms, expels the dead birth: It is excellent good for the griefs of the sinews, itch, stone and toothach, the biting of mad dogs and venemous beasts, and purgeth choler very gently.

Alkanet.

BESIDES the common name, it is called Orchanet, and Spanish Bugloss, and by apothecaries, Enchusa.

Descript.] Of the many sorts of this herb, there is but one known to grow commonly in this nation; of which one takes this description. It hath a great and thick root, of a reddish colour, long, narrow, hairy leaves, green like the leaves of Bugloss, which lie very thick upon the ground;

the stalks rise up compassed round about, thick with leaves, which are lesser and narrower than the former; they are tender, and slender, the flowers are hollow, small, and of a reddish colour.

Place.] It grows in Kent near Rochester, and in many places in the West Country, both in Devonshire and Cornwall.

Time] They flower in July, and the beginning of August, and the seed is ripe soon after, but the root is in its prime, as carrots and parsnips are, before the herb runs up to stalk.

Government and Virtues] It is an herb under the dominion of Venus, and indeed one of her darlings, though somewhat hard to come by. It helps old ulcers, hot inflammations, burnings by common fire, and St Anthony's fire, by antipathy to mars: for these uses, your best way is to make it into an ointment; also, if you make a vinegar of it, as you make vinegar of roses, it helps the morphew and leprosy; if you apply the herb to the privities, it draws forth the dead child. It helps the yellow jaundice, spleen, and gravel in the kidneys. Dioscordes saith, it helps such as are bitten by venomous beasts, whether it be taken inwardly, or applied to the wound; nay, he saith further, if any one that hath newly eaten it, do but spit into the mouth of a serpent, it instantly dies. It stays the flux of the belly, kills worms, helps the fits of the mother. Its decoction made in wine, and drank, strengthens the back, and easeth the pains thereof: It helps bruises and falls, and is as gallant a remedy to drive out the small pox and measles as any is, an ointment made of it, is excellent for green wounds, pricks or thrusts.

Adder's Tongue, or Serpent's Tongue.

Descript.] THIS herb hath but one leaf, which grows with the stalk a finger's length above the ground, being flat and of a fresh green colour; broad like Water Plantane, but less, without any rib in it; from the bottom of which leaf, on the inside, riseth up (ordinarily) one, sometimes two or three slender stalks, the upper half whereof is somewhat bigger, and dented with small dents of a yellowish green colour, like the tongue of an adder serpent (only this is as useful as they are formidable). The roots continue all the year.

Place] It grows in moist meadows, and such like places

Time.] It is to be found in May or April, for it quickly perisheth with a little heat.

Government and Virtues] It is an herb under the dominion of the Moon and Cancer, and therefore, if the weakness of the retentive faculty be caused by an evil influence of Saturn in any part of the body governed by the moon, or under the dominion of Cancer, this herb cures it by sympathy: It cures these diseases after specified, in any part of the body under the influence of Saturn, by antipathy.

It is temperate in respect of heat, but dry in the second degree. The juice of the leaves drank with the distilled water of horse tail, is a singular remedy for all manner of wounds in the breasts, bowels, or other parts of the body, and is given with good success unto those that are troubled with casting, vomiting, or bleeding at the mouth or nose, or otherwise downwards. The said juice given in the distilled water of Oaken buds, is very good for women who have their usual courses, or the whites flowing down too abundantly. It helps sore eyes. Of the leaves infused or boiled in oil, omphanine, or unripe olives, set in the sun for certain days, or the green leaves sufficiently boiled in the said oil, is made an excellent green balsam, not only for green and fresh wounds, but also for old and inveterate ulcers, especially if a little fine clear turpentine be dissolved therein. It also stayeth and refresheth all inflammations that arise upon pains by hurts and wounds.

What parts of the body are under each planet and sign, and also what disease may be found in my astrological judgment of diseases, and for the internal work of nature in the body of man, as vital, animal, natural and procreative spirits of man; the apprehension, judgment, memory, the external senses viz. Seeing, hearing, smelling, tasting, and feeling, the virtues attractive, retentive, digestive, expulsive, &c. under the dominion of what planets they are, may be found in my *Ephemeris* for the year 1651. In both which you shall find the chaff of authors blown away by the fame of Dr Reason, and nothing but rational truths left for the ingenious to feed upon.

Lastly, To avoid blotting paper with one thing many times, and also to ease your purses in the price of the book, and withal to make you studious in physic; you have at the latter end of the book, the way of preserving all herbs

either

either in juice, conserve, oil, ointment or plaister, electuary, pills or troches.

Agrimony.

Descript.] THIS hath divers long leaves (some greater, some smaller) set upon a stalk, all of them dented about the edges, green above, and greyish underneath, and a little hairy withal. Among which ariseth up usually but one strong, round, hairy, brown stalk, two or three feet high, with smaller leaves set here and there upon it. At the top hereof grow many small yellow flowers, one above another, in long spikes; after which come rough heads of seed, hanging downwards, which will cleave to and stick upon garments, or any thing that shall rub against them. The knot is black, long, and somewhat woody, abiding many years, and shooting afresh every Spring, which root, though small, hath a reasonable good scent.

Place] It groweth upon banks, near the sides of hedges.

Time] It flowereth in July and August, the seed being ripe shortly after.

Government and Virtues] It is an herb under Jupiter, and the sign Cancer; and strengthens those parts under the planet and sign, and removes diseases in them by sympathy, and those under Saturn, Mars and Mercury by antipathy, if they happen in any part of the body governed by Jupiter, or under the signs Cancer, Sagittary, or Pisces, and therefore must needs be good for the gout, either used outwardly in oil or ointment, or inwardly in an electuary, or syrup, or concerted juice; for which see the latter end of this book.

It is of a cleansing and cutting faculty, without any manifest heat, moderately drying and binding. It openeth and cleanseth the liver, helpeth the jaundice, and is very beneficial to the bowels, healing all inward wounds, bruises, hurts, and other distempers. The decoction of the herb made with wine, and drank is good against the biting and stinging of serpents, and helps them that make foul, troubled or bloody water, and makes them piss clear speedily. It also helpeth the colic, cleanseth the breast, and rids away the cough. A draught of the decoction taken warm before the fit, first removes, and, in time rids away the tertian or quartan agues. The leaves and seeds taken in wine stays the bloody flux; outwardly applied, being stamped with old swines grease,

grease, it helpeth old sores, cancers, and inveterate ulcers; and draweth forth thorns and splinters of wood, nails, or any other such things gotten into the flesh. It helpeth to strengthen the members that be out of joint; and being bruised and applied, or the juice dropped in it, helpeth foul and imposthumed ears.

The distilled water of the herb is good to all the said purposes, either inward or outward, but a great deal weaker.

It is a most admirable remedy for such whose lives are annoyed either by heat or cold. The liver is the former of blood, and blood the nourisher of the body, and Agrimony a strengthener of the liver.

I cannot stand to give you a reason in every herb, why it cureth such diseases; but if you please to peruse my judgment in the herb Wormwood, you shall find them there, and it will be well worth your while to consider it in every herb, you shall find them true throughout the book.

Water Agrimony.

IT is called in some countries Water Hemp, Bastard Hemp, and Bastard Agrimony, Eupatorium, and Hepatorium, because it strengthens the liver.

Descript] The root continues a long time, having many long slender strings. The stalk grows up about two feet high, sometimes higher. They are of a dark purple colour. The branches are many, growing at distances the one from the other, the one from the one side of the stalk, the other from the opposite point. The leaves are winged, and much indented at the edges. The flowers grow at the top of the branches, of a brown yellow colour, spotted with black spots, having a substance within the midst of them like that of a Daisy. If you rub them between your fingers, they smell like rosin or cedar when it is burnt. The seeds are long, and easily stick to any woollen thing they touch.

Place] They delight not in heat, and therefore they are not so frequently found in the southern parts of England, as in the northern, where they grow frequently: You may look for them in cold grounds, by ponds and ditches sides, as also by running waters; sometimes you shall find them grow in the midst of the waters.

Time] They all flower in July or August, and the seed is ripe presently after.

Government

Government and Virtues.] It is a plant of Jupiter, as well as the other Agrimony, only this belongs to the celestial sign Cancer. It healeth and drieth, cutteth and cleanseth thick and tough humours of the breast, and for this I hold it inferior to but few herbs that grow. It helps the cachexia or evil disposition of the body, the dropsy and yellow jaundice. It opens obstructions of the liver, mollifies the hardness of the spleen, being applied outwardly. It breaks imposthumes, taken inwardly. It is an excellent remedy for the third day ague. It provokes urine and the terms; it kills worms, and cleanseth the body of sharp humours, which are the cause of itch and scabs, the herb being burnt, the smoke thereof drives away flies, wasps, &c. It strengthen the lungs exceedingly. Country people give it to their cattle when they are troubled with the cough, or broken winded.

Alehoof, or Ground-ivy.

SEVERAL counties give it several names, so that there is scarce an herb growing of that bigness that has got so many: It is called Cats-foot, Ground-ivy, Gill go-by-ground, and Gill creep by ground, Turnhoof, Haymaids, and Alehoof.

Descript.] This well known herb lieth, spreadeth, and creepeth upon the ground, shooteth forth roots, at the corners of tender jointed stalks, set with two round leaves at every joint somewhat hairy, crumpled, and unevenly dented about the edges with round dents; at the joints likewise, with the leaves towards the end of the branches, come forth hollow, long flowers, of a bluish purple colour, with small white spots upon the lips that hang down. The root is small with strings.

Place.] It is commonly found under hedges, and on the sides of ditches, under houses, or in shadowed lanes, and other waste grounds, in almost every part of this land.

Time.] They flower somewhat early, and abide a great while; the leaves continue green until Winter, and sometimes abide, except the Winter be very sharp and cold.

Government and Virtues.] It is an herb of Venus, and therefore cures the diseases she causes by sympathy, and those of Mars by antipathy; you may usually find it all the year long, except the year be extremely frosty; it is quick,

sharp,

sharp, and bitter in taste, and is thereby found to be hot and dry; a singular herb for all inward wounds, exulcerated lungs, or other parts, either by itself, or boiled with other the like herbs; and being drank, in a short time it easeth all griping pains, windy and choleric humours in the stomach, spleen, or belly; helps the yellow jaundice, by opening the stoppings of the gall and liver, and melancholy, by opening the stoppings of the spleen; expelleth venom or poison, and also the plague; it provokes urine and womens courses; the decoction of it in wine drank for some time together, procureth ease unto them that are troubled with the sciatica, or hip gout; as also the gout in hands, knees, or feet; if you put to the decoction some honey and a little burnt allum, it is excellent good to gargle any sore mouth or throat, and to wash the sores and ulcers in the privy parts of man or woman, it speedily helpeth green wounds, being bruised and bound thereto. The juice of it boiled with a little honey and verdigrease, both wonderfully cleanse fistulas, ulcers, and stayeth the spreading or eating of cancers and ulcers; it helpeth the itch, scabs, wheals, and other breakings out in any part of the body. The juice of Celandine, Field daisies, and Ground ivy clarified, and a little fine sugar dissolved therein, and dropped into the eyes, is a sovereign remedy for all pains, redness, and watering of them; as also for the pin and web, skins and films growing over the sight; it helpeth beasts as well as men. The juice dropped into the ears doth wonderfully help the noise and singing of them, and helpeth the hearing which is decayed. It is good to tun up with new drink, for it will clarify it in a night, that it will be the fitter to be drank the next morning; or if any drink be thick with removing, or any other accident, it will do the like in a few hours.

Alexander.

IT is also called Alisander, Horse parsley, and Wild parsley, and the Black Pot herb, the seed of it is that which is usually sold in apothecaries shops for Macedonian Parsleyseed.

Descript] It is usually sown in all the gardens in Europe, and so well known, that it needs no farther description.

Time.] It flowereth in June and July; the seed is ripe in August.

Govern.

Government and Virtues.] It is an herb of Jupiter, and therefore friendly to nature, for it warmeth a cold stomach, and openeth a stoppage to the liver and spleen; it is good to move womens courses, to expel the after-birth, to break wind, to provoke urine, and helpeth the stranguary; and these things the seeds will do likewise. If either of them be boiled in wine, or being bruised and taken in wine, is also effectual against the biting of serpents. And you know what Alexander Pottage is good for, that you may no longer eat it out of ignorance, but out of knowledge.

The Black Alder-tree.

Descript.] THIS tree seldom groweth to any great bigness, but for the most part abideth like a hedge bush, or a tree spreading its branches, the woods of the body being white, and a dark red coal, or heart; the outward bark is of a blackish colour, with many whitish spots therein; but the inner bark next the wood is yellow, which being chewed, will turn the spittle near unto a saffron colour. The leaves are somewhat like those of an ordinary Alder-tree, or the Female Cornel, or Dogberry-tree, called in Sussex Dogwood, but blacker, and not so long. The flowers are white, coming forth with the leaves at the joints, which turn into small round berries, first green, afterwards red, but blackish when they are thorough ripe, divided, as it were, into two parts, wherein is contained two small round and flat seeds. The root runneth not deep into the ground, but spreads rather under the upper crust of the earth.

Place.] This tree or shrub may be found plentifully in St John's wood by Hornsey, and the woods upon Hamstead-Heath; as also a wood called the Old Park in Barcomb in Essex, near the brooks sides.

Time.] It floweth in May, and the berries are ripe in September.

Government and Virtues] It is a tree of Venus, and perhaps under the celestial sign Cancer. The inner yellow bark hereof purgeth downwards both choler and phlegm, and the watery humours of such that have the dropsy, and strengthens the inward parts again by binding. If the bark hereof be boiled with Agrimony, Wormwood, Dodder, Hops and some Fennel, with Smallage, Endive, and Succory roots, and a reasonable draught taken every morning

for

for some time together, it is very effectual against the jaundice, dropsy, and the evil disposition of the body, especially if some suitable purging medicines have been taken before, to void the grosser excrements. It purgeth and strengtheneth the liver and spleen, cleansing them from such evil humours and hardness as they are afflicted with. It is to be understood that these things are performed by the dried bark; for the fresh green bark taken inwardly provokes strong vomitings, pains in the stomach, and gripings in the belly; yet if the decoction may stand and settle two or three days, until the yellow colour be changed black, it will not work so strongly as before, but will strengthen the stomach, and procure an appetite to meat. The outward bark contrariwise doth bind the body, and is helpful for all lasks and fluxes thereof, but this also must be dried first, whereby it will work the better. The inner bark thereof boiled in vinegar is an approved remedy to kill lice, to cure the itch, and take away scabs, by drying them up in a short time. It is singularly good to wash the teeth, to take away the pains, to fasten those that are loose, to cleanse them, and keep them sound. The leaves are good fodder for kine, to make them give more milk.

In the Spring-time you use the herbs before-mentioned, and will take but a handful of each of them, and to them add an handful of Elder buds, and having bruised them all, boil them in a gallon of ordinary beer, when it is new; and having boiled them half an hour, add to this three gallons more, and let them work together, and drink a draught of it every morning, half a pint, or thereabouts, it is an excellent purge for the Spring, to consume the phlegmatic quality the Winter hath left behind it, and withal to keep your body in health, and consume those evil humours which the heat of Summer will readily stir up. Esteem it as a jewel.

The Common Alder-tree.

Descript.] GROWETH to a reasonable height, and spreads much if it like the place. It is so generally well known unto country people, that I conceive it needless to tell that which is no news.

Place and Time.] It delighteth to grow in moist woods, and watery places; flowering in April or May, and yielding ripe seed in September.

Government

Government and Use.] It is a tree under the dominion of Venus, and of some watery sign or other, I suppose Pisces; and therefore the decoction, or distilled water of the leaves, is excellent against burnings and inflammations, either with wounds or without, to bathe the place grieved with, and especially for that inflammation in the breast, which the vulgar call an ague.

If you cannot get the leaves (as in Winter 'tis impossible) make use of the bark in the same manner.

The leaves and bark of the Alder tree are cooling, drying, and binding. The fresh leaves laid upon swellings dissolve them, and stay the inflammations. The leaves put under the bare feet gauled with travelling, are a great refreshing to them. The said leaves gathered while the morning dew is on them, and brought into a chamber troubled with fleas, will gather them thereunto, which being suddenly cast out, will rid the chamber of those troublesome bed fellows.

Angelica.

TO write a description of that which is so well known to be growing almost in every garden, I suppose is altogether needless; yet for its virtues it is of admirable use.

In time of Heathenism, when men had found out any excellent herb, they dedicated it to their gods; as the Bay-tree to Apollo, the Oak to Jupiter, the Vine to Bacchus, the Poplar to Hercules. These the Papists following as the Patriarchs, they dedicated to their Saints; as our Lady's Thistle to the Blessed Virgin, St John's Wort to St John, and another Wort to St Peter, &c. Our physicians must imitate like apes (though they cannot come off half so cleverly) for they blasphemously call Phansies or Hearts-ease, *an herb of the Trinity,* because it is of three colours: And a certain ointment, *an ointment of the Apostles,* because it consists of twelve ingredients: Alas, I am sorry for their folly, and grieved at their blasphemy God send them wisdom the rest of their age, for they have their share of ignorance already. Oh! Why must ours be blasphemous, because the Heathens and Papists were idolatrous? Certainly they have read so much in old rusty authors that they have lost all their divinity; for unless it were amongst the Ranters, I never read or heard of such blasphemy. The Heathens
and

and Papists were bad, and ours worse; the Papists giving idolatrous names to herbs for their virtues sake, not for their fair looks; and therefore some called this an herb of the *Holy Ghost;* others more moderate called it Angelica, because of its angelical virtues, and that name it retains still, and all nations follow it so near as their dialect will permit

Government and Virtues] It is an herb of the Sun in Leo, let it be gathered when he is there. the Moon applying to his good aspect; let it be gathered either in his hour, or in the hour of Jupiter, let Sol be angular; observe the like in gathering the herbs of other planets, and you may happen to do wonders. In all epidemical diseases caused by Saturn, that is as good a preservative as grows It resists poison, by defending and comforting the heart, blood, and spirits; it doth the like against the plague and all epidemical diseases, if the root be taken in powder to the weight of half a dram at a time, with some good treacle in Carduus water, and the party thereupon laid to sweat in his bed, if treacle is not to be had, take it alone in Carduus or Angelica water. The stalks or roots canned and eaten fasting, are good preservatives in time of infection, and at other times to warm and comfort a cold stomach The root also steeped in vinegar, and a little of that vinegar taken sometimes fasting, and the root smelled unto, is good for the same purpose. A water distilled from the root simply, as steeped in wine, and distilled in a glass, is much more effectual than the water of the leaves; and this water, drank two or three spoonfuls at a time, easeth all pains and torments coming of cold and wind, so that the body be not bound; and taken with some of the root in powder at the beginning, helpeth the pleurisy, as also all other diseases of the lungs and breast, as coughs, phthysic, and shortness of breath, and a syrup of the stalks doth the like It helps pains of the colic the stranguary and stoppage of the urine, procureth womens courses, and expelleth the after-birth, openeth the stoppings of the liver and spleen, and briefly easeth and discusseth all windiness and inward swellings The decoction drunk before the fit of an ague, that they may sweat (if possible) before the fit comes, will, in two or three times taking, rid it quite away; it helps digestion, and is a remedy for a surfeit. The juice, or the water, being dropped into the eyes or ears, helps dimness of sight and deafness; the juice put into the hollow teeth, easeth their pains. The root in powder, made up into a plaister with a little pitch, and laid on the biting of mad dogs, or any other venomous creature, doth wonderfully help. The juice or the water dropped, or tents wet therein, and put into filthy dead ulcers, or the powder of the root (in want of either) doth cleanse and cause them to heal quickly, by covering the naked bones with flesh; the distilled water applied to places pained with the gout, or sciatica, doth give a great deal of ease.

The wild Angelica is not so effectual as the garden; although it may be safely used to all the purposes aforesaid.

Amaranthus.

BESIDES its common name, by which it is best known by the florists of our days, it is called Flower Gentle, Flower Velure, Floramor, and Velvet Flower.

Descript.] It being a garden flower, and well known to every one that keeps it, I might forbear the description; yet, notwithstanding, because some desire it, I shall give it. It runneth up with a stalk a cubit high, streaked, and somewhat reddish toward the root, but very smooth, divided towards the top with small branches, among which stand long broad leaves of a reddish green colour, slippery; the flowers are not properly flowers, but tufts, very beautiful to behold, but of no smell, of reddish colour; if you bruise them, they yield juice of the same colour: being gathered, they keep their beauty a long time; the seed is of a shining black colour.

Time] They continue in flower from August till the time the frost nip them.

Government and Virtues] It is under the dominion of Saturn, and is an excellent qualifier of the unruly actions and passions of Venus, though Mars also should join with her. The flowers dried and beaten into powder stop the terms in women, and so do almost all other red things. And by the icon, or image of every herb, the ancients at first found out their virtues. Modern writers laugh at them for it; but I wonder in my heart, how the virtue of herbs came at first to be known, if not by their signatures; the moderns have them from the writings of the ancients; the ancients had no writings to have them from. But to proceed. The flowers stop all fluxes of blood: whether in man or woman bleeding either at the nose or wound. There is also a sort of Amaranthus that bears a white flower, which stops the whites in women, and the running of the reins in men, and is a most gallant antivenereal, and a singular remedy for the French pox.

Anemone.

CALLED also Wind Flower, because they say the flowers never open but when the wind bloweth. Pliny is my author; if it be not so, blame him. The seed also (if it bears any at all) flies away with the wind.

Place and Time] They are sown usually in the gardens of the curious, and flower in the Spring time. As for description I shall pass it, being well known to all those that sow them.

Government and Virtues] It is under the dominion of Mars, being supposed to be a kind of Crow-foot. The leaves provoke the terms mightily, being boiled, and the decoction drunk. The body being bathed with the decoction of them, cures the leprosy. The leaves being stamped, and the juice snuffed up in the nose, purgeth the head mightily, so doth the root, being chewed in the mouth, for it procureth much spitting, and bringeth away many watery and phlegmatic humours, and is therefore excellent for the lethargy. And when all is done, let physicians prate what they please, all the pills in the dispensatory purge not the head like to hot things held in the mouth. Being made into an ointment, and the eye lids anointed with it, it helps inflammation of the eyes, whereby it is palpable, that every stronger draweth its weaker like. The same ointment is excellent good to cleanse malignant and corroding ulcers.

Garden Arrach.

CALLED also Orach and Arage.

Descrip.] It is so commonly known to every house-wife, it were labour lost to describe it.

Time] It flowereth and seedeth from June to the end of August.

Government and Virtues.] It is under the government of

the Moon; in quality cold and moist like unto her. It softeneth and looseneth the body of man being eaten, and fortifieth the expulsive faculty in him. The herb, whether it be bruised and applied to the throat, or boiled, and in like manner applied, it matters not much, it is excellent good for swellings in the throat; the best way, I suppose, is to boil it, and having drunk the decoction inwardly, apply the herb outwardly: The decoction of it besides is an excellent remedy for the yellow jaundice.

Arrach, wild and stinking.

CALLED also Vulvaria, from that part of the body upon which the operation is most; also Dogs Arrach, Goats Arrach, and Stinking Motherwort.

Descript] This hath small and almost round leaves, yet a little pointed and without dent or cut, of a dusky mealy colour, growing on the slender stalks and branches that spread on the ground, with small flowers in clusters set with the leaves, and small seeds succeeding like the rest, perishing yearly, and rising again with its own sowing. It smells like rotten fish, or something worse.

Place] It grows usually upon dunghills.

Time] They flower in June and July, and their seed is ripe quickly after.

Government and Virtues.] Stinking Arrach is used as a remedy to help women pained, and almost strangled with the mother, by smelling to it; but inwardly taken there is no better remedy under the moon for that disease. I would be large in commendation of this herb, were I but eloquent. It is an herb under the dominion of Venus, and under the sign Scorpio; it is common almost upon every dunghill. The works of God are given freely to man, his medicines are common and cheap, and easy to be found: ('Tis the medicines of the College of Physicians that are so dear and scarce to find.) I commend it for an universal medicine for the womb, and such a medicine as will easily, safely, and speedily cure any disease thereof, as the fits of the mother, dislocation, or falling out thereof; it cools the womb being over-heated. And let me tell you this, and I will tell you the truth, heat of the womb is one of the greatest causes of hard labour in child birth. It makes barren women fruitful. It cleanseth the womb if it be foul, and strengthens it

exceedingly;

exceedingly, it provokes the terms if they be stopped, and stops them if they flow immoderately. you can desire no good to your womb, but this herb will effect it; therefore if you love children, if you love health, if you love ease, keep a syrup always by you, made of the juice of this herb, and sugar, (or honey, if it be to cleanse the womb) and let such as be rich keep it for their poor neighbours; and bestow it as freely as I bestow my studies upon them, or else let them look to answer it another day, when the Lord shall come to make inquisition of blood.

Archangel.

TO put a gloss upon their practice, the physicians call an herb which country people vulgarly know by the name of Dead Nettle Archangel, whether they favour more of superstition or folly, I leave to the judicious reader. There is more curiosity than courtesy to my countrymen used by others in the explanation as well of the names, as description of this so well known herb; which, that I may not also be guilty of, take this short description, first of the Red Archangel.

Descript.] This has divers square stalks, somewhat hairy, at the joints whereof grow two sad green leaves dented about the edges, opposite to one another to the lowermost upon long foot stalks, but without any toward the tops, which are somewhat round, yet pointed, and a little crumpled and hairy; round about the upper joints, where the leaves grow thick, are sundry gaping flowers of a pale reddish colour; after which come the seeds three or four in a husk. The root is smaller and thready, perishing every year; the whole plant hath a strong scent but not stinking.

White Archangel hath divers square stalks, none standing straight upward, but bending downward, whereon stand two leaves at a joint, larger and more pointed than the other dented about the edges, and greener also, more like unto Nettle leaves, but not stinking, yet hairy. At the joints with the leaves stand larger and more open gaping white flowers, husks round about the stalks, but not with such a bush of leaves as flowers set in the top, as is on the other, wherein stand small roundish black seeds, the root is white, with many strings at it, not growing downward, but lying under the upper crust of the earth, and abideth many years increasing, this hath not so strong a scent as the former.

Yellow Archangel is like the White in the stalks and leaves; but that the stalks are more straight and upright, and the joints with leaves are farther asunder, having longer leaves than the former, and the flowers a little larger and more gaping, of a fair yellow colour in most, in some paler. The roots are like white, only they creep not so much under the ground.

Place] They grow almost every where, unless it be in the middle of the street, the yellow most usually in the wet grounds of woods, and sometimes in the drier, in divers counties of this nation.

Time] They flower from the beginning of the Spring all the Summer long.

Virtues and Use.] The Archangels are somewhat hot and drier than the stinging Nettles, and used with better success for the stopping and hardness of the spleen, than they, by using the decoction of the herb in wine, and afterwards applying the herb hot unto the region of the spleen as a plaister, or the decoction with spunges. Flowers of the White Archangel are preserved or conserved to be used to stay the whites, and the flowers of the red to stay the reds in women. It makes the heart merry, drives away melancholy, quickens the spirits, is good against quartian agues, stauncheth bleeding at mouth and nose, if it be stamped and applied to the nape of the neck, the herb also bruised, and with some salt and vinegar and hogs grease, laid upon an hard tumour or swelling, or that vulgarly called the King's evil, do help to dissolve or discuss them; and being in like manner applied, doth much allay the pains, and give ease to the gout, sciatica, and other pains of the joints and sinews. It is also very effectual to heal green wounds, and old ulcers; also to stay their fretting, gnawing and spreading. It draweth forth splinters, and such like things gotten into the flesh, and is very good against bruises and burnings. But the yellow Archangel is most commended for old, filthy, corrupt sores and ulcers, yea although they grow to be hollow; and to dissolve tumours. The chief use of them is for women, it being a herb of Venus, and may be found in my *Guide for Women.*

Arssmart.

Arssmart.

THE hot Arssmart is called also Water pepper, or Cul-rage. The mild Arssmart is called dead Arssmart Persicaria, or Peach-wort, because the leaves are so like the leaves of a peach-tree; it is also called Plumbago.

Description of the Mild] This hath broad leaves set at the great red joint of the stalks, with semi-circular blackish marks on them, usually either bluish or whitish, with such like seed following. The root is long, with many strings thereat, perishing yearly; this hath no sharp taste (as another sort hath, which is quick and biting) but rather sour like sorrel, or else a little drying, or without taste.

Place] It groweth in watery places, ditches, and the like, which for the most part are dry in Summer.

Time.] It flowereth in June, and the seed is ripe in August.

Government and Virtues] As the virtue of both these is various, so is also their government, for that which is hot and biting, is under the dominion of Mars, but Saturn challengeth the other, as appears by that leaden coloured spot he hath placed upon the leaf.

It is of a cooling and drying quality, and very effectual for putrified ulcers in man or beast, to kill worms, and cleanse the putrified places. The juice thereof dropped in, or otherwise applied, consumeth all cold swellings, and dissolveth the congealed blood of bruises, by strokes, falls, &c. A piece of the root, or some of the seeds bruised, and held to an aching tooth, taketh away the pain. The leaves bruised and laid to the joint that hath a felon thereon taketh it away. The juice destroyeth worms in the ears, being dropped into them; if the hot Arssmart be strewed in a chamber, it will soon kill all the fleas; and the herb or juice of the cold Arssmart, put to a horse, or other cattle's sores, will drive away the fly in the hottest time of Summer; a good handful of the hot biting Arssmart put under a horse's saddle will make him travel the better, although he were half tired before. The mild Arssmart is good against all imposthumes and inflammations at the beginning, and to heal green wounds.

All authors chop the virtues of both sorts of Arssmart together,

together, as men chop herbs to the pot, when both of them are of clean contrary qualities. The hot Arsmart groweth not so high or tall as the mild doth, but hath many leaves of the colour of peach leaves, very seldom or never spotted; in other particulars it is like the former, but may easily be known from it, if you will be but pleased to break a leaf of it cross your tongue, for the hot will make your tongue to smart, so will not the cold. If you see them both together, you may easily distinguish them, because the mild hath far broader leaves; and our College of Physicians, out of the learned care of the public good, Anglice, their own gain, mistake the one for the other in their *New Master-piece,* whereby they discover, 1. Their ignorance. 2. Their carelessness; and he that hath but half an eye, may see their pride without a pair of spectacles. I have done what I could to distinguish them in their virtues, and when you find not the contrary named, use the cold. The truth is, I have not yet spoken with Dr Reason, nor his brother Dr Experience concerning either of them.

Asarabacca.

Descript.] ASARABACCA hath many heads rising from the roots, from whence come many smooth leaves, every one upon his own foot-stalks, which are rounder and bigger than Violet leaves, thicker also, and of a dark green shining colour on the upper side, and of a pale yellow green underneath, little or nothing dented about the edges, from among which rise small, round, hollow, brown, green husks upon short stalks, about an inch long, divided at the brims into five divisions, very like the cups or heads of the Henbane seed, but that they are smaller and these be all the flowers it carrieth, which are somewhat sweet, being smelled unto, and wherein, when they are ripe, is contained small cornered rough seeds, very like the kernels or stones of grapes or raisins. The roots are small and whitish, spreading divers ways in the ground, increasing into divers heads, but not running or creeping under the ground, as some other creeping herbs do. They are somewhat sweet in smell, resembling Nardus, but more when they are dry than green, and of a sharp but not unpleasant taste.

Place] It groweth frequently in gardens.

Time.]

Time] They keep their leaves green all Winter; but shoot forth new in the Spring, and with them come forth those heads or flowers which give ripe seed about Midsummer, or somewhat after.

Government and Virtues] 'Tis a plant under the dominion of Mars, and therefore inimical to nature. This herb being drank, not only provoketh vomiting, but purgeth downward, and by urine also, purgeth both choler and phlegm. If you add to it some spikenard, with the whey of goat's milk, or honeyed water, it is made more strong; but it purgeth phlegm more manifestly than choler, and therefore doth much help pains in the hips, and other parts; being boiled in whey, they wonderfully help the obstructions of the liver and spleen, and therefore profitable for the dropsy and jaundice; being steeped in wine and drank, it helps those continual agues that come by the plenty of stubborn humours, an oil made thereof by setting in the sun, with some laudanum added to it, provoketh sweating, (the ridge of the back being anointed therewith) and thereby driveth away the shaking fits of the ague. It will not abide any long boiling, for it looseth its chief strength thereby; nor much beating, for the finer powder doth provoke vomits and urine, and the coarser purgeth downwards.

The common use hereof is, to take the juice of five or seven leaves in a little drink to cause vomiting: the roots have also the same virtue, though they do not operate so forcibly; they are very effectual against the biting of serpents, and therefore are put as an ingredient both into Mithridate and Venice treacle. The leaves and roots being boiled in lee, and the head often washed therewith while it was warm, comforteth the head and brain that is ill affected by taking cold, and helpeth the memory.

I shall desire ignorant people to forbear the use of the leaves; the roots purge more gently, and may prove beneficial in such as have cancers, or old putrified ulcers, or fistulas upon their bodies, to take a dram of them in powder in a quarter of a pint of white wine in the morning. The truth is, I fancy purging and vomiting medicines as little as any man breathing doth, for they weaken nature, nor shall ever advise them to be used, unless upon urgent necessity. If a physician be nature's servant, it is his duty to strengthen his mistress as much as he can, and weaken her as little as may be.

Asparagus, Sparagus, or Sperage.

Descript.] IT riseth up at first with divers white and green scaly heads, very brittle or easy to break while they are young, which afterwards rise up in very long and slender green stalks, of the bigness of an ordinary riding wand, at the bottom of most, or bigger or lesser, as the roots are of growth; on which are set divers branches of green leaves shorter and smaller than fennel to the top; at the joints whereof come forth small yellowish flowers, which run into round berries, green at first, and of an excellent red colour when they are ripe, shewing like bead or coral, wherein are contained exceeding hard black seeds, the roots are dispersed from a spongeous head into many long, thick, and round strings, wherein is sucked much nourishment out of the ground, and increaseth plentifully thereby.

Prickly Asparagus, or Sperage.

Descript] IT groweth usually in gardens, and some of it grows wild in Appleton meadows in Gloucestershire, where the poor people do gather the buds of young shoots, and sell them cheaper than our garden Asparagus is sold at London.

Time] They do for the most part flower and bear their berries late in the year, or not at all, although they are housed in Winter.

Government and Virtue] They are both under the dominion of Jupiter. The young buds or branches boiled in ordinary broth, make the belly soluble and open, and boiled in white wine, provoke urine, being stopped, and is good against the stranguary or difficulty of making water; it expelleth the gravel and stone out of the kidneys, and helpeth pains in the reins. And boiled in white wine or vinegar, it is prevalent for them that have their arteries loosened, or are troubled with the hip gout or sciatica. The decoction of the roots boiled in wine and taken, is good to clear the sight, and being held in the mouth easeth the tooth-ach; and being taken fasting several mornings together, stirreth up bodily lust in man or woman (whatever some have written to the contrary)

trary.) The garden Asparagus nourisheth more than the wild, yet it hath the same effects in all the afore-mentioned diseases. The decoction of the roots in white wine, and the back and belly bathed therewith, or kneeling or lying down in the same, or sitting therein as a bath, hath been found effectual against pains of the reins and bladder, pains of the mother and cholic, and generally against all pains that happen to the lower parts of the body, and no less effectual against stiff and benumbed sinews, or those that are shrunk by cramps and convulsions, and helpeth the sciatica.

Ash Tree.

THIS is so well known, that time will be misspent in writing a description of it; and therefore I shall only insist upon the virtues of it.

Government and Virtues.] It is governed by the Sun; and the young tender tops, with the leaves taken inwardly, and some of them outwardly applied, are singularly good against the biting of viper, adder, or any other venomous beast; and the water distilled therefrom being taken a small quantity every morning fasting, is a singular medicine for those that are subject to dropsy, or to abate the greatness of those that are too gross or fat. The decoction of the leaves in white wine helpeth to break the stone, and expel it, and cureth the jaundice. The ashes of the bark of the Ash made into lee, and those heads bathed therewith, which are leprous, scabby, or scald, they are thereby cured. The kernels within the husks, commonly called Ashen Keys, prevail against stitches and pains in the sides, proceeding of wind, and voideth away the stone by provoking urine.

I can justly except against none of this, save only the first, viz. That Ash tree top and leaves are good against the biting of serpents and vipers. I suppose this had its rise from Gerard or Pliny, both which hold, That there is such an antipathy between an adder and an Ash tree, that if an adder be encompassed round with Ash tree leaves, she will sooner run through the fire than through the leaves. The contrary to which is the truth, as both my eyes are witness. The rest are virtues something likely, only if it be in Winter when you cannot get the leaves, you may safely use the bark instead of them. The keys you may easily keep all the year, gathering them when they are ripe.

Avens, called also Colewort, and Herb bonet.

Descript.] THE ordinary Avens hath many long, rough, dark green winged leaves, rising from the root, every one made of many leaves set on each side of the middle rib, the largest three whereof grow at the end, and are snipped or dented round about the edges; the other being small pieces, sometimes two and sometimes four, standing on each side of the middle rib underneath them. Among which do rise up divers rough or hairy stalks about two feet high, branching forth with leaves at every joint, not so long as those below, but almost as much cut in on the edges, some into three parts, some into more. On the tops of the branches stand small pale yellow flowers, consisting of five leaves, like the flowers of Cinquefoil, but large, in the middle whereof standeth a small green herb which when the flower is fallen, groweth to be round, being made of many long greenish purple seeds (like grains) which will stick upon your cloaths. The root consists of many brownish strings or fibres, smelling somewhat like unto cloves, especially those which grow in the higher, hotter, and drier grounds, and in free and clear air.

Place] They grow wild in many places under hedges sides, and by the path ways in fields; yet they rather delight to grow in shadowy than sunny places.

Time] They flower in May and June for the most part, and their seed is ripe in July at the farthest.

Government and Virtues] It is governed by Jupiter, and that gives hopes of a wholesome healthful herb. It is good for the diseases of the chest or breast, for pains, and stitches in the side, and to expel crude and raw humours from the belly and stomach, by the sweet savour and warming quality. It dissolves the inward congealed blood happening by falls or bruises, and the spitting of blood, if the root, either green or dry, be boiled in wine and drank, as also all manner of inward wounds or outward, if washed or bathed therewith. The decoction also being drank, comforts the heart, and strengthens the stomach and a cold brain, and therefore is good in the
Spring-

Spring-time to open obstructions of the liver, and helpeth the wind colic; it also helps those that have fluxes, or are bursten, or have a rupture, it taketh away spots or marks in the face, being washed therewith. The juice of the fresh root, or powder of the dried root, hath the same effect with the decoction. The root in the Spring time, steeped in wine doth give it a delicate savour and taste, and being drank fasting every morning, comforteth the heart, and is a good preservative against the plague, or any other poison. It helpeth digestion, and warmeth a cold stomach, and openeth obstructions of the liver and spleen.

It is very safe; you need have no dose prescribed; and is very fit to be kept in every body's house.

Balm.

THIS herb is so well known to be an inhabitant almost in every garden, that I shall not need to write any description thereof, although the virtues thereof, which are many, should not be omitted.

Government and Virtues.] It is an herb of Jupiter, and under Cancer, and strengthens nature much in all its actions. Let a syrup made with the juice of it and sugar (as you shall be taught at the latter end of the book) be kept in every gentlewoman's house, to relieve the weak stomachs and sick bodies of their poor sickly neighbours; as also the herb kept dry in the house, that so with other convenient simples, you may make it into an electuary with honey, according as the disease is, you shall be taught at the latter end of my book. The Arabian physicians have extolled the virtues thereof to the skies; although the Greeks thought it not worth mentioning. Seraphio saith, it causeth the mind and heart to become merry, and reviveth the heart, faintings and swoonings, especially of such who are overtaken in sleep, and driveth away all troublesome cares and thoughts out of the mind, arising from melancholy or black choler, which Avicen also confirmeth. It is very good to help digestion, and open obstructions of the brain, and hath so much purging quality in it (saith Avicen) as to expel those melancholy vapours from the spirits and blood which are in the heart and arteries, although it cannot do so in other parts of the body. Dioscorides saith, That the leaves steeped in wine, and the wine drank, and the leaves externally applied, is a remedy against

against the stings of a scorpion, and the bitings of mad dogs; and commendeth the decoction thereof for women to bathe or sit in to procure their courses; it is good to wash aching teeth therewith, and profitable for those that have the bloody flux. The leaves also, with a little nitre taken in drink, are good against the surfeit of mushrooms, help the griping pains of the belly; and being made into an electuary, it is good for them that cannot fetch their breath: Used with salt, it takes away wens, kernels, or hard swellings in the flesh or throat; it cleanseth foul sores, and easeth pains of the gout. It is good for the liver and spleen. A tansy or caudle made with eggs, and juice thereof while it is young, putting to it some sugar and rose water, is good for a woman in child bed, when the after birth is not thoroughly voided, and for their faintings upon or in their sore travel. The herb bruised and boiled in a little wine and oil, and laid warm on a boil, will ripen it, and break it.

Barberry.

THE shrub is so well known by every boy and girl that hath but attained to the age of seven years, that it needs no description.

Government and Virtues] Mars owns the shrub, and presents it to the use of my countrymen, to purge their bodies of choler. The inner rind of the Barberry tree boiled in white wine, and a quarter of a pint drank each morning, is an excellent remedy to cleanse the body of choleric humours, and free it from such diseases as choler causeth, such as scabs, itch, tetters, ringworms, yellow jaundice, boils, &c. It is excellent for hot agues, burnings, scaldings, heat of the blood, heat of the liver, bloody flux, for the berries are as good as the bark, and more pleasing; they get a man a good stomach to his victuals, by strengthening the attractive faculty which is under Mars, as you may see more at large at the latter end of my *Ephemeris* for the year 1651. The hair washed with the lee made of ashes of the tree and water, will make it turn yellow, viz. of Mars' own colour. The fruit and rind of the shrub, the flowers of broom and of heath, or furz, cleanse the body of choler by sympathy, as the flowers, leaves, and bark of the peach tree do by antipathy; because these are under Mars, that under Venus.

Bailey.

Barley.

THE continual usefulness hereof hath made all in general so acquainted herewith, that it is altogether needless to describe it, several kinds hereof plentifully growing, being yearly sown in this land. The virtues thereof take as followeth.

Government and Virtues.] It is a notable plant of Saturn: if you view diligently its effects by sympathy and antipathy, you may easily perceive a reason of them; and also why barley bread is so unwholesome for melancholy people. Barley in all the parts and compositions thereof, (except malt) is more cooling than wheat, and a little cleansing; and all the preparations thereof, as Barley water and other things made thereof, do give great nourishment to persons troubled with fevers, agues, and heats in the stomach. A poultice made of barley meal or flower boiled in vinegar and honey, and a few dry figs put into them, dissolveth all hard imposthumes, and assuageth inflammations, being thereto applied. And being boiled with melilot and camomile flowers, and some lintseed, fenugreek and rue in powder, and applied warm, it easeth pains in the side and stomach, and windiness of the spleen. The meal of barley and flowers boiled in water, and made a poultice with honey and oil of lilies applied warm, cureth swellings under the ears, throat, neck and such like; and a plaister made thereof with tar, wax, and oil, helpeth the king's evil in the throat, boiled with sharp vinegar into a poultice, and laid on hot, helpeth the leprosy; being boiled in red wine with pomegranate rind, and myrtles, stayeth the lask or other flux of the belly. boiled with vinegar and quince, it easeth the pains of the gout; barley flour, white salt, honey and vinegar mingled together, taketh away the itch speedily and certainly. The Water distilled from the green barley in the end of May, is very good for those that have defluctions of humours fallen into their eyes, and easeth the pain being dropped into them; or white bread steeped therein, and bound on the eyes, doth the same.

Garden Bazil, or Sweet Bazil.

Descript] THE greater or ordinary Bazil riseth up usually with one upright stalk diversely branching

ing forth on all sides, with two leaves at every joint, which are somewhat broad and round, yet pointed of a pale green colour, but fresh; a little snipped about the edges, and of a strong healthy scent. The flowers are small and white, and standing at the tops of the branches, with two small leaves at the joints, in some places green, in others brown, after which come black seed. The root perisheth at the approach of Winter, and therefore must be new sown every year.

Place] It groweth in gardens.

Time.] It must be sowed late, and flowers in the heart of Summer, being a very tender plant.

Government and Virtues.] This is the herb which all authors are together by the ears about, and rail at one another (like lawyers). Galen and Dioscorides hold it not fitting to be taken inwardly; and Chrysippus rails at it with down right Billingsgate rhetoric, Pliny, and the Arabian physicians defend it.

For mine own part, I presently found that speech true;
Non nostrum inter nos tantas componere lites.
And away to Dr Reason went I, who told me it was an herb of Mars, and under the Scorpion, and perhaps therefore called Basilicon, and it is no marvel if it carry a kind of virulent quality with it. Being applied to the place bitten by venomous beasts, or stung by a wasp or hornet, it speedily draws the poison to it. *Every like draws his like.* Mizaldus affirms, that, being laid to rot in horse dung, it will breed venomous beasts. Hilarius, a French physician, affirms upon his own knowledge, that an acquaintance of his, by common smelling to it, had a scorpion bred in his brain. Something is the matter, this herb and rue will never grow together, no, nor near one another; and we know rue is as great an enemy to poison as any that grows.

To conclude it expelleth both birth and after birth; and as it helps the deficiency of Venus in one kind, so it spoils all her actions in another. I dare write no more of it.

The Bay Tree.

THIS is so well known, that it needs no description; I shall therefore only write the virtues thereof, which are many.

Government and Virtues.] I shall but only add a word or two

two to what my friend hath written, viz. That it is a tree of the Sun, and under the celestial sign Leo, and resisteth witchcraft very potently, as also all the evils old Saturn can do to the body of man, and they are not a few; for it is the speech of one, and I am mistaken if it were not Mizaldus, that neither witch nor devil, thunder nor lightning, will hurt a man in the place where a bay tree is. Galen said, that the leaves or bark do dry and heal very much, and the berries more than leaves; the bark of the root is less sharp and hot, but more bitter, and hath some astriction withal, whereby it is effectual to break the stone, and good to open obstructions of the liver, spleen, and other inward parts, which bring the jaundice, dropsy, &c. The berries are very effectual against all poison of venomous creatures, and the sting of wasps and bees; as also against the pestilence, or other infectious diseases, and therefore, put into sundry treacles for that purpose: they likewise procure women's courses; and seven of them given to a woman in sore travel of childbirth, do cause a speedy delivery, and expel the after birth, and therefore not to be taken by such as have not gone out their time, lest they procure abortion, or cause labour too soon. They wonderfully help all cold and rheumatic distillations from the brain to the eyes, lungs, or other parts; and being made into an electuary with honey, do help the consumption, old coughs, shortness of breath, and thin rheums; as also the megrum. They mightily expel the wind, and provoke urine; help the mother, and kill the worms. The leaves also work the like effects. A bath of the decoction of the leaves and berries, is singularly good for women to sit in, that are troubled with the mother, or the diseases thereof, or the stoppings of their courses, or for the diseases of the bladder, pains in the bowels by wind and stopping of urine. A decoction likewise of equal parts of Bay berries, cummin seed, hyssop, origanum, and euphorbium, with some honey, and the head bathed therewith, doth wonderfully help distillations and rheums, and settleth the palate of the mouth into its place. The oil made of the berries is very comfortable in all cold griefs of the joints, nerves, arteries, stomach, belly, or womb, and helpeth palsies, convulsions, cramp, aches, tremblings and numbness in any part, weariness also, and pains that come by sore travelling. All griefs and pains proceeding from wind, either in the head, stomach, back,

belly,

belly, or womb, by anointing the parts affected therewith. And pains in the ears are also cured by dropping in some of the oil, or by receiving into the ears the fume of the decoction of the berries through a funnel. The oil takes away the marks of the skin and flesh by bruises, falls, &c. and dissolveth the congealed blood in them: It helpeth also the itch, scabs and weals in the skin.

Beans.

BOTH the garden and field beans are so well known, that it saveth me the labour of writing any description of them. Their virtues follow.

Government and Virtues.] They are plants of Venus, and the distilled water of the flower of garden beans is good to clean the face and skin from spots and wrinkles, and the meal or flour of them, or the small beans doth the same. The water distilled from the green husks, is held to be very effectual against the stone, and to provoke urine. Bean flour is used in poultices to assuage inflammations rising upon wounds, and the swelling of women's breasts, caused by the curdling of their milk, and represseth their milk: Flour of beans and fenugreek mixed with honey, and applied to felons, boils, bruises, or blue marks by blows, or the imposthumes in the kernels of the ears, helpeth them all; and with rose leaves, frankincense, and the white of an egg, being applied to the eyes, helpeth them that are swollen or do water, or have received any blow upon them, if used with wine. If a Bean be parted in two, the skin being taken away, and laid on the place where the leech hath been set that bleedeth too much, stayeth the bleeding. Bean flour boiled to a poultice with wine and vinegar, and some oil put thereto, easeth both pains and swelling of the cods. The husks boiled in water to the consumption of a third part thereof, stayeth a lask: And the ashes of the husks, made up with old hog's grease, helpeth the old pains, contusions, and wounds of the sinew, the sciatica and gout. The field Beans have all the afore-mentioned virtues as the garden Beans.

Beans eaten are extremely windy meat; but if after the Dutch fashion, when they are half boiled you husk them and then stew them (I cannot tell you how, for I never was cook in all my life,) they are wholesome food.

French

French Beans.

Descript.] THIS French or Kidney-Bean ariseth at first but with one stalk, which afterwards divides itself into many arms or branches, but all so weak, that if they be not sustained with sticks or poles, they will be fruitless upon the ground. At several places of these branches grow foot stalks, each with three broad round and pointed green leaves at the end of them; towards the top comes forth divers flowers made like unto peas blossoms, of the same colour for the most part that the fruit will be of; that is to say, white, yellow, red, blackish, or of a deeper purple, but white is the most usual; after which come long and slender flat cods, some crooked, some strait, with a string running down the back thereof, wherein is flattish round fruit made like a kidney; the root long, spreadeth with many strings annexed to it, and perisheth every year.

There is another sort of French Beans commonly growing with us in this land, which is called the scarlet flowered Bean.

This ariseth with sundry branches as the other, but runs higher to the length of hop poles, about which they grow twining, but turning contrary to the sun, having foot-stalks with three leaves on each, as on the other; the flowers also are like the other, and of a most orient scarlet colour. The Beans are larger than the ordinary kind, of a dead purple colour, turning black when ripe and dry: The root perisheth in Winter.

Government and Virtues] These also belong to Dame Venus, and being dried and beat to powder, are as great strengtheners of the kidneys as any are; neither is there a better remedy than it; a dram at a time taken in white wine, doth prevent the stone, or do cleanse the kidneys of gravel or stoppage. The ordinary French Beans are of an easy digestion; they move the belly, provoke urine, enlarge the breast that is straitened with shortness of breath, engender sperm, and incite to venery. And the scarlet coloured Beans, in regard of the glorious beauty of their colour, being set near a quickset hedge, will bravely adorn the same by climbing up thereon, so that they may be discerned a great way, not without admiration of the beholders at a distance. But they
will

will go near to kill the quickets by cloathing them in scarlet.

Ladies Bed-Straw.

BESIDES the common name above written, it is called Cheese Renner, because it performs the same office, as also Gallion, Pettimugget, and Maid-Hair; and by some Wild Rosemary.

Descript.] This riseth up with divers small, brown and square upright stalks a yard high, or more: sometimes branches forth into divers parts, full of joints, and with divers very fine small leaves at every one of them little or nothing rough at all: at the tops of the branches grow many long tufts or branches of yellow flowers very thick set together, from the several joints which consist of four leaves a piece, which smell somewhat strong, but not unpleasant. The seed is small and black like poppy seed, two for the most part joined together: The root is reddish, with many small threads fastened into it, which take strong hold of the ground, and creepeth a little; and the branches leaning a little down to the ground, take root at the joints thereof, whereby it is easily increased.

There is another sort of Ladies Bed-straw growing frequently in England which beareth white flowers as the other doth yellow; but the branches of this are so weak, that unless it be sustained by the hedges, or other things near which it groweth, it will lie down to the ground: The leaves a little bigger than the former, and the flowers not so plentiful as these; and the root hereof is also thready and abiding.

Place.] They grow in meadows and pastures both wet and dry, and by the hedges.

Time] They flower in May for the most part, and the seed is ripe in July and August.

Government and Virtues] They are both herbs of Venus, and therefore strengthening the parts both internal and external, which she rules. The decoction of the former of those being drank, is good to fret and break the stone, provoke urine, stayeth inward bleeding, and healeth inward wounds. The herb or flower bruised and put up into the nostrils, stayeth their bleeding likewise: The flowers and herbs being made into an oil, by being set in the sun, and
changed

changed after it hath stood ten or twelve days; or into an ointment being boiled in *Axunga*, or sallet oil, with some wax melted therein, after it is strained; either the oil made thereof, or the ointment, do help burnings with fire, or scaldings with water: The same also, or the decoction of the herb and flower, is good to bathe the feet of travellers and lacquies, whose long running causeth weariness and stiffness in their sinews and joints. If the decoction be used warm, and the joints afterwards anointed with ointment, it helpeth the dry scab, and the itch in children; and the herb with the white flower is also very good for the sinews, arteries, and joints, to comfort and strengthen them after travel, cold, and pains.

Beets.

OF Beets there are two sorts, which are best known generally, and whereof I shall principally treat at this time, viz. the white and red Beets, and their virtues.

Descript] The common white Beet hath many great leaves next the ground, somewhat large, and of a whitish green colour. The stalk is great, strong and ribbed, bearing great store of leaves upon it, almost to the very top of it. The flowers grow in very long tufts, small at the end, and turning down their heads, which are small, pale, greenish, yellow buds, giving cornered prickly seed. The root is great, long, and hard, and when it hath given seed, is of no use at all.

The common red Beet differeth not from the white, but only it is lesser, and the leaves and the roots are somewhat red: The leaves are differently red, some only with red stalks or veins; some of a fresh red, and others of a dark red. The root thereof is red, spungy, and not used to be eaten.

Government and Virtues] The government of these two sorts of beets are far different; the red Beet being under Saturn, and the white under Jupiter. therefore take the virtues of them apart, each by itself The white Beet doth much loosen the belly, and is of a cleansing, digesting quality, and provoketh urine. The juice of it openeth obstructions both of the liver and spleen, and is good for the head-ach and swimmings therein, and turnings of the brain; and is effectual also against all venomous creatures; and applied

unto

unto the temples, stayeth inflammations in the eyes; helpeth burnings, being used without oil, and with a little allum put to it, is good for St Anthony's fire. It is good for all wheals, pushes, blisters, and blains in the skin: the herb boiled and laid upon chilblains or kibes helpeth them. The decoction thereof in water and some vinegar healeth the itch, if bathed therewith, and cleanseth the head of dandruff, scurf, and dry scabs, and doth much good for fretting and running sores, ulcers, and cankers in the head, legs, or other parts, and is much commended against baldness and shedding the hair.

The red Beet is good to stay the bloody flux, women's courses, and the whites, and do help the yellow jaundice: the juice of the root put into the nostrils, purgeth the head, helpeth the noise in the ears, and the tooth-ach; the juice snuffed up the nose, helps a stinking breath, if the cause lies in the nose, as many times it doth, if any bruise hath been there; as also want of smell coming that way.

Water Betony.

CALLED also Brown wort, and in Yorkshire, Bishops-leaves.

Descript] First, of the Water Betony, which riseth up with square, hard, greenish stalks, sometimes brown, set with broad dark green leaves dented about the edges with notches somewhat resembling the leaves of the Wood Betony, but much larger too, for the most part set at a joint. The flowers are many, set at the tops of the stalks and branches, being round bellied and opened at the brims, and divided into two parts, the uppermost being like a hood, and the lowermost like a hip hanging down, of a dark red colour, which passing, there come in their places small round heads with small points at the ends, wherein lie small and brownish seeds the root is a thick bush of strings and shreds growing from the head.

Place.] It groweth by the ditch side, brooks, and other water-courses, generally through this land, and is seldom found far from the water side.

Time.] It flowereth about July, and the seed is ripe in August.

Government and Virtues.] Water Betony is an herb of Jupiter in Cancer, and is appropriated more to wounds and

hurts

hurts in the breasts than Wood Betony, which follows: It is an excellent remedy for sick hogs. It is of a cleansing quality: The leaves bruised and applied are effectual for all old and filthy ulcers; and especially if the juice of the leaves be boiled with a little honey, and dipped therein, and the sores dressed therewith; as also for bruises or hurts, whether inward or outward: The distilled water of the leaves is used for the same purpose; as also to bathe the face and hands spotted or blemished, or discoloured by sun burning.

I confess I do not much fancy distilled waters, I mean such waters as are distilled cold; some virtues of the herb they may happily have (it were a strange thing else); but this I am confident of, that being distilled in a pewter still, as the vulgar and apish fashion is, both chymical oil and salt is left behind, unless you burn them, and then all is spoiled, water and all, which was good for as little as can be by such a distillation in my translation of the London Dispensatory.

Wood Betony.

Descript] COMMON or Wood Betony hath many leaves rising from the root, which are somewhat broad and round at the end, roundly dented about the edges, standing upon long foot stalks, from among which arise up small, square, slender, but upright hairy stalks, with some leaves thereon to a piece at the joints, smaller than the lower, whereon are set several spiked heads of flowers like lavender, but thicker and shorter for the most part, and of a reddish or purple colour, spotted with white spots both in the upper and lower part, the seeds being contained within the husks that hold the flowers, are blackish, somewhat long and uneven. The roots are many white thready strings; the stalk perisheth, but the roots, with some leaves thereon, abide all the Winter. The whole plant is something small.

Place] It groweth frequently in woods, and delighteth in shady places

Time] And it flowereth in July; after which the seed is quickly ripe, yet in its prime in May.

Government and Virtues] The herb is appropriated to the planet Jupiter, and the sign Aries. Antonius Musa, physician

cian to the Emperor Auguſtus Cæſar, wrote a peculiar book of the virtues of this herb; and among other virtues, ſaith of it, that it preſerveth the liver and bodies of men from the danger of epidemical diſeaſes, and from witchcrafts alſo, it helpeth thoſe that loath or cannot digeſt their meat, thoſe that have weak ſtomachs, or ſour belchings, or continual riſing in their ſtomach, uſing it familiarly, either green or dry; either the herb or root, or the flowers in broth, drink, or meat, or made into conſerve, ſyrup water, electuary, or powder, as every one may beſt frame themſelves unto, or as the time or ſeaſon requireth; taken any of the aforeſaid ways, it helpeth the jaundice, falling ſickneſs, the palſy, convulſions, or ſhrinking of the ſinews, the gout, and thoſe that are inclined to dropſy, thoſe that have continual pains in their heads, although it turn to phrenſy. The powder mixed with pure honey, is no leſs available for all ſorts of coughs or colds, wheeſing, or ſhortneſs of breath, diſtillations of thin rheum upon the lungs, which cauſeth conſumptions. The decoction made with mead, and a little penny-royal, is good for thoſe that are troubled with putrid agues, whether quotidian, tertian, or quartan, and to draw down and evacuate the blood and humours, that by falling into the eyes, do hinder the ſight; the decoction thereof made in wine, and taken, killeth the worms in the belly openeth obſtructions both of the ſpleen and liver, cureth ſtitches, and the pains in the back or ſides, the torments and griping pains of the bowels, and the wind colic; and mixed with honey purgeth the belly, helpeth to bring down women's courſes, and is of ſpecial uſe for thoſe that are troubled with the falling down of the mother, and pains thereof, and cauſeth an eaſy and ſpeedy delivery of women in child birth. It helpeth alſo to break and expel the ſtone either in the bladder or kidneys. The decoction with wine gargled in the mouth, eaſeth the toothach It is commended againſt the ſtinging or biting of venomous ſerpents, or mad dogs, being uſed inwardly and applied outwardly to the place. A dram of the powder of Betony, taken with a little honey in ſome vinegar, doth wonderfully refreſh thoſe that are over wearied by travel. It ſtayeth bleeding at the mouth or noſe, and helpeth thoſe that piſs or ſpit blood, and thoſe that are burſten or have a rupture, and is good for ſuch as are bruiſed by any fall or otherwiſe. The green herb bruiſed, or the juice applied to any inward hurt, or outward green wound in the head or body, will quickly heal and close it up, as also any veins or sinews that are cut; and will draw forth any broken bone or splinter, thorn or other things got into the flesh. It is no less profitable for old sores or filthy ulcers; yea, though they be fistulous and hollow. But some do advise to put a little salt to this purpose, being applied with a little hog's lard, it helpeth a plague sore, and other boils and pushes. The fume of the decoction while it is warm, received by a funnel into the ears, easeth the pains of them, destroys the worms, and cureth the running sores in them. The juice dropped into them doth the same. The root of Betony is displeasing both to the taste and stomach, whereas the leaves and flowers, by their sweet and spicy taste, are comfortable both to meat and medicine.

These are some of the many virtues Antony Muse, an expert physician (for it was not the practice of Octavius Cæsar to keep fools about him) appropriates to Betony; it is a very precious herb, that is certain, and most fitting to be kept in a man's house, both in syrup, conserve, oil, ointment, and plaister. The flowers are usually conserved.

The Beech Tree.

IN treating of this tree, you must understand that I mean the green Mast beech, which is, by way of distinction from that other small rough sort, called in Sussex the smaller Beech, but in Essex Horn bean.

I suppose it is needless to describe it, being already too well known to my countrymen.

Place.] It groweth in woods amongst oaks and other trees, and in parks, forests, and chaces, to feed deer; and in other places to fatten swine.

Time] It bloometh in the end of April, or beginning of May, for the most part, and the fruit is ripe in September.

Government and Virtues] It is a plant of Saturn, and therefore performs his qualities and proportion in these operations. The leaves of the Beech Tree are cooling and binding, and therefore good to be applied to hot swellings to discuss them; the nuts do much nourish such beasts as feed thereon. The water that is found in the hollow places of decaying Beeches will cure both man and beast of any scurf, scab, or running tetters, if they be washed therewith; you may boil the leaves into a poultice, or make an ointment of them when time of year serves.

Bilberries, called by some Whorts, and Whortle-Berries.

Descript.] OF these I shall only speak of two sorts which are common in England, viz. the black and red berries. And first of the black.

The small bush creepeth along upon the ground, scarce rising half a yard high, with divers small dark green leaves set on the green branches, not always one against the other, and a little dented about the edges; at the foot of the leaves come forth small, hollow, pale, bluish coloured flowers, the brims ending in five points, with a reddish thread in the middle, which pass into small round berries of the bigness and colour of juniper berries, but of a purple, sweetish, sharp taste; the juice of them giveth a purplish colour in their hands and lips that eat and handle them, especially if they break them. The root groweth aslope under ground, shooting forth in sundry places as it creepeth. This loses its leaves in Winter.

The Red Bilberry, or Whortle Bush, riseth up like the former, having sundry hard leaves, like the Box tree leaves, green and round pointed, standing on the several branches, at the top whereof only, and not from the sides, as in the former, come forth divers round, reddish, sappy berries, when they are ripe, of a sharp taste. The root runneth in the ground, as in the former, but the leaves of this abide all the Winter.

Place] The first groweth in forests, on the heaths, and such like barren places. The red grows in the north parts of this land, as Lancashire, Yorkshire, &c.

Time.] They flower in March and April, and the fruit of the black is ripe in July and August.

Government and Virtues.] They are under the dominion of Jupiter. It is a pity they are used no more in physic than they are. The Black Bilberries are good in hot agues, and to cool the heat of the liver and stomach; they do somewhat bind the belly, and stay vomitings and loathings; the juice of the berries made in a syrup, or the pulp made into a conserve with sugar, is good for the purposes aforesaid, as also for an old cough, or an ulcer in the lungs, or other

diseases

diseases therein. The red Whorts are more binding, and stop women's courses, spitting of blood, or any other flux of blood or humours, being used as well outwardly as inwardly.

Bifoil, or Twablade.

Descript.] THIS small herb, from a root somewhat sweet, shooting downwards many long strings, riseth up a round green stalk, bare or naked next the ground for an inch, two or three to the middle thereof, as it is in age or growth; as also from the middle upward to the flowers, having only two broad plantain-like leaves (but whiter) set at the middle of the stalk, one against another, compasseth it round at the bottom of them.

Place.] It is an usual inhabitant in woods, copses, and in many other places in this land.

There is another sort groweth in wet grounds and marshes, which is somewhat different from the former. It is a smaller plant, and greener, having sometimes three leaves; the spike of the flowers is less than the former, and the roots of this do run or creep in the ground.

They are much and often used by many to good purpose for wounds, both green and old, and to consolidate or knit ruptures, as well it may, being a plant of Saturn.

The Birch Tree.

Descript.] THIS groweth a goodly tall straight tree, fraught with many boughs, and slender branches bending downward, the old being covered with a discoloured chipped bark, and the younger being browner by much. The leaves at the first breaking out are crumpled, and afterwards like beech leaves, but smaller and greener, and dented about the edges. It beareth small short cat skins, somewhat like those of the hazel nut tree, which abide on the branches a long time, until growing ripe, they fall on the ground, and then seed with them.

Place.] It usually groweth in woods.

Government and Virtues.] It is a tree of Venus; the juice of the leaves, while they are young, or the distilled water of them, or the water that comes from the tree being bored with an augur, and distilled afterwards; any of these being drank for some days together, is available to break the stone in the kidneys and bladder, and is good also to wash sore mouths.

Bird's Foot.

THIS small herb groweth not above a span high, with many branches spread upon the ground, set with many wings of small leaves. The flowers grow upon the branches, many small ones of a pale yellow colour being set a head together, which afterwards turneth into small jointed cods, well resembling the claws of small birds, whence it took its name.

There is another sort of Bird's-foot in all things like the former, but a little larger; the flower of a pale whitish red colour, and the cods distinct by joints like the other, but a little more crooked; and the roots do carry many small white knots or kernels amongst the strings.

Place.] These grow on heaths, and many open untilled places of this land.

Time.] They flower and seed in the end of Summer.

Government and Virtues.] They belong to Saturn, and are of a drying, binding quality, and thereby very good to be used in wound drinks; as also to apply outwardly for the same purpose. But the latter Bird's-foot is found by experience to break the stone in the back or kidneys, and drives them forth, if the decoction thereof be taken; and it wonderfully helpeth the rupture, being taken inwardly, and outwardly applied to the place.

All salts have best operation upon the stone, as ointments and plaisters have upon wounds; and therefore you may make a salt of this for the stone, the way how to do so may be found in my translation of the London Dispensatory, and it may be I may give you it again in plainer terms at the latter end of this book.

Bishop's-weed.

BESIDES the common name Bishop-weed, it is usually known by the Greek name *Ammi* and *Ammios*; some call it Ethiopian Cummin-seed, and others Cummin royal, as also Herb-William, and Bull-wort.

Descript.] Common Bishop's weed riseth up with a round straight stalk, sometimes as high as a man, but usually three or four feet high, beset with divers small, long, somewhat broad leaves, cut in some places, and dented about the edges, growing one against another, of a dark green colour, having sundry

sundry branches on them, at the top small umbels of white flowers, which turn into small round seeds, little bigger than parsley-seeds, of a quick hot scent and taste: the root is white and stringy, perishing yearly, and usually riseth again on its own sowing.

Place] It groweth wild in many places in England and Wales, as between Greenhith and Grave end.

Government and Virtues] It is hot and dry in the third degree, of a bitter taste, and somewhat sharp withal; it provokes lust to purpose. I suppose Venus owns it. It digesteth humours, provoketh urine and women's courses, dissolveth wind, and being taken in wine it easeth pain and gripping in the bowels, and is good against the biting of serpents. It is used to good effects in those medicines which are given to hinder the poisonous operation of Cantharides upon the passage of the urine, being mixed with honey and applied to black and blue marks, coming of blows or bruises, it takes them away, and being drank or outwardly applied, it abateth an high colour, and makes it pale; and the fumes thereof taken with rosin or raisins, cleanseth the mother.

Bistort, or Snakeweed.

IT is called Snakeweed, English Serpentary, Dragon wort, Osteric, and Passions.

Descript] This hath a thick short knobbed root, blackish without, and somewhat reddish within, a little crooked or turned together, of a hard astringent taste, with divers black threads hanging there, from whence spring up every year divers leaves standing upon long foot stalks, being somewhat broad and long like a dock leaf, and a little pointed at the ends, but that it is of a bluish green colour on the upper side, and of an ash colour grey, and a little purplish underneath, with divers veins therein, from among which rise up divers small and slender stalks, two feet high, and almost naked and without leaves, or with a very few, and narrow, bearing a spikey bush of pale coloured flowers, which being past, there abideth small seed, like unto sorrel seed, but greater.

There are other sorts of Bistort growing in this land, but smaller, both in height, root, and stalks, and especially in the leaves. The root blackish without, and somewhat whitish within, of an austere binding taste, as the former.

Place.] They grow in shadowy moist woods, and at the foot of hills, but are chiefly nourished up in gardens. The narrow leafed Bistort groweth in the north, in Lancashire, Yorkshire, and Cumberland.

Time] They flower about the end of May, and the seed is ripe about the beginning of July.

Government and Virtues] It belongs to Saturn, and is in operation cold and dry; both the leaves and roots have a powerful faculty to resist all poison. The root in powder taken in drink expelleth the venom of the plague, the small pox, measles, purples, or any other infectious disease, driving it out by sweating. The root in powder, the decoction thereof in wine being drank, stayeth all manner of inward bleeding, or spitting of blood, and any fluxes in the body of either man or woman, or vomiting. It is also very available against ruptures, or burstings, or all bruises, or falls, dissolving the congealed blood, and easing the pains that happen thereupon, it also helpeth the jaundice.

The water distilled from both leaves and roots, is a singular remedy to wash any place bitten or stung by any venomous creature, as also for any of the purposes before spoken of, and is very good to wash any running sores or ulcers. The decoction of the root in wine being drank hindereth abortion or miscarriage in child bearing. The leaves also kill the worms in children, and is a great help to them that cannot keep their water; if the juice of plantain be added thereto, and outwardly applied, it much helpeth the gonorrhea, or running of the reins. A dram of the powder of the root taken in water thereof, wherein some red hot iron or steel hath been quenched, is also an admirable help thereto, so as the body be first prepared and purged from the offensive humours. The leaves, seed, or roots, are all very good in decoctions, drinks, or lotions, for inward or outward wounds, or other sores. And the powder strewed upon any cut or wound in a vein stayeth the immoderate bleeding thereof. The decoction of the root in water, whereunto some pomegranate-peels and flowers are added, injected into the matrix, stayeth the immoderate flux of the courses. The root thereof with pellitory of Spain, and burnt allum, of each a little quantity, beaten small and made into paste, with some honey, and a little piece thereof put into an hollow tooth, or held between the teeth, if there be no hollowness in them stayeth the defluxion of rheum upon them, which causeth pains, and helps to cleanse the head, and void much offensive water. The distilled water is very effectual to wash sores or cankers in the nose, or any other part, if the powder of the root be applied thereunto afterwards. It is good also to fasten the gums, and to take away the heat and inflammations that happen in the jaws, almonds of the throat, or mouth, if the decoction of the leaves, roots, or seeds bruised, or the juice of them be applied; but the roots are most effectual to the purposes aforesaid.

One-Blade.

Descript] THIS small plant never beareth more than one leaf, but only when it riseth up with its stalk, when thereon beareth another, and seldom more, which are of a bluish green colour, broad at the bottom, and pointed with many ribs or veins like plantain, at the top of the stalk grows many small flowers star-fashion, smelling somewhat sweet, after which cometh small reddish berries when they are ripe. The root small, of the bigness of a rush, lying and creeping under the upper crust of the earth, shooting forth in divers places.

Place] It grows in moist, shadowy, grassy places of wood, in many places of this realm.

Time] It flowereth about May, and the berries are ripe in June, and then quickly perisheth, until the next year it springeth from the same again.

Government and Virtues.] It is an herb of the Sun, and therefore cordial; half a dram, or a dram at most, of the roots hereof in powder, taken in wine and vinegar, of each a like quantity, and the party presently laid to sweat, is held to be a sovereign remedy for those that are infected with the plague, and have a sore upon them, by expelling the poison, and defending the heart and spirits from danger. It is also accounted a singular good wound herb, and therefore used with other herbs in making such balms as are necessary for curing of wounds, either green or old, and especially if the nerves be hurt.

The Bramble, or Black berry Bush.

IT is so well known that it needeth no description. The virtues thereof are as follow.

Government and Virtues.] It is a plant of Venus in Aries. You shall have some directions at the latter end of the book for the gathering of all herbs and plants, &c. If any ask the reason why Venus is so prickly? Tell them it is because she is in the house of Mars. The buds, leaves, and branches, while they are green, are of a good use in the ulcers and putrid sores of the mouth and throat, and of the quinsy, and likewise to heal other fresh wounds and sores; but the flowers and fruits unripe are very binding, and so profitable for the bloody flux, lasks, and are a fit remedy for spitting of blood. Either the decoction or powder of the root being taken, is good to break or drive forth gravel, and the stone in the reins and kidneys. The leaves and brambles, as well green as dry, are excellent good lotions for sores in the mouth, or secret parts. The decoction of them, and of the dryed branches, do much bind the belly, and are good for too much flowing of women's courses; the berries of the flowers are a powerful remedy against the poison of the most venomous serpents as well drank as outwardly applied. It helpeth the sores of the fundament, and the piles, the juice of the berries mixed with the juice of mulberries, do bind more effectually, and help all fretting and eating sores and ulcers whatsoever. The distilled water of the branches, leaves, and flowers, or of the fruit, is very pleasant in taste, and very effectual in fevers, and hot distempers of the body, head, eyes, and other parts, and for the purposes aforesaid. The leaves boiled in lee, and the head washed therewith, healeth the itch, and the running sores thereof, and maketh the hair black. The powder of the leaves strewed on cankers and running ulcers, wonderfully helps to heal them. Some use to condensate the juice of the leaves, and some the juice of the berries, to keep for their use all the year, for the purposes aforesaid.

Blites.

Descript] OF these there are two sorts commonly known, viz. White and Red. The White hath leaves somewhat like unto beets, but smaller, rounder, and of a whitish green colour, every one standing upon a small long foot stalk, the stalk rises up two or three feet high, with such like leaves thereon, the flowers grow at the top in long round tufts or clusters, wherein are contained
small

small and round seeds; the root is very full of threads or strings.

The red Blite is in all things like the white, but that his leaves and tufted heads are exceeding red at first, and after turn more purplish.

There are other kinds of Blites which grow, differing from the two former sorts but little, but only the wild are smaller in every part.

Place] They grow in gardens, and wild in many places in this land.

Time.] They seed in August and September.

Government and Virtues] They are all of them cooling, drying, and binding, serving to restrain the fluxes or blood in either man or woman, especially the red, which also stayeth the overflowing of the woman's red, as the white Blites stayeth the whites in women. It is an excellent secret, you cannot well fail in the use: They are all under the dominion of Venus.

There is another sort of wild Blites like the other wild kinds, but have long and spikey heads of green ish seeds, seeming by the thick setting together to be all seed.

This sort the fishers are delighted with, and it is a good and usual bait, for fishes will bite fast enough at them, if you have but wit enough to catch them when they bite.

Borage and Bugloss.

THESE are so well known to the inhabitants in every garden, that I hold it needless to describe them.

To these I may add a third sort, which is not so common, nor yet so well known, and therefore I shall give you its name and description.

It is called *Langue de Beuf,* but why then should they call one herb by the name Bugloss, and another by the name *Langue de Beuf?* It is some question to me, seeing one signifies Ox tongue in Greek, and the other signifies the same in French.

Descript.] The leaves whereof are smaller than those of Bugloss, but much rougher, the stalks arising up about a foot and a half high, and is most commonly of a red colour; the flowers stand in scaly rough heads, being composed of many small yellow flowers, not much unlike to those of Dandelions, and the seed flieth away in down, as that doth; you may easily know the flowers by their taste, for they are very bitter.

Place] It groweth wild in many places of this land, and may be plentifully found near London, as between Rotherhithe and Deptford, by the ditch-side. Its virtues are held to be the same with Borage and Bugloss, only this is somewhat hotter.

Time] They flower in June and July, and the seed is ripe shortly after.

Government and Virtues.] They are all three herbs of Jupiter, and under Leo, all great cordials and great strengtheners of nature. The leaves and roots are to very good purpose used in putrid and pestilential fevers, to defend the heart, and help to resist and expel the poison, or the venom of other creatures, the seed is of the like effects, and the seed and leaves are good to increase milk in women's breasts, the leaves, flowers, and seed, all or any of them, are good to expel pensiveness and melancholy; it helpeth to clarify the blood, and mitigate heat in fevers. The juice made into a syrup, prevaileth much to all the purposes aforesaid, either in put with other cooling, opening and cleansing herbs, to open obstructions and help the yellow jaundice, and mixed with fumitory, to cool, cleanse, and temper the blood thereby; it helpeth the itch, ringworm, and tetters, or other spreading scabs or sores. The flowers candied or made into a conserve are helpful in the former cases, but are chiefly used as a cordial, and are good for those that are weak in long sickness, and to comfort the heart and spirits of those that are in a consumption, or troubled with often swoonings, or passions of the heart. The distilled water is no less effectual to all the purposes aforesaid, and helpeth the redness and inflammations of the eyes, being washed therewith; the dried herb is never used, but the green, yet the ashes thereof, boiled in mead, or honied water, is available against the inflammations and ulcers in the mouth or throat to gargle it therewith; the roots of Bugloss are effectual, being made into a licking electuary for the cough, and to condensate thick phlegm, and the rheumatic distillations upon the lungs.

Blue-Bottle.

IT is called Cyanus, I suppose from the colour of it, Huntsickle, because it turns the edge of the sickles that reap the corn; Blue blow, Corn flower, and Blue bottle

Descript]

Descript.] I shall only describe that which is commonest, and in my opinion most useful; its leaves spread upon the ground, being of a whitish green colour, somewhat on the edges like those of Cornscabions, amongst which ariseth up a stalk divided into divers branches, beset with long leaves of a greenish colour, either but very little indented, or not at all, the flowers are of a blue colour, from whence it took its name, consisting of an innumerable company of small flowers set in a scaly head, not much unlike those of knap-weed; the seed is smooth, bright and shining, wrapped up in a wooly mantle, the root perisheth every year.

Place.] They grow in corn fields, amongst all sorts of corn (peas, beans, and tares excepted). If you please to take them up from thence, and transplant them in your garden, especially towards the full of the moon, they will grow more double than they are, and many times change colour.

Time.] They flower from the beginning of May to the end of harvest.

Government and Virtues.] As they are naturally cold, dry, and binding, so they are under the dominion of Saturn. The powder or dried leaves of the Blue-bottle, or Corn flower, is given with good success to those that are bruised by a fall, or have broken a vein inwardly and void much blood at the mouth, being taken in the water of plantain, horsetail, or the greater comfrey, it is a remedy against the poison of the scorpion, and resisteth all venoms and poison. The seed or leaves taken in wine, is very good against the plague, and all infectious diseases, and is very good in pestilential fevers. The juice put into fresh or green wounds, doth quickly solder up the lips of them together, and is very effectual to heal all ulcers and sores in the mouth. The juice dropped into the eyes takes away the heat and inflammation of them. The distilled water of this herb hath the same properties, and may be used for the effects aforesaid.

Brank Ursine.

BESIDE the common name Brank Ursine, it is also called Bears breech, and Acanthus, though I think our English names to be more proper; for the Greek word *Acanthus* signifies any thistle whatsoever.

Descript.] This thistle shooteth forth very many large,

thick, sad green smooth leaves upon the ground, with a very thick and juicy middle rib; the leaves are parted with sundry deep gashes on the edges; the leaves remain a long time before any stalk appears, afterwards riseth up a reasonable big stalk, three or four feet high, and bravely decked with flowers from the middle of the stalk upwards; for on the lower part of the stalk there is neither branches nor leaf. The flowers are hooded and gaping, being white in colour, and standing in brownish husks, with a long small undivided leaf under each leaf; they seldom seed in our country. Its roots are many, great and thick, blackish without, and whitish within, full of a clammy sap; a piece of them, if you set in the garden, and defend it from the first Winter cold, will grow and flourish.

Place] They are only nursed up in the gardens in England, where they will grow very well.

Time] It flowereth in June and July.

Government and Virtues] It is an excellent plant under the dominion of the Moon. I could wish such as are studious would labour to keep it in their garden. The leaves being boiled and used in clisters, are excellent good to mollify the belly, and make the passage slippery. The decoction drank inwardly, is excellent and good for the bloody flux. The leaves being bruised, or rather boiled, and applied like a poultice, are excellent good to unite broken bones, and strengthen joints that have been put out. The decoction of either leaves or roots being drank, and the decoction of leaves applied to the place, is excellent good for the king's evil that is broken and runneth; for by the influence of the Moon, it reviveth the ends of the veins which are relaxed. There is scarce a better remedy to be applied to such places as are burnt with fire than this is, for it fetches out the fire, and heals it without a scar. This is an excellent remedy for such as are bursten, being either taken inwardly, or applied to the place. In like manner used it helps the cramp and the gout. It is excellent good in hectic fevers, and restores radical moisture to such as are in consumptions.

Briony, or Wild Vine.

IT is called Wild, and Wood Vine, Tamus or Ladies Seal. The white is called White Vine by some; and the black, Black Vine.

Descript.]

Descript] The common White Briony groweth ramping upon the hedges, sending forth many long rough, very tender branches at the beginning, with many very rough and broad leaves thereon, cut (for the most part) into five partitions, in form very like a vine leaf, but smaller, rough, and of a whitish hoary green colour, spreading very far spreading and twining with his small claspers (that come forth at the joints with the leaves) very far on whatsoever standeth next to it. At the several joints also (especially towards the top of the branches) cometh forth a long stalk bearing many whitish flowers together on a long tuft, consisting of five small leaves a piece, laid open like a star, after which come the berries separated one from another, more than a cluster of grapes, green at the first, and very red when they are thorough ripe, of no good scent. but of a most loathsome taste, provoking vomit. The root groweth to be exceeding great, with many long twines or branches going from it, of a pale whitish colour on the outside, and more white within, and of a sharp, bitter, loathsome taste.

Place] It groweth on banks, or under hedges, through this land: the roots lie very deep.

Time] It flowereth in July and August, some earlier, and some later than the other.

Government and Virtues] They are furious martial plants. The root of Briony purges the belly with great violence, troubling the stomach and burning the liver, and therefore not rashly to be taken; but being corrected, is very profitable for the diseases of the head, as falling sickness, giddiness and swimmings, by drawing away much phlegm and rheumatic humours that oppress the head, as also the joints and sinews; and is therefore good for palsies, convulsions, cramps, and stitches in the sides, and the dropsy and in provoking urine; it cleanseth the reins and kidneys from gravel and stone, by opening the obstruction of the spleen, and consumeth the hardness and swelling thereof. The decoction of the root in wine, drunk once a week at going to bed, cleanseth the mother, and helpeth the rising thereof, expelleth the dead child, a dram of the root in powder taken in white wine, bringeth down their courses. An electuary made of the roots and honey, doth mightily cleanse the chest of rotten phlegm, and wonderfully helps any old strong cough, to those that are troubled with shortness of breath, and is very

good

good for them that are bruised inwardly, to help to expel the clotted or congealed blood. The leaves, fruit and root do cleanse old and filthy sores, are good against all fretting and running cankers, gangreens, and tetters, and therefore the berries are by some country people called tetter-berries. The root cleanseth the skin wonderfully from all black and blue spots, freckles, morphew, leprosy, foul scars, or other deformity whatsoever; also all running scabs and manginess are healed by the powder of the dried root, or the juice thereof, but especially by the fine white hardened juice. The distilled water of the root worketh the same effects, but more weakly; the root bruised and applied of itself to any place where the bones are broken, helpeth to draw them forth, as also splinters and thorns in the flesh, and being applied with a little wine mixed therewith it breaketh boils, and helpeth whitlows on the joints—For all these latter beginning at sores, cancers, &c. apply it outwardly, and take my advice in my translation of the London Dispensatory, among the preparations at the latter end, where you have a medicine called *Fæcula Brionia*, which take and use, mixing it with a little hog's grease, or other convenient ointment.

As for the former diseases where it must be taken inwardly, it purgeth very violently, and needs an abler hand to correct it than most country people have, therefore it is a better way for them in my opinion to let the simple alone, and take the compound water of it mentioned in my Dispensatory, and that is far more safe, being wisely corrected.

Brook Lime, or Water Pimpernal.

Descript] THIS sendeth forth from a creeping root that shooteth forth strings at every joint, as it runneth, divers and sundry green stalks round and sappy, with some branches on them, somewhat broad, round, deep green and thick leaves, set by couples thereon; from the bottom whereof shoot forth long foot-stalks, with sundry small blue flowers on them, that consist of five small round pointed leaves a-piece.

There is another sort nothing differing from the former, but that it is greater, and the flowers of a paler green colour.

Place.] They grow in small standing waters, and usually near water cresses.

Time] And flowers in June and July, giving seed the next month after.

Govern-

Government and Virtues.] It is a hot and biting martial plant. Brook-lime and water cresses are generally used together in diet drink, with other things serving to purge the blood and body from all ill humours that would destroy health, and are helpful to the scurvy. They do all provoke urine, and help to break the stone and pass it away; they procure women's courses, and expel the dead child. Being fried with butter and vinegar, and applied warm, it helpeth all manner of tumours, swellings, and inflammations.

Such drinks ought to be made of sundry herbs, according to the malady. I shall give a plain and easy rule at the latter end of this book.

Butchers Broom.

IT is called Ruscus, and Bruscus, Kneecrolm, Kneeholy, Kneehulver, and Pettigree.

Descript.] The first shoots that sprout from the root of Butchers Broom, are thick, whitish, and short, somewhat like those of asparagus, but greater they rising up to be a foot and a half high, are spread into divers branches, green, and somewhat crested with the roundness, tough and flexible, whereon are set somewhat broad and almost round hard leaves, and prickly, pointed at the end, of a dark green colour, two for the most part set at a place, very close and near together, about the middle of the leaf, on the back and lower side from the middle rib, breaketh forth a small whitish green flower, consisting of four small round pointed leaves, standing upon little or no foot-stalk, and in the place whereof cometh a small round berry, green at the first, and red when it is ripe, wherein are two or three white, hard, round seeds contained. The root is thick, white, and great at the head, and from thence sendeth forth divers thick, white, long, tough strings.

Place.] It groweth in copses, and upon heaths and waste grounds, and oftentimes under or near the holly bushes.

Time.] It shooteth forth its young buds in the Spring, and the berries are ripe about September, the branches of leaves abiding green all the Winter.

Government and Virtues.] 'Tis a plant of Mars, being of a gallant cleansing and opening quality. The decoction of the root made with wine, openeth obstructions, provoketh urine, helpeth to expel gravel and the stone, the stranguary
and

and women's courses, also the yellow jaundice and the head-ach. And with some honey or sugar put thereunto, cleanseth the breast of phlegm, and the chest of such clammy humours gathered therein. The decoction of the root drank, and a poultice made of the berries and leaves being applied, are effectual in knitting and consolidating broken bones or parts out of joint. The common way of using it, is to boil the root of it, with parsley and fennel, and smallage in white wine, and drink the decoction, adding the like quantity of grass root to them: The more of the root you boil, the stronger will the decoction be, it works no ill effects, yet I hope you have wit enough to give the strongest decoction to the strongest bodies.

Broom, and Broom-Rape.

TO spend time in writing a description hereof is altogether needless, it being so generally used by all the good housewives almost through this land to sweep their houses with, and therefore very well known to all sorts of people.

The Broom rape springeth up on many places from the roots of the broom (but more often in fields, as by hedgesides and on heaths). The stalk whereof is of the bigness of a finger or thumb, above two feet high, having a shew of leaves on them, and many flowers at the top, of a reddish yellow colour, as also the stalks and leaves are.

Place] They grow in many places of this land commonly, and as commonly spoil all the land they grow in.

Time.] And flower in the Summer months, and give their seed before Winter.

Government and Virtues] The juice or decoction of the young branches, or seed, or the powder of the seed taken in drink, purgeth downwards, and draweth phlegmatick and watery humours from the joints, whereby it helpeth the dropsy, gout, sciatica, and pains of the hips and joints, it also provoketh strong vomits, and helpeth the pains of the sides, and swelling of the spleen, cleanseth also the reins or kidneys and bladder of the stone, provoketh urine abundantly, and hindereth the growing again of the stone in the body. The continual use of the powder of the leaves and seed doth cure the black jaundice. The distilled water of the flowers is profitable for all the same purposes; it also

helpeth

helpeth surfeits, and altereth the fits of agues, if three or four ounces thereof, with as much of the water of the lesser centaury, and a little sugar put therein, be taken a little before the fit cometh, and the party be laid down to sweat in his bed. The oil or water that is drawn from the end of the green sticks heated in the fire, helpeth the tooth ach. The juice of young branches made into an ointment of old hog's grease, and anointed, or the young branches bruised and heated in oil or hog's grease and laid to the sides pained by wind, as in stitches, or the spleen, easeth them in once or twice using it. The same boiled in oil is the safest and surest medicine to kill lice in the head or body of any; and is an especial remedy for joint aches, and swollen knees, that come by the falling down of humours.

The *Broom-rape* also is not without its virtues.

The decoction thereof in wine, is thought to be as effectual to void the stone in the kidneys and bladder, and to provoke urine, as the Broom itself. The juice thereof is a singular good help to cure as well green wounds, as old and filthy sores and malignant ulcers. The insolate oil, wherein there hath been three or four repetitions of infusion of the top stalks, with flowers strained and cleared, cleanseth the skin from all manner of spots, marks, and freckles that rise either by the heat of the sun, or the malignity of humours. As for the Broom and Broom rape, Mars owns them, and is exceeding prejudicial to the liver; I suppose by reason of the antipathy between Jupiter and Mars, therefore if the liver be disaffected, administer none of it.

Bucks-Horn Plantain.

Descript.] THIS being sown of seed, riseth up at first with small, long narrow, hairy, dark green leaves like grass, without any division or gash in them, but those that follow are gashed in on both sides the leaves into three or four gashes, and pointed at the ends, resembling the knags of a buck's horn, (whereof it took its name) and being well ground round about the root upon the ground, or order one by another, thereby resembling the form of a star, from among which rise up divers hairy stalks about a hand's breadth high, bearing every one a small, long, spikey head, like to those of the common plantain, having such like bloomings and seed after them. The root is single, long and small, with divers strings at it.

Place]

Place] They grow in sandy grounds, as in Tothil fields, by Westminster, and divers other places of this land.

Time] They flower and seed in May, June, and July, and their green leaves do in a manner abide fresh all the Winter.

Government and Virtues] It is under the dominion of Saturn, and is of a gallant drying and binding quality. This boiled in wine and drank, and some of the leaves put to the hurt place, is an excellent remedy for the biting of the viper or adder, which I take to be one and the same. The same being also drank, helpeth those that are troubled with the stone in the reins or kidneys, by cooling the heat of the part afflicted, and strengthening them; also weak stomachs that cannot retain, but cast up their meat. It stayeth all bleeding both at mouth and nose; bloody urine or the bloody flux, and stoppeth the lask of the belly and bowels. The leaves hereof bruised and laid to their sides that have an ague, suddenly easeth the fit; and the leaves and roots being beaten with some bay salt and applied to the wrists, worketh the same effects. The herb boiled in ale or wine, and given for some mornings and evenings together, stayeth the distillation of hot and sharp rheums falling into the eyes from the head, and helpeth all sorts of sore eyes.

Bucks Horn.

IT is called Harts-horn, Herb Stella, and Herba-stellaria, Sanguinaria, Herb Eve, Herb Ivy, Wort-Cresses, and Swine Cresses.

Descript] They have many small and weak straggling branches trailing here and there upon the ground. The leaves are many, small and jagged, not much unlike to those of Bucks-horn Plantain, but much smaller, and not so hairy. The flowers grow among the leaves in small, rough, whitish clusters: The seeds are smaller and brownish, of a bitter taste.

Place.] They grow in dry barren sandy grounds.

Time.] They flower and seed when the rest of the plantains do.

Government and Virtues] This is also under the dominion of Saturn, the virtues are held to be the same as Bucks-horn Plantain, and therefore by all authors it is joined with it. The leaves bruised and applied to the place, stops bleeding,

bleeding; the herb bruised and applied to warts, will make them consume and waste away in a short time.

Bugle.

BESIDES the name Bugle, it is called Middle Confound and Middle Comfrey, Brown Bugle, and of some Sicklewort, and Herb Carpenter; though in Essex we call another herb by that name.

Descript.] This hath larger leaves than those of the Self-heal, but else of the same fashion, or rather longer, in some green on the upper side, and in others more brownish, dented about the edges, somewhat hairy, as the square stalk is also, which riseth up to be half a yard high sometimes, with the leaves set by couples, from the middle almost, whereof upward stand the flowers, together with many smaller and browner leaves than the rest, on the stalk below set at distance, and the stalk bare between them; among which flowers are also small ones of a bluish and sometimes of an ash colour, fashioned like the flowers of ground ivy, after which come small, round, blackish seeds. The root is composed of many strings, and spreadeth upon the ground.

The white flowered Bugle differeth not in form or greatness from the former, saving that the leaves and stalks are always green, and never brown, like the other, and the flowers thereof are white.

Place] They grow in woods, copses, and fields, generally throughout England, but the white flowered Bugle is not so plentiful as the former.

Time] They flower from May until July, and in the mean time perfect their seed. The roots and leaves next thereunto upon the ground abiding all the Winter.

Government and Virtues] This herb belongeth to Dame Venus. If the virtues of it make you fall in love with it (as they will if you be wise) keep a syrup of it to take inwardly, and an ointment and plaister of it to use outwardly, always by you.

The decoction of the leaves and flowers made in wine, and taken, dissolveth the congealed blood in those that are bruised inwardly by a fall, or otherwise, and is very effectual for any inward wounds, thrusts or stabs in the body or bowels, and is an especial help in all wound drinks, and for those that are liver grown, (as they call it). It is wonderful

derful in curing all manner of ulcers and sores, whether new and fresh, or old and inveterate; yea, gangrenes and fistulas also, if the leaves bruised and applied, or their juice be used to wash and bathe the place, and the same made into a lotion, and some honey and allum, cureth all sores in the mouth and gums, be they never so foul, or of long continuance; and worketh no less powerfully and effectually for such ulcers and sores as happen in the secret parts of men and women. Being also taken inwardly, or outwardly applied, it helpeth those that have broken any bone, or have any member out of joint. An ointment made with the leaves of Bugle, Scabious and Sanicle bruised and boiled in hog's grease, until the herbs be dry, and then strained forth into a pot for such occasions as shall require; it is so singular good for all sorts of hurts in the body, that none that know its usefulness will be without it.

The truth is, I have known this herb cure some diseases of Saturn, of which I thought good to quote one. Many times such as give themselves much to drinking are troubled with strange fancies, strange sights in the night time, and some with voices, as also with the disease ephialtes, or the mare. I take the reason of this to be (according to Fernelius) a melancholy vapour made thin by excessive drinking strong liquor, and so flies up and disturbs the fancy, and breeds imaginations like itself, viz. fearful and troublesome. These I have known cured by taking only too spoonfuls of the syrup of this herb, after supper two hours, when you go to bed. But whether this does it by sympathy or antipathy, is some doubt in astrology. I know there is a great antipathy between Saturn and Venus in matter of procreation; yea, such a one, that the barrenness of Saturn can be removed by none but Venus; nor the lust of Venus be repelled by none but Saturn; but I am not of opinion this is done this way, and my reason is, because these vapours, though in quality melancholy, yet by their flying upward, seem to be something arial, therefore I rather think it is done by sympathy; Saturn being exalted in libra, in the house of Venus.

Burnet.

IT is called Sanguisorbia, Pimpinella, Bipula Solbegrella, &c. The common garden Burnet is so well known, that it needeth no description.—There is another sort which is wild, the description whereof take as followeth.

Descript] The great wild Burnet hath winged leaves rising from the roots like the garden Burnet, but not so many; yet each of these leaves are at the least twice as large as the other, and nicked in the same manner about the edges, of a greyish colour on the under side; the stalks are greater, and rise higher, with many such like leaves set thereon, and greater heads at the top, of a brownish colour, and out of them come small dark purple flowers like the former, but greater. The root is black, and long like the other, but great also: It hath almost neither scent nor taste therein, like the garden kind.

Place] The first grows frequently in gardens. The wild kind groweth in divers counties of this island, especially in Huntingdon and Northamptonshires, in the meadows there: as also near London, by Pancras church, and by a causey-side in the middle of a field by Paddington.

Time] They flower about the end of June, and beginning of July, and their seed is ripe in August.

Government and Virtues.] This is an herb the sun challengeth dominion over, and is a most precious herb, little inferior to Betony; the continual use of it preserves the body in health, and the spirit in vigour; for if the sun be the preserver of life under God, his herbs are the best in the world to do it. They are accounted to be both of one property, but the lesser is more effectual, because quicker and more aromatical. It is a friend to the heart, liver, and other principal parts of a man's body. Two or three of the stalks, with leaves put into a cup of wine, especially claret, are known to quicken the spirits, refresh and clear the heart, and drive away melancholy. It is a special help to defend the heart from noisome vapours, and from infection of the pestilence, the juice thereof being taken in some drink, and the party laid to sweat thereupon. They have also a drying and astringent quality, whereby they are available in all manner of fluxes of blood or humours, to staunch bleedings inward or outward, lasks, scourgings, the bloody flux, women's too abundant flux of courses, the whites, and the choleric belchings and castings of the stomach, and is a singular wound herb for all sorts of wounds, both of the head and body, either inward or outward; for all old ulcers, running cankers, and moist sores, to be used either by the juice or decoction of the herb, or by the powder of the herb or root, or the water of the distilled herb or ointment by itself, or with other things to be kept. The seed is also no less effectual both to fluxes and drying up moist sores, being taken in powder inwardly in wine, or steeled water, that is, wherein hot gads of steel have been quenched, or the powder or the seed mixed with the ointments.

The Butter-Bur, or Petasitis.

Descript.] THIS riseth up in February, with a thick stalk about a foot high, whereon are set a few small leaves, or rather pieces, and at the top a long spike head; flowers of a bluish or deep red colour, according to the soil where it groweth, and before the stalk with the flowers have abidden a month above ground, it will be withered and gone, and blown away with the wind, and the leaves will begin to spring, which being full grown, are very large and broad, being somewhat thin and almost round, whose thick red foot stalks above a foot long stand towards the middle of the leaves. The lower part being divided into two round parts, close almost one to another, and are of a pale green colour, and hairy underneath. The root is long, and spreadeth underground, being in some places no bigger than ones finger, in others much bigger, blackish on the outside, and whitish within, of a bitter and unpleasant taste.

Place and Time.] They grow in low and wet grounds by rivers and water-sides. Their flower (as is said) rising and decaying in February and March, before their leaves, which appear in April.

Government and Virtues.] It is under the dominion of the Sun, and therefore is a great strengthener of the heart, and chearer of the vital spirits. The roots thereof are by long experience found to be very available against the plague and pestilential fevers by provoking sweat; if the powder thereof be taken in wine, it also resisteth the force of any other poison. The root hereof taken with zedoary and angelica, or without them, helps the rising of the mother. The decoction of the root in wine is singular good for those that wheeze much, or are short winded. It provoketh urine also, and women's courses, and killeth the flat and broad worms in the belly. The powder of the root doth
wonderfully

wonderfully help to dry up the moisture of the sores that are hard to be cured, and taketh away all spots and blemishes of the skin. It were well if gentlewomen would keep this root preserved, to help their poor neighbours. *It is fit the rich should help the poor, for the poor cannot help themselves.*

The Burdock.

THEY are also called Perionata, and Loppy-major, great Burdock, and Clodbur; it is so well known, even by the little boys, who pull the Burs to throw and stick upon one another, that I shall spare to write any description of it.

Place.] They grow plentifully by ditches and water-sides, and by the highways almost every where thro' this land.

Government and Virtues.] Venus challengeth this herb for her own, and by its leaf and seed you may draw the womb which way you please, either upwards by applying it to the crown of the head, in case it falls out; or downwards in fits of the mother, by applying it to the soles of the feet; or if you would stay it in its place, apply it to the navel, and that is one good way to stay the child in it. (See more of it in my *Guide for Women.*) The Burdock leaves are cooling, moderately drying, and discussing withal, whereby it is good for old ulcers and sores. A dram of the roots taken with pine kernels, helpeth them that spit foul, mattery, and bloody phlegm. The leaves applied to the places troubled with the shrinking of the sinews or arteries, give much ease. The juice of the leaves, or rather the roots themselves, given to drink with old wine, doth wonderfully help the biting of any serpents: And the root beaten with a little salt, and laid on the place, suddenly easeth the pain thereof, and helpeth those that are bit by a mad dog. The juice of the leaves being drank with honey, provoketh urine, and remedieth the pain of the bladder. The seed being drank in wine forty days together, doth wonderfully help the sciatica. The leaves bruised with the white of an egg, and applied to any place burnt with fire, taketh out the fire, gives sudden ease, and heals it up afterwards. The decoction of them fomented on any fretting sore or canker, stayeth the corroding quality, which must be afterwards anointed with an ointment made of the same liquor, hogs-grease, nitre and vinegar boiled together.

together. The roots may be preserved with sugar, and taken fasting, or at other times, for the same purposes, and for consumptions, the stone, and the lask. The seed is much commended to break the stone, and cause it to be expelled by urine, and is often used with other seeds and things to that purpose.

Cabbages and Coleworts.

I SHALL spare labour in writing a description of these, since almost every one that can but write at all, may describe them from his own knowledge, they being generally so well known, that descriptions are altogether needless.

Place.] They are generally planted in gardens

Time] Their flower time is towards the middle or end of July, and the seed is ripe in August.

Government and Virtues] The Cabbages or Coleworts boiled gently in broth, and eaten, do open the body, but the second decoction doth bind the body. The juice thereof drank in wine, helpeth those that are bitten by an adder, and the decoction of the flowers bringeth down women's courses: Being taken with honey, it recovereth hoarseness, or loss of the voice. The often eating of them well boiled, helpeth those that are entering into a consumption. The pulp of the middle ribs of Coleworts boiled in almond milk, and made up into an electuary with honey, being taken often, is very profitable for those that are pursy and short winded. Being boiled twice, an old cock boiled in the broth and drank, it helpeth the pains, and the obstructions of the liver and spleen, and the stone in the kidneys. The juice boiled with honey, and dropped into the corner of the eyes, cleareth the sight, by consuming any film or cloud beginning to dim it; it also consumeth the canker growing therein. They are much commended, being eaten before meat to keep one from surfeiting, as also from being drunk with too much wine, or quickly make a man sober again that is drunk before. For (as they say) there is such an antipathy or enmity between the Vine and the Coleworts, that the one will die where the other groweth. The decoction of Coleworts taketh away the pain and ach, and allayeth the swellings of sores and gouty legs and knees, wherein many gross and watery humours are fallen, the place being bathed therewith warm. It helpeth also old and filthy sores, being bathed ed therewith, and healeth all small scabs, pushes and wheals, that break out in the skin. The ashes of Colewort stalks mixed with old hogs grease, are very effectual to anoint the sides of those that have had long pains therein, or any other place pained with melancholy and windy humours. This was surely Chrysippus's God, and therefore he wrote a whole volume of them and their virtues, and that none of the least neither, for he would be no small fool. He appropriates them to every part of the body, and to every disease in every part, and honest old Cato (they say) used no other physic. I know not what metal their bodies were made of, this I am sure, Cabbages are extreme windy, whether you take them as meat or as medicine. Yea, as windy meat as can be eaten, unless you eat bag pipes or bellows, and they are but seldom eaten in our days, and Colewort flowers are something more tolerable, and the wholesomer food of the two. The moon challengeth the dominion of the herb.

The Sea Coleworts.

Descript.] THIS hath divers somewhat long and broad, large and thick wrinkled leaves, somewhat crumpled about the edges, and growing each upon a thick footstalk, very brittle, of a greyish green colour; from among which riseth up a strong thick stalk, two feet high, and better, with some leaves thereon to the top, where it branches forth much; and on every branch standeth a large bush of pale whitish flowers, consisting of four leaves a-piece: The root is somewhat great, shooteth forth many branches under ground, keeping the leaves green all the Winter.

Place.] They grow in many places upon the sea coasts, as well on the Kentish as Essex shores, as at Lid in Kent, Colchester in Essex, and divers other places, and in other counties of this land.

Time.] They flower and seed about the time that other kinds do.

Government and Virtues.] The moon claims the dominion of these also. The broth, on first decoction of the Sea Colewort, doth by the sharp, nitrous, and bitter qualities therein, open the belly and purge the body, it cleanseth and digests more powerfully than the other kind: The seed hereof bruised and drank killeth worms. The leaves or the juice of them applied to sores or ulcers, cleanseth and healeth them, and dissolveth swellings, and taketh away inflammations.

Calamint, or Mountain-Mint.

Descript.] THIS is a small herb, seldom rising above a foot high, with square, hairy, and woody stalks, and two small hoary leaves set at a joint, about the bigness of marjoram, or not much bigger, a little dented about the edges, and of a very fierce or quick scent, as the whole herb is. The flowers stand at several spaces of the stalks, from the middle almost upwards, which are small and gaping like to those of Mints, and of a pale bluish colour. After which follow small, round, blackish seed. The root is small and woody, with divers small strings spreading within the ground, and dieth not, but abideth many years.

Place.] It groweth on heaths, and uplands, and dry ground in many places of this land.

Time] They flower in July, and their seed is ripe quickly after.

Government and Virtues.] It is an herb of Mercury, and a strong one too, therefore excellent good in all afflictions of the brain; the decoction of the herb being drank, bringeth down womens courses, and provoketh urine. It is profitable for those that are bursten, or troubled with convulsions or cramps, with shortness of breath, or choleric torments and pains in their bellies or stomach; it also helpeth the yellow jaundice, and stayeth vomiting, being taken in wine: Taken with salt and honey, it killeth all manner of worms in the body. It helpeth such as have the leprosy, either taken inwardly, drinking whey after it, or the green herb outwardly applied. It hindereth conception in women, but either burned or strewed in the chamber, it driveth away venomous serpents. It takes away black and blue marks in the face, and maketh black scars become well coloured, if the green herb (not the dry) be boiled in wine, and laid to the place, or the place washed therewith. Being applied to the huckle bone, by continuance of time, it spends the humours, which cause the pain of the sciatica. The juice being dropped into the ears, killeth the worms in them. The leave boiled in wine and drank, provoke sweat, and open obstructions of the liver and spleen. It helpeth them that have a cretian ague, (the body being first purged) by taking away the cold fits. The decoction hereof, with some sugar put thereto afterwards, is very profitable for those that be troubled with the overflowing of the gall, and that have an old cough, and that are scarce able to breathe by shortness of their wind; that have any cold distemper in their bowels, and are troubled with the hardness of the spleen, for all which purposes, both the powder, called Diacalamintlies, and the compound syrup of Calamint (which are to be had at the apothecaries) are the most effectual. Let not women be too busy with it, for it works very violently upon the feminine part.

Camomile.

IT is so well known every where, that it is but lost time and labour to describe it. The virtues thereof are as followeth.

A decoction made of Camomile, and drank, taketh away all pains and stitches in the side. The flowers of Camomile beaten, and made up into balls with Oil, drive away all sorts of agues, if the part grieved be anointed with that oil taken from the flowers, from the crown of the head to the sole of the foot, and afterwards laid to sweat in his bed, and that he sweats well. This is Nechessor an Egyptian's medicine. It is profitable for all sorts of agues that come either from phlegm, or melancholy or from an inflammation of the bowels, being applied when the humours causing them shall be concocted; and there is nothing more profitable to the sides and region of the liver and spleen than it. The bathing with a decoction of Camomile taketh away weariness, easeth pains, to what part of the body soever they be applied. It comforteth the sinews that are over strained, mollifieth all swellings: It moderately comforteth all parts that have need of warmth, digesteth and dissolveth whatsoever hath need thereof, by a wonderful speedy property. It easeth all the pains of the cholic and stone, and all pains and torments of the belly, and gently provoketh urine. The flowers boiled in posset drink provoke sweat, and help to expel all cold

aches

aches and pains whatsoever, and is an excellent help to bring down womens courses. Syrup made of the juice of Camomile, with the flowers in white wine, is a remedy against the jaundice and dropsy. The flowers boiled in lee, are good to wash the head, and comfort both it and the brain. The oil made of the flowers of Camomile, is much used against all hard swellings, pains or aches, shrinking of the sinews, or cramps, or pains in the joints, or any other part of the body. Being used in glysters, it helps to dissolve the wind and pains in the belly; anointed also it helpeth stitches and pains in the sides.

Nichessor saith, the Egyptians dedicated it to the sun, because it cured agues, and they were like enough to do it, for they were the arrantest apes in their religion I ever read of. Bachinus, Bena, and Lobel, commend the syrup made of the juice of it and sugar, taken inwardly, to be excellent for the spleen. Also this is certain, that it most wonderfully breaks the stone. Some take it in syrup or decoction, others inject the juice of it into the bladder with a syringe. My opinion is, that the salt of it taken half a dram in the morning in a little white or rhenish wine is better than either; that it is excellent for the stone, appears in this which I have tried, viz. That a stone that hath been taken out of the body of a man, being wrapped in Camomile, will in time dissolve, and in a little time too.

Water Caltrops.

THEY are called also Tribulus Aquaticus, Tribulus Lacustris, Tribulus Marinus, Caltrops, Saligos, Water Nuts, and Water Chesnuts.

Descript.] As for the greater sort of Water Caltrop it is not found here, or very rarely. Two other sorts there are, which I here shall describe. The first hath a long creeping and jointed root, sending forth tufts at each joint, from which joints arise long, flat, slender knotted stalks, even to the top of the water, divided towards the top into many branches, each carrying two leaves on both sides, being about two inches long, and half an inch broad, thin and almost transparent, they look as tho' they were torn; the flowers are long, thick and whitish, set together almost like a bunch of grapes, which being gone, there succeed for the most part sharp-pointed grains altogether, containing a small white kernel in them

The second differs not much from this, save that it delights in more clear water; its stalks are not flat, but round; its leaves are not so long, but more pointed. As for the place we need not determine, for their name sheweth they grow in the water.

Government and Virtues] They are under the dominion of the Moon, and being made into a poultice are excellent good for hot inflammations, swellings, cankers, sore mouths and throats, being washed with the decoction. It cleanseth and strengtheneth the neck and throat, and helps those swellings which when people have, they say the almonds of their ears are fallen down; it is excellent good for the king's evil; they are excellent good for the stone and gravel, especially the last being dried; they also resist poison, and bitings of venomous beasts.

Campion Wild.

Descript] THE wild White Campion hath many long and somewhat broad dark green leaves lying upon the ground, and divers ribs therein, somewhat like plantain, but somewhat hairy; broader, and not so long: The hairy stalks rise up in the middle of them three or four feet high, and sometimes more, with divers great white joints at several places thereon, and two such like leaves thereat up to the top, sending forth branches at several joints also. All which bear on several foot-stalks white flowers at the top of them, consisting of five broad pointed leaves, every one cut in on the end unto the middle, making them seem to be two a piece, smelling somewhat sweet, and each of them standing in a large green striped hairy husk, large and round below next to the stalk. The seed is small and greyish in the hard heads that come up afterwards. The root is white and long, spreading divers fangs in the ground.

This red Wild Campion groweth in the same manner as the white, but his leaves are not so plainly ribbed, somewhat shorter, rounder, and more woolly in handling. The flowers are of the same form and bigness, but in some of a pale, in others of a bright red colour, cut in at the ends more finely, which makes the leaves look more in number than the other. The seeds and the roots are alike, the roots of both sorts abiding many years.

There are forty five kinds of Campion more, those of them which are of a physical use, having the like virtues with those above described, which I take to be the two chiefest kind.

Place] They grow commonly through this land by fields and hedge sides and ditches.

Time] They flower in Summer, some earlier than others, and some abiding longer than others.

Government and Virtues] They belong unto Saturn, and it is found by experience, that the decoction of the herb, either in white or red wine being drank, doth stay inward bleedings, and applied outwardly it doth the like; and being drank helpeth to expel urine being stopped, and gravel and stone in the reins or kidneys. Two drams of the seed drank in wine, purgeth the body of choleric humours, and helpeth those that are stung by scorpions, or other venomous beasts, and may be as effectual for the plague. It is of very good use in old sores, ulcers, cankers, fistulas, and the like, to cleanse and heat them, by consuming the moist humours falling into them, and correcting the putrefaction of humours offending them.

Carduus Benedictus.

It is called Carduus Benedictus, or Blessed Thistle, or Holy Thistle, I suppose the name was put upon it by some that had little holiness in themselves.

I shall spare labour in writing a description of this, as almost every one that can but write at all may describe them from his own knowledge.

Time] They flower in August, and seed not long after.

Government and Virtues] It is an herb of Mars, and under the sign Aries. Now, in handling this herb, I shall give you a rational pattern of all the rest: and if you please to view them throughout the book, you shall to your content find it true. It helps swimmings and giddiness of the head, or the disease called Vertigo, because Aries is in the house of Mars. It is an excellent remedy against the yellow jaundice, and other infirmities of the gall, because Mars governs choler. It strengthens the attractive faculty in man, and clarifies the blood, because the one is ruled by Mars. The continual drinking the decoction of it, helps red faces, tetters, and ring-worms, because Mars causeth them. It helps the plague, sores, boils, and itch, the bitings

of

of mad dogs and venomous beasts, all which infirmities are under Mars; thus you see what it doth by sympathy.

By antipathy to other planets it cures the French pox. By antipathy to Venus, who governs it, it strengthens the memory, and cures deafness by antipathy to Saturn, who hath his fall in Aries which rules the head. It cures quartian agues, and other diseases of melancholy and adust choler, by sympathy to Saturn, Mars being exalted in Capricorn. Also it provokes urine, the stopping of which is usually caused by Mars or the Moon.

Carrots.

GARDEN Carrots are so well known, that they need no description, but because they are of less physical use than the wild kind (as indeed almost in all herbs the wild are most effectual in physic, as being more powerful in operations than the garden kind), I shall therefore briefly describe the Wild Carrot.

Descript] It groweth in a manner altogether like the tame, but that the leaves and stalks are somewhat whiter and rougher. The stalks bear large tufts of white flowers, with a deep purple spot in the middle, which are contracted together when the seed begins to ripen, that the middle part being hollow and low, and the outward stalk rising high, maketh the whole umbel shew like a bird's nest. The roots small, long and hard, and unfit for meat, being somewhat sharp and strong.

Place] The wild kind groweth in divers parts of this land plentifully by the field-sides and untilled places.

Time] They flower and seed in the end of Summer.

Government and Virtues] Wild Carrots belong to Mercury, and therefore break wind and remove stitches in the sides, provoke urine and womens courses, and helpeth to break and expel the stone; the seed also of the same worketh the like effect, and is good for the dropsy, and those whose bellies are swollen with wind, helpeth the colic, the stone in the kidneys, and rising of the mother, being taken in wine, or boiled, in wine and taken, it helpeth conception. The leaves being applied with honey to running sores or ulcers, do cleanse them.

I suppose the seeds of them perform this better than the roots; and tho' Galen commended garden Carrots highly to break wind, yet experience teacheth they breed it first, and we may thank nature for expelling it, not they; the seeds of them expel wind indeed, and so mend what the root marreth.

Carraway.

Descript.] IT beareth divers stalks of fine cut leaves, lying upon the ground, somewhat like to the leaves of carrots, but not bushing so thick, of a little quick taste in them, from among which riseth up a square stalk, not so high as the carrot, at whose joints are set the like leaves, but smaller and finer, and at the top small open tufts, or umbels of white flowers, which turn into small blackish seed, smaller than the Anniseed, and of a quicker and better taste. The root is whitish, small and long, somewhat like unto a parsnip, but with more wrinkled bark, and much less, of a little hot and quick taste, and stronger than the parsnip, and abideth after seed-time.

Place.] It is usually sown with us in gardens.

Time.] They flower in June and July, and seed quickly after.

Government and Virtues] This is also a Mercurial plant. Carraway seed hath a moderate sharp quality, whereby it breaketh wind, and provoketh urine, which also the herb doth. The root is better food than the parsnips; it is pleasant and comfortable to the stomach, and helpeth digestion. The seed is conducing to all cold griefs of the head and stomach, bowels, or mother, as also the wind in them, and helpeth to sharpen the eye-sight. The powder of the seed put into a poultice, taketh away black and blue spots of blows and bruises. The herb itself, or with some of the seed bruised and fried, laid hot in a bag or double cloth, to the lower parts of the belly, easeth the pains of the wind and colic.

The roots of Carraways eaten as men eat parsnips, strengthen the stomachs of ancient people exceedingly, and they need not to make a whole meal of them neither, and are fit to be planted in every garden.

Carraway comfits, once only dipped in sugar, and half a spoonful of them eaten in the morning fasting, and as many after each meal, is a most admirable remedy for those that are troubled with wind.

Celandine

Celandine.

Descript.] THIS hath divers tender, round, whitish green stalks, with greater joints than ordinary in other herbs, as it were knees, very brittle and easy to break, from whence grow branches with large tender broad leaves, divided into many parts, each of them cut in on the edges, set at the joint on both sides of the branches, of a dark bluish green colour, on the upper side like columbine, and of a more pale bluish green underneath, full of yellow sap, when any part is broken, of a bitter taste, and strong scent. At the flowers of four leaves a-piece, after which come small long pods, with blackish seed therein. The root is somewhat great at the head, shooting forth divers long roots and small strings, reddish on the out side, and yellow within, full of yellow sap therein.

Place.] They grow in many places by old walls, hedges and way sides in untilled places; and being once planted in a garden, especially some shady places, it will remain there.

Time.] They flower all the summer long, and the seed ripeneth in the mean time.

Government and Virtues.] This is an herb of the Sun, and under the celestial Lion, and is one of the best cures for the eyes; for, all that know any thing in astrology, know that the eyes are subject to the luminaries, let it then be gathered when the Sun is in Leo, and the Moon in Aries, applying to this time, let Leo arise, then may you make it into an oil or ointment, which you please, to anoint your sore eyes with. I can prove it doth both by my own experience, and the experience of those to whom I have taught it, that most desperate sore eyes have been cured by this only medicine, and then I pray, is not this far better than endangering the eyes by the art of the needle? For if this doth not absolutely take away the film, it will so facilitate the work, that it may be done without danger. The herb or root boiled in white wine and drunk, a few aniseeds being boiled therewith, openeth obstructions of the liver and gall, helpeth the yellow jaundice; and often using it, helps the dropsy and the itch, and those that have old sores in their legs, or other parts of the body. The juice thereof taken fasting, is held to be of singular good use against the pestilence. The distilled water, with a little sugar and a little good treacle mixed therewith (the party upon the taking being laid down to sweat a little) hath the same effect. The juice dropped in the eyes, cleanseth them from films and cloudiness which darken the sight, but it is best to allay the sharpness of the juice with a little breast-milk. It is good in old filthy corroding creeping ulcers wheresoever, to stay their malignity of fretting and running, and to cause them to heal more speedily. The juice often applied to tetters, ring worms, or other such like spreading cankers, will quickly heal them, and rubbed often upon warts, will take them away. The herb with the roots bruised and bathed with oil of camomile, and applied to the navel, taketh away the griping pains in the belly and bowels, and all the pains of the mother, and applied to womens breasts, stayeth the overmuch flowing of the courses. The juice or decoction of the herb gargled between the teeth that ach easeth the pain, and the powder of the dried root laid upon any aching, hollow or loose tooth, will cause it to fall out. The juice mixed with some powder of brimstone is not only good against the itch, but taketh away all discolourings of the skin whatsoever; and if it chance that in a tender body it causeth any itchings or inflammations, by bathing the place with a little vinegar, it is helped.

Another ill favoured trick have physicians got to use to the eye, and that is worse than the needle; which is to take away films by corroding or gnawing medicines. This I absolutely protest against.

1. Because the tunicles of the eyes are very thin, and therefore soon eaten asunder.

2. The callus or film that they would eat away, is seldom of an equal thickness in every place, and then the tunicle may be eaten asunder in one place, before the film be consumed in another, and so be a readier way to extinguish the sight than to restore it.

It is called Chelidonium, from the Greek word *chelidon*, which signifies a swallow, because they say, that if you put out the eyes of young swallows when they are in the nest, the old ones will recover their eyes again with this herb. This I am confident, for I have tried it, that if we mar the very apple of their eyes with a needle, she will recover them again; but whether with this herb or not, I know not.

Also I have read (and it seems to be somewhat probable,) that

that the herb being gathered as I shewed before, and the elements drawn apart from it by art of the alchymist, and after they are drawn apart rectified, the earthly quality, still receiving them, added to the *Terra damnata* (as alchymists call it) or *Terra sacratissima* (as some philosophers call it) the elements so rectifie are sufficient for the cure of all diseases, the humours offending being known, and the contrary element given: It is an experiment worth the trying, and can do no harm.

The Lesser Celandine, usually known by the name of Pilewort and Fogwort.

I WONDER what ailed the ancients to give this the name of Celandine, which resembles it neither in nature or form; it required the name of Pilewort from its virtues, and it being no great matter where I set it down, so I set it down at all, I humoured Dr Tradition so much, as to set him down here.

Descript.] This Celandine or Pilewort (which you please) doth spread many round pale green leaves, set on weak and trailing branches, which lie upon the ground, and are flat, smooth, and somewhat shining, and in some places (though seldom) marked with black spots, each standing on a long foot stalk, among which rise small yellow flowers, consisting of nine or ten small narrow leaves, upon slender foot stalks, very like unto Crowsfoot, whereunto the seed also is not unlike, being many small kernels like a grain of corn, sometimes twice as long as others, of a whitish colour, with some fibres at the end of them.

Place.] It groweth for the most part in moist corners of fields and places that are near water sides, yet will abide in drier ground if they be but a little shady.

Time] It flowereth betimes about March or April, is quite gone by May; so it cannot be found till it spring again.

Government and Virtues] It is under the dominion of Mars, and behold here another verification of the learning of the ancients, viz. that the virtue of an herb may be known by its signature, as plainly appears in this; for if you dig up the root of it, you shall perceive the perfect image of the disease which they commonly call the piles. It is certain by good experience, that the decoction of the leaves and roots doth wonderfully help piles and hæmorrhoids, also kernels by the ears and throat, called the kings evil, or any other hard wens or tumours.

Here is another secret for my countrymen and women a couple of them together, Pilewort made into an oil, ointment, or plaister, readily cures both the piles, or hæmorrhoids, and the king's evil. The very herb borne about one's body next the skin helps in such diseases, though it never touch the place grieved; let poor people make much of it for their uses, with this I cured my own daughter of the king's evil, broke the sore, drew out a quarter of a pint of corruption, cured without any scar at all in one week's time.

The ordinary small Centaury.

Descript.] THIS groweth up most usually but with one round and somewhat crusted stalk, about a foot high or better, branching forth at the top into many sprigs, and some also from the joints of the stalks below, the flowers thus stand at the tops as it were in one umbel or tuft, are of a pale red, tending to carnation colour, consisting of five, sometimes six small leaves, very like those of St John's Wort, opening themselves in the day time and closing at night, after which come seeds in little short husks, in form like unto wheat corn. The leaves are small and somewhat round; the root small and hard, perishing every year. The whole plant is of an exceeding bitter taste.

There is another sort in all things like the former, save only it beareth white flowers.

Place] They grow ordinary in fields, pastures and woods, but that with the white flowers not so frequently as the other.

Time] They flower in July or thereabouts, and seed within a month after.

Government and Virtues] They are under the dominion of the Sun, as appears in that their flowers open and shut as the sun either sheweth or hideth his face. This herb, boiled and drank, purgeth all choleric and gross humours, and helpeth the sciatica; it openeth obstructions of the liver, gall, and spleen, helpeth the jaundice, and easeth the pains in the sides, and hardness of the spleen, used outwardly, and is given with very good effect in agues. It helpeth those that have the dropsy, or the green-sickness, being much used by the Italians in powder for that purpose. It killeth the worms in the belly, as is found by experience. The decoction thereof, viz. the tops of the stalks,

stalks, with the leaves and flowers, is good against the colic, and to bring down womens courses, helpeth to void the dead birth, and easeth pains of the mother, and is very effectual in old pains of the joints, as the gout, cramps, or convulsions. A dram of the powder thereof taken in wine, is a wonderful good help against the biting and poison of an adder. The juice of the herb with a little honey put to it, is good to clear the eyes from dimness, mists and clouds that offend or hinder sight. It is singular good both for green and fresh wounds, as also for old ulcers and sores, to close up the one, and cleanse the other, and perfectly to cure them both, although they are hollow or fistulous, the green herb especially being bruised and laid thereto. The decoction therefore dropped into the ears, cleanseth them from worms, cleanseth the foul ulcers and spreading scabs of the head, and taketh away all freckles, spots, and marks in the skin, being washed with it. The herb is so safe you cannot fail in the using of it, only giving it inwardly for inward diseases. 'Tis very wholesome, but not very toothsome.

There is, besides these, another small Centaury, which beareth a yellow flower; in all other respects it is like the former, save that the leaves are bigger, and of a darker green, and the stalk passeth through the midst of them, as it doth the herb Thorowax. They are all of them, as I told you, under the government of the Sun; yet this, if you observe it, you shall find an excellent truth; in diseases of the blood, use the red Centaury, if of choler, use the yellow; but if phlegm or water, you will find the white best.

The Cherry-Tree.

I SUPPOSE there are few but know this tree, for its fruit's sake; and therefore I shall spare writing a description thereof.

Place] For the place of its growth, it is afforded room in every orchard.

Government and Virtues] It is a tree of Venus. Cherries, as they are of different tastes, so they are of different qualities. The sweet pass through the stomach and the belly more speedily, but are of little nourishment, the tart or sour are more pleasing to an hot stomach, procure appetite to meat, and help to cut tough phlegm, and gross humours;

but

but when these are dried, they are more binding to the belly than when they are fresh, being cooling in hot diseases, and welcome to the stomach, and provoke urine. The gum of the Cherry-tree, dissolved in wine, is good for a cold, cough, and hoarseness of the throat; mendeth the colour in the face, sharpeneth the eye-sight, provoketh appetite, and helpeth to break and expel the stone; the Black Cherries bruised with the stones, and dissolved, the water thereof is much used to break the stone, and to expel gravel and wind.

Winter-Cherries.

Descript] THE Winter Cherry hath a running or creeping root in the ground, of the bigness many times of one's little finger, shooting forth at several joints in several places, whereby it quickly spreads a great compass of ground. The stalk riseth not above a yard high, whereon are set many broad and long green leaves, somewhat like nigh shade, but larger, at the joints whereof come forth whitish flowers made of five leaves a piece, which afterwards turn into green berries inclosed with thin skins, which change to be reddish when they grow ripe, the berries likewise being reddish, and as large as a cherry, wherein are contained many flat and yellowish seeds lying within the pulp, which being gathered and strung up, are kept all the year to be used upon occasion.

Place.] They grow not naturally in this land, but are cherished in gardens for their virtues.

Time] They flower not until the middle or latter end of July, and the fruit is ripe about August, or the beginning of September.

Government and Virtues] This also is a plant of Venus. They are of great use in physic. The leaves being cooling, may be used in inflammations, but not opening as the berries and fruit are, which by drawing down the urine provoke it to be voided plentifully when it is stopped or grown hot, sharp, and painful in the passage; it is good also to expel the stone and gravel out of the reins, kidneys, and bladder, helping to dissolve the stone, and voiding it by grit or gravel sent forth in the urine, it also helpeth much to cleanse inward imposthumes or ulcers in the reins or bladder, or in those that void a bloody or foul urine. The distilled water of the fruit, or the leaves together with them, or the berries, green or dry, distilled with a little milk, and drank morning and evening with a little sugar, is effectual to all the purposes before specified, and especially against the heat and sharpness of the urine. I shall only mention one way, amongst many others, which might be used for ordering the berries, to be helpful for the urine and stone; which is this. Take three or four good handfuls of the berries, either green or fresh, or dried, and having bruised them, put them into so many gallons of beer or ale when it is new tunned up. This drink, taken daily, hath been found to do much good to many, both to ease the pains, and expel urine and the stone, and to cause the stone not to engender. The decoction of the berries in wine and water is the most usual way, but the powder of them taken in drink is more effectual.

Chervil.

IT is called Cerefolium, Mirrhis, and Mirra, Chervil, Sweet Chervil, and Sweet Cicely.

Descript] The garden Chervil doth at first somewhat resemble Parsley, but after it is better grown, the leaves are much cut in and jagged, resembling hemlock, being a little hairy and of a whitish green colour, sometimes turning reddish in the Summer, with the stalks also; it riseth a little above half a foot high, bearing white flowers in spiked tufts, which turn into long and round seeds pointed at the ends and blackish when they are ripe, of a sweet taste, but no smell, though the herb itself smelleth reasonably well. The root is small and long, and perisheth every year, and must be sown anew in Spring, as seed after July or Autumn fails.

The wild Chervil groweth two or three feet high, with yellow stalks and joints, set with broader and more hairy leaves, divided into sundry parts, nicked about the edges, and of a dark green colour, which likewise grow reddish with the stalks; at the tops whereof stand small white tufts of flowers, afterwards smaller and longer seed. The root is white, hard and endureth long. This hath little or no scent.

Place] The first is sown in gardens for a sallet herb, the second groweth wild in many of the meadows of this land, and by the hedge sides, and on heaths.

Time] They flower and seed yearly, and thereupon are down again in the end of Summer.

Govern-

but when these are dried, they are more binding to the belly than when they are fresh, being cooling in hot diseases, and welcome to the stomach, and provoke urine. The gum of the Cherry-tree, dissolved in wine, is good for a cold, cough, and hoarseness of the throat; mendeth the colour in the face, sharpeneth the eye-sight, provoketh appetite, and helpeth to break and expel the stone; the Black Cherries bruised with the stones, and dissolved, the water thereof is much used to break the stone, and to expel gravel and wind.

Winter-Cherries.

Descript] THE Winter Cherry hath a running or creeping root in the ground, of the bigness many times of one's little finger, shooting forth at several joints in several places, whereby it quickly spreads a great compass of ground. The stalk riseth not above a yard high, whereon are set many broad and long green leaves, somewhat like nightshade, but larger; at the joints whereof come forth whitish flowers made of five leaves a piece, which afterwards turn into green berries inclosed with thin skins, which change to be reddish when they grow ripe, the berries likewise being reddish, and as large as a cherry, wherein are contained many flat and yellowish seeds lying within the pulp, which being gathered and strung up, are kept all the year to be used upon occasion.

Place.] They grow not naturally in this land, but are cherished in gardens for their virtues.

Time.] They flower not until the middle or latter end of July; and the fruit is ripe about August or the beginning of September.

Government and Virtues] This also is a plant of Venus. They are of great use in physic. The leaves being cooling, may be used in inflammations, but not opening as the berries and fruit are; which by drawing down the urine provoke it to be voided plentifully when it is stopped or grown hot, sharp, and painful in the passage, it is good also to expel the stone and gravel out of the reins, kidneys, and bladder, helping to dissolve the stone, and voiding it by grit or gravel sent forth in the urine; it also helpeth much to cleanse inward imposthumes or ulcers in the reins or bladder, or in those that void a bloody or foul urine. The distilled water of the fruit, or the leaves together with them, or the berries, green or dry, distilled with a little milk, and drank morning and evening with a little sugar, is effectual to all the purposes before specified, and especially against the heat and sharpness of the urine. I shall only mention one way, amongst many others, which might be used for ordering the berries, to be helpful for the urine and stone; which is this. Take three or four good handfuls of the berries, either green or fresh, or dried, and having bruised them, put them into so many gallons of beer or ale when it is new tunned up. This drink, taken daily, hath been found to do much good to many, both to ease the pains, and expel urine and the stone, and to cause the stone not to engender. The decoction of the berries in wine and water is the most usual way; but the powder of them taken in drink is more effectual.

Chervil.

IT is called Cerefolium, Mirrhis, and Mura, Chervil, Sweet Chervil, and Sweet Cicely.

Descript] The garden Chervil doth at first somewhat resemble Parsley, but after it is better grown, the leaves are much cut in and jagged, resembling hemlock, being a little hairy and of a whitish green colour, sometimes turning reddish in the Summer, with the stalks also; it riseth a little above half a foot high, bearing white flowers in spiked tufts, which turn into long and round seeds pointed at the ends and blackish when they are ripe; of a sweet taste, but no smell, though the herb itself smelleth reasonably well. The root is small and long, and perisheth every year, and must be sown anew in Spring, as seed after July or Autumn fails.

The wild Chervil groweth two or three feet high, with yellow stalks and joints, set with broader and more hairy leaves, divided into sundry parts, nicked about the edges, and of a dark green colour, which likewise grow reddish with the stalks; at the top, whereof stand small white tufts of flowers, afterwards smaller and longer seed. The root is white, hard and endureth long. This hath little or no scent.

Place] The first is sown in gardens for a sallet herb; the second groweth wild in many of the meadows of this land, and by the hedge sides, and on heaths.

Time] They flower and seed yearly, and thereupon are down again in the end of Summer.

Govern.-

Government and Virtues] The garden Chervil being eaten, doth moderately warm the stomach, and is a certain remedy (saith Tragus) to dissolve congealed or clotted blood in the body, or that which is clotted by bruises, falls, &c. The juice or distilled water thereof being drank, and the bruised leaves laid to the place, being taken either in meat or drink, is good to help to provoke urine, or expel the stone in the kidneys, to send down womens courses, and to help the pleurisy and pricking of the sides.

The wild Chervil bruised and applied, dissolveth swellings in any part, or the marks of congealed blood by bruises or blows, in a little space.

Sweet Chervil, or Sweet Cicely.

Descript.] THIS groweth very like the great hemlock, having large spread leaves cut into divers parts, but of a fresher green colour than the hemlock, tasting as sweet as the anniseed. The stalks rise up a yard high, or better, being crested or hollow, having leaves at the joints, but lesser; and at the tops of the branched stalks, umbels or tufts of white flowers, after which comes large and long crested black shining seed, pointed at both ends, tasting quick, yet sweet and pleasant. The root is great and white, growing deep in the ground, and spreading sundry long branches therein, in taste and smell stronger than the leaves or seeds, and continuing many years.

Place] This groweth in gardens.

Government and Virtues] These are all three of them of the nature of Jupiter, and under his dominion. This whole plant, besides its pleasantness in sallets, hath its physical virtue. The root boiled, and eaten with oil and vinegar, (or without oil) does much please and warm old and cold stomachs oppressed with wind or phlegm, or those that have the phthisic or consumption of the lungs. The same drank with wine is a preservation from the plague. It provoketh womens courses, and expelleth the after birth, procureth an appetite to meat, and expelleth wind. The juice is good to heal the ulcers of the head and face; the candied roots hereof are held as effectual as Angelica, to preserve from infection in the time of a plague, and to warm and comfort a cold weak stomach. It is so harmless, you cannot use it amiss.

Chesnut Tree.

IT were as needless to describe a tree so commonly known, as to tell a man he had gotten a mouth; therefore take the government and virtues of them thus:

The tree is abundantly under the dominion of Jupiter, and therefore the fruit must needs breed good blood, and yield commendable nourishment to the body; yet, if eaten overmuch, they make the blood thick, procure head ach, and bind the body; the inner skin, that covereth the nut, is of so binding a quality, that a scruple of it been taken by a man, or ten grains by a child, soon stops any flux whatsoever: The whole nut being dried and beaten into powder, and a dram taken at a time, is a good remedy to stop the terms in women. If you dry Chesnuts, (only the kernels I mean) both the barks being taken away, beat them into powder, and make the powder up into an electuary with honey, so have you an admirable remedy for the cough and spitting of blood.

Earth Chesnuts.

THEY are called Earth nuts, Earth Chesnuts, Ground Nuts, Cipper-nuts, and in Sussex Pig-nuts. A description of them were needless, for every child knows them.

Government and Virtues] They are something hot and dry in quality, under the dominion of Venus, they provoke lust exceedingly, and stir up those sports she is mistress of; the seed is excellent good to provoke urine, and so also is the root, but it doth not perform it so forcibly as the seed doth. The root being dried and beaten into powder, and the powder made into an electuary, is as singular a remedy for spitting and pissing of blood, as the former Chesnut was for coughs.

Chickweed.

IT is so generally known to most people, that I shall not trouble you with the description thereof, nor myself with setting forth the several kinds, since but only two or three are considerable for their usefulness.

Place] They are usually found in moist and watery places, by wood sides, and elsewhere.

Time] They flower about June, and their seed is ripe in July.

Government and Virtues.] It is a fine soft pleasing herb under the dominion of the Moon. It is found to be effectual as Purflain to all the purposes whereunto it serveth, except for meat only. The herb bruised, or the juice applied (with cloths or spunges dipped therein) to the region of the liver, and as they dry, to have it fresh applied, doth wonderfully temperate the heat of the liver, and is effectual for all imposthumes and swellings whatsoever, for all redness in the face, wheals, pushes, itch, scabs; the juice either simply used, or boiled with hogs grease and applied helpeth cramps, convulsions, and palsy. The juice, or distilled water, is of much good use for all heats and redness in the eyes, to drop some thereof into them; as also into the ears, to ease pains in them; and is of good effect to ease pains from the heat and sharpness of the blood in the piles, and generally all pains in the body that arise of heat. It is used also in hot and virulent ulcers and sores in the privy parts of men and women, or on the legs, or elsewhere. The leaves boiled with marsh mallows, and made into a poultice with fenugreek and lint seed, applied to swellings and imposthumes, ripen and break them, or assuage the swelling and ease the pains. It helpeth the sinews when they are shrunk by cramps, or otherwise, and to extend and make them pliable again by this medicine. Boil a handful of Chickweed, and a handful of red rose leaves dried, in a quart of mascadine, until a fourth part be consumed; then put to them a pint of oil of trotters or sheep's feet; let them boil a good while still stirring them well; which being strained, anoint the grieved place therewith, warm against the fire, rubbing it well with one hand; and bind also some of the herb (if you will) to the place, and with God's blessing, it will help it in three times dressing.

Chick-Pease, or Cicers.

Descript.] THE garden sorts, whether red, black, or white, bring forth stalks a yard long whereon do grow many small and almost round leaves dented about the edges, set on both sides of a middle rib. At the joints come forth one or two flowers, upon sharp foot stalks, pease fashion, either white or whitish, or purplish red, lighter or deeper, according as the pease that follow will be that are contained in small, thick, and short pods, wherein be one or two pease, more usually pointed at the lower end, and
almost

almost round at the head, yet a little cornered or sharp; the root is small, and perisheth yearly.

Place and Time] They are sown in gardens, or fields, as pease, being sown later than pease, and gathered at the same time with them, or presently after.

Government and Virtues] They are both under the dominion of Venus. They are less windy than beans, but nourish more, they provoke urine, and are thought to increase sperm; they have a cleansing faculty, whereby they break the stone in the kidneys. To drink the cream of them, being boiled in water, is the best way. It moves the belly downwards, provokes womens courses and urine, increases both milk and seed. One ounce of Cicers, two ounces of French barley, and a small handful of marsh-mallow roots, clean washed and cut, being boiled in the broth of a chicken, and four ounces taken in the morning, and fasting two hours after, is a good medicine for a pain in the side. The white Cicers are used more for meat than medicine, yet have the same effects, and are thought more powerful to increase milk and seed. The wild Cicers are so much more powerful than the garden kinds, by how much they exceed them in heat and dryness, whereby they do more open obstructions, break the stone, and have all the properties of cutting, opening, digesting and dissolving; and this more speedily and certainly than the former.

Cinquefoil, or Five-leaved Grass; called in some Counties Five-fingered Grass.

Descript] IT spreads and creeps far upon the ground, with long slender strings like strawberries, which take root again, and shoot forth many leaves made of five parts, and sometimes of seven, dented about the edges, and somewhat hard. The stalks are slender, leaning downwards, and bear many small yellow flowers thereon, with some yellow threads in the middle standing about a smooth green head, which, when it is ripe, is a little rough, and containeth small brownish seed. The root is of a blackish brown colour, as big as one's little finger, but growing long, with some threads thereat; and by the small strings it quickly spreadeth over the ground.

Place.] It groweth by wood sides, hedge sides, the pathway in fields, and in the borders and corners of them, almost through all this land.

Time]

Time.] It flowereth in Summer, some sooner, some later.

Government and Virtues] This is an herb of Jupiter, and therefore strengthens the part of the body it rules; let Jupiter be angular and strong when it is gathered; and if you give but a scruple (which is but twenty grains) of it at a time either in white wine, or in white wine vinegar, you shall very seldom miss the cure of an ague, be it what ague soever, in three fits, as I have often proved, to the admiration both of myself and others; let no man despise it because it is plain and easy, the ways of God are all such. It is an especial herb used in all inflammations and fevers, whether infectious or pestilential; or among other herbs to cool and temper the blood and humours in the body. As also for all lotions, gargles, infections, and the like, for sore mouths, ulcers, cancers, fistulas, and other corrupt, foul, or running sores. The juice hereof drank about four ounces at a time, for certain days together, cureth the quinsy and yellow jaundice, and taken for thirty days together, cureth the falling sickness. The roots boiled in milk and drunk, is a more effectual remedy for all fluxes in man or woman, whether the white or red, as also the bloody flux. The roots boiled in vinegar, and the decoction thereof held in the mouth, easeth the pains of the tooth ach. The juice or decoction taken with a little honey, helpeth the hoarseness of the throat, and is very good for the cough of the lungs. The distilled water of both roots and leaves is also effectual to all the purposes aforesaid, and if the hands be often washed therein, and suffered at every time to dry in of itself without wiping, it will in a short time help the palsy, or shaking in them. The root boiled in vinegar helpeth all knots, kernels, hard swellings, and lumps growing in any part of the flesh, being thereto applied, as also inflammations, and St Anthony's fire, all imposthumes, and painful sores with heat and putrefaction, the shingles also, and all other sorts of running and foul scabs, sores and itch. The same also boiled in wine, and applied to any joint full of pain ach, or the gout in the hands or feet, or the hip gout, called the Sciatica, and the decoction thereof drank the while doth cure them, and easeth much pain in the bowels. The roots are likewise effectual to help ruptures or burstings, being used with other things available to that purpose, taken either inwardly or outwardly, or both, as

also

to bruises or hurts by blows, falls, or the like, and to stay the bleeding of wounds in any parts inward or outward.

Some hold that one leaf cures a quotidian, three a tertian, and four a quartan ague, and a hundred to one if it be not Dioscorides; for he is full of whims. The truth is, I never stood so much upon the number of the leaves, nor whether I give it in powder or decoction: If Jupiter were strong, and the Moon applying to him, or his good aspect at the gathering, I never knew it miss the desired effects.

Cives.

CALLED also Rush Leeks, Chives, Civet, and Sweth.
Temperature and Virtues] I confess I had not added these, had it not been for a country gentleman, who by a letter certified me, that amongst other herbs, I had left these out; they are indeed a kind of Leeks, hot and dry in the fourth degree as they are, and so under the dominion of Mars: if they be eaten raw, (I do not mean raw, opposite to roasted or boiled, but raw, opposite to chymical preparation) they send up very hurtful vapours to the brain, causing troublesome sleep, and spoiling the eye sight, yet of them, prepared by the art of the alchymist, may be made an excellent remedy for the stoppage of urine.

Clary, or, more properly, Clear-Eye.

Descript] OUR ordinary garden Clary hath four square stalks, with broad, rough, wrinkled, whitish, or hoary green leaves, somewhat evenly cut in on the edges, and of a strong sweet scent growing some near the ground and some by couples upon the stalks. The flowers grow at certain distances, with two small leaves at the joints under them, somewhat like unto the flowers of sage, but smaller, and of a whitish blue colour. The seed is brownish, and somewhat flat, or not so round as the wild. The roots are blackish, and spread not far, and perish after the seed time. It is usually sown, for it seldom rises of its own sowing.

Place] This groweth in gardens.

Time] It flowers in June and July, some a little later than others, and their seed is ripe in August or thereabouts.

Government and Virtues] It is under the dominion of the Moon. The seed put into the eyes clears them from motes

and

and such like things gotten within the lids to offend them, as also clears them from white and red spots on them. The mucilage of the seed made with water, and applied to tumours, or swellings, disperseth and taketh them away; as also draweth forth splinters, thorns, or other things gotten into the flesh. The leaves used with vinegar, either by itself, or with a little honey, doth help boils, felons, and the hot inflammations that are gathered by their pains, if applied before it be grown too great. The powder of the dried root put into the nose, provoketh sneezing, and thereby purgeth the head and brain of much rheum and corruption. The seed or leaves taken in wine, provoketh to venery. It is of much use both for men and women that have weak backs, and helpeth to strengthen the reins, used either by itself, or with other herbs conducing to the same effect, and in tansies often. The fresh leaves dipped in a batter of flour, eggs, and a little milk, and fried in butter, and served to the table, is not unpleasant to any, but exceeding profitable for those that are troubled with weak backs, and the effects thereof. The juice of the herb put into ale or beer, and drank, bringeth down women's courses, and expelleth the after-birth.

It is an usual course with many men, when they have gotten the running of the reins, or women the whites, they run to the bush of Clary: Maid, bring hither the frying pan, fetch me some butter quickly, then for eating fried Clary, just as hogs eat acorns; and this they think will cure their disease (forsooth), whereas when they have devoured as much Clary as will grow upon an acre of ground, their back are as much the better, as though they had pissed in their shoes; nay, perhaps much worse.

We will grant that Clary strengthens the back; but this we deny, that the cause of the running of the reins in men, or the whites in women, lies in the back (though the back sometimes be weakened by them): and therefore the medicine is as proper, as for me when my toe is sore, to lay a plaister on my nose.

Wild Clary.

WILD Clary is most blasphemously called Christ's Eye, because it cures diseases of the eyes. I could wish from my soul blasphemy, ignorance, and tyranny were ceased among physicians, that they may be happy, and I joyful.

Descript.] It is like the other Clary, but lesser, with many stalks about a foot and a half high. The stalks are square and somewhat hairy; the flowers of a bluish colour. He that knows the common Clary cannot be ignorant of this.

Place] It grows commonly in this nation in barren places; you may find it plentifully, if you look in the fields near Gray's Inn, and the fields near Chelsea.

Time] They flower from the beginning of June, till the latter end of August.

Government and Virtues.] It is something hotter and drier than the garden Clary is, yet nevertheless under the dominion of the Moon, as well as that: the seeds of it being beaten to powder, and drank with wine, is an admirable help to provoke lust. A decoction of the leaves being drank, warm the stomach, and it is a wonder if it should not, the stomach being under Cancer, the house of the Moon. Also it helps digestion, scatters congealed blood in any part of the body. The distilled water hereof cleanseth the eyes of redness, waterishness and heat. It is a gallant remedy for dimness of sight, to take one of the seeds of it, and put into the eyes, and there let it remain till it drops out of itself, the pain will be nothing to speak on; it will cleanse the eyes of all filthy and putrified matter, and in often repeating it, will take off a film which covereth the sight; a handsomer, safer and easier remedy by a great deal, than to tear it off with a needle.

Cleavers.

IT is also called Aparine, Goose-share, Goose-grass, and Cleavers.

Descript] The common Cleavers have divers very rough square stalks, not so big as the top of a point, but raised up to be two or three yards high sometimes, if it meet with any tall bushes or trees, whereon it may climb, yet without any claspers, or else much lower and lying on the ground, full of joints, and at every one of them shooteth forth a branch, besides the leaves thereat which are usually six, set in a round compass like a star, or a rowel of a spur: From between the leaves or the joints towards the tops of the branches, come forth very small white flowers, at every one upon small thready foot stalks, which after they have fallen, there do shew two small round and rough seeds joined together

together like two testicles, which, when they are ripe, grow hard and whitish, having a little hole on the side, something like unto a navel. Both stalks, leaves, and seeds are so rough, that they will cleave to any thing that shall touch them. The root is small and thready, spreading much to the ground, but dieth every year.

Place] It groweth by the hedge and ditch-sides in many places of this land, and is so troublesome an inhabitant in gardens, that it rampeth upon, and is ready to choak whatever grows near it.

Time] It flowereth in June or July, and the seed is ripe and falleth again in the end of July or August, from whence it springeth up again and not from the old roots.

Government and Virtues] It is under the dominion of the Moon. The juice of the herb and the seed together taken in wine helpeth those bitten with an adder, by preserving the heart from the venom. It is familiarly taken in broth to keep them lean and lank, that are apt to grow fat. The distilled water drank twice a day, helpeth the yellow jaundice, and the decoction of the herb, in experience, is found to do the same, and stayeth lasks and bloody-fluxes. The juice of the leaves, or they a little bruised and applied to any bleeding wounds, stayeth the bleeding. The juice also is very good to close up the lips of green wounds, and the powder of the dried herb strewed thereupon doth the same, and likewise helpeth old ulcers. Being boiled in hogs grease it helpeth all sorts of hard swellings or kernels in the throat, being anointed therewith. The juice dropped into the ears, taketh away the pain of them.

It is a good remedy in the Spring, eaten (being first chopped small and boiled well) in water gruel, to cleanse the blood, and strengthen the liver, thereby to keep the body in health, and fitting it for that change of season that is coming.

Clowns Woodwort.

Descript.] IT groweth up sometimes to two or three feet high, but usually about two feet, with square, green, rough stalks, but slender, joined somewhat far asunder, and two very long, somewhat narrow dark green leaves bluntly dented about the edges thereof, ending in a long point. The flowers stand towards the tops, compassing the stalks at the joints with the leaves, and end likewise in a
spiked

spiked top, having long and much gaping hoods of a purplish red colour, with whitish spots in them standing in somewhat round husks, wherein afterwards stand blackish round seeds. The root is composed of many long strings, with some tuberous long knobs growing among them, of a pale yellowish or whitish colour, yet sometimes of the year these knobby roots in many places are not seen in this plant: The plant smelleth somewhat strong.

Place] It groweth in sundry counties of this land, both north and west, and frequently by both sides in the fields near about London, and within three or four miles distance about it, yet it usually grows in or near ditches.

Time] It flowereth in June or July, and the seed is ripe soon after.

Government and Virtues] It is under the dominion of the planet Saturn. It is singularly effectual in all fresh and green wounds, and therefore beareth not this name for nought. And it is very available in staunching of blood, and to dry up the fluxes of humours in old fretting ulcers, cankers, &c. that hinder the healing of them.

A syrup made of the juice of it is inferior to none for inward wounds, ruptures of veins, bloody flux, vessels broken, spitting, pissing or vomiting blood. Ruptures are excellently and speedily, even to admiration cured by taking now and then a little of the syrup, and applying an ointment or plaister of this herb to the place. Also, if an vein or muscle be swelled, apply a plaister of this herb to it, and if you add a little Comfrey to it, it will not do amiss. I assure thee the herb deserves commendations, though it has gotten such a clownish name: and whosoever reads this, (if he try it as I have done) will commend it; only take notice that it is of a dry earthy quality.

Cock's Head, Red Fitching, or Medic Fetch.

Descript] This hath divers weak but rough stalks, half a yard long, leaning downward, but set with winged leaves, longer and more pointed than those of lintels, and whitish underneath: from the tops of these stalks arise up other slender stalks, naked without leaves up to the tops, where there grow many small flowers in manner of a spike, of a pale reddish colour, with some blueness among them; after which rise up in their places, round, rough and somewhat flat heads. The root is tough, and somewhat woody, yet liveth and shooteth a new every year.

Place] It groweth under hedges, and sometimes in the open fields, in divers places of this land.

Time.] They flower all the months of July and August, and the seed ripeneth in the mean while.

Government and Virtues.] It is under the dominion of Venus. It hath power to rarify and digest; and therefore the green leaves bruised and laid as a plaister, disperse knots, nodes, or kernels in the flesh; and if when dry it be taken in wine, it helpeth the stranguary; and being anointed with oil, it provoketh sweat. It is a singular food for cattle, to cause them to give store of milk; and why then may it not do the like, being boiled in ordinary drink, for nurses?

Columbines.

THESE are so well known, growing almost in every garden, that I think I may save the expence of time in writing a description of them.

Time] They flower in May, and abide not for the most part when June is past, perfecting their seed in the mean time.

Government and Virtues] It is also an herb of Venus. The leaves of Columbines are commonly used in lotions with good success for sore mouths and throats. Tragus saith, that a dram of the seed taken in wine with a little saffron, openeth obstructions of the liver, and is good for the yellow jaundice, if the party after the taking thereof be laid to sweat well in bed. The seed also taken in wine causeth a speedy delivery of women in child-birth; if one draught suffice not, let her drink the second, and it is effectual. The Spaniards used to eat a piece of the root thereof in a morning fasting many days together, to help them when troubled with the stone in the reins or kidneys.

Coltsfoot.

CALLED also Coughwort, Foals foot, Horse hoof, and Bulls foot.

Descript] This shooteth up a slender stalk, with small yellowish flowers somewhat earlier, which fall away quickly, and after they are past, come up somewhat round leaves, sometimes dented about the edges, much lesser, thicker, and greener than those of butter-bur, with a little down or frieze over the green leaf on the upper side, which may be rubbed away, and whitish or meally underneath. The root is small and white, spreading much under ground, so that where it taketh it will hardly be driven away again, if any little piece be abiding therein; and from thence spring fresh leaves.

Place] It groweth as well in wet grounds as in drier places

Time] And flowereth in the end of February, the leaves begin to appear in March

Government and Virtues] The plant is under Venus, the fresh leaves or juice, or a syrup thereof is good for a hot dry cough, or wheesing, and shortness of breath. The dry leaves are best for those that have thin rheums and distillations upon their lungs, causing a cough, for which also the dried leaves taken as tobacco, or the root is very good The distilled water hereof simply, or with elder flowers and nightshade, is a singular good remedy against all hot agues, to drink two ounces at a time, and apply cloths wet therein to the head and stomach, which also does much good, being applied to any hot swellings and inflammations: It helpeth St Anthony's fire and burnings, and is singular good to take away wheals and small pushes that arise through heat; as also the burning heat of the piles, or privy parts, cloths wet therein being thereunto applied.

Comfrey.

Descript.] THE common Great Comfrey hath divers very large hairy green leaves lying on the ground, so hairy or prickly, that if they touch any tender part of the hands, face, or body, it will cause it to itch; the stalk that riseth from among them, being two or three feet high, hollow and cornered, is very hairy also, having many such like leaves as grow below, but lesser and lesser up to the top, at the joints of the stalks it is divided into many branches, with some leaves thereon, and at the ends stand many flowers in order one above another, which are somewhat long and hollow like the finger of a glove, of a pale whitish colour, after which come small black seeds. The roots are great and long, spreading great thick branches under ground. black on the outside, and whitish within, short and easy to break, and full of glutinous or clammy juice, of little or no taste at all.

There is another sort in all things like this, only somewhat less, and beareth flowers of a pale purple colour.

Place.] They grow by ditches and water sides, and in divers fields that are moist, for therein they chiefly delight to grow. The first generally through all the land, and the other but in some places. By the leave of my authors, I know the first grows often in dry places.

Time.] They flower in June or July, and give their seed in August.

Government and Virtues.] This is an herb of Saturn, and I suppose under the sign Capricorn, cold, dry, and earthly in quality. What was spoken of Clowns Woundwort, may be said of this. The Great Comfrey helpeth those that spit blood, or make a bloody urine. The root boiled in water or wine, and the decoction drank, helps all inward hurts, bruises, wounds, and ulcers of the lungs, and causeth the phlegm that oppresseth them to be easily spit forth: It helpeth the defluction of rheum from the head upon the lungs, the fluxes of blood or humours by the belly, womens immoderate courses, as well the reds as the whites, and the running of the reins, happening by what cause soever. A syrup made thereof is very effectual for all those inward griefs and hurts, and the distilled water for the same purpose also, and for outward wounds and sores in the fleshy or sinewy part of the body whatsoever, as also to take away the fits of agues, and to allay the sharpness of humours. A decoction of the leaves hereof is available to all the purposes, though not so effectual as the roots. The roots being outwardly applied, help fresh wounds or cuts immediately, being bruised and laid thereto; and is special good for ruptures and broken bones; yea, it is said to be so powerful to consolidate and knit together, that if they be boiled with dissevered pieces of flesh in a pot, it will join them together again. It is good to be applied to womens breasts that grow sore by the abundance of milk coming into them; also, to repress the overmuch bleeding of the hæmorrhoids, to cool the inflammation of the parts thereabouts, and to give ease of pains. The roots of Comfrey taken fresh, beaten small, and spread upon leather, and laid upon any place troubled with the gout, doth presently give ease of the pains, and applied in the same manner, giveth ease to pained joints, and profiteth very much for running and moist ulcers, gangrenes, and cations, and the like, for which it hath by often experience been found helpful.

Coralwort.

IT is also called by some Toothwort, Tooth Violet, Dog-Teeth Violet, and Dentaria.

Descript.] Of the many sorts of this herb two of them may be seen growing in this nation, the first of which sproweth forth one or two winged leaves upon long brownish foot-stalks, which are doubled down at their first coming out of the ground; when they are fully opened they consist of seven leaves, most commonly of a sad green colour, dented about the edges, set on both sides the middle rib one against another as the leaves of the ash tree; the stalk beareth no leaves on the lower half of it, the upper half beareth sometimes three or four, each consisting of five leaves, sometimes of three; on the top stand four or five flowers upon short foot stalks, with long husks; the flowers are very like the flowers of stock-gilliflower, of a pale purplish colour, consisting of four leaves a piece, after which come small cods which contain the seed; the root is very smooth, white, and shining; it doth not grow downwards, but creeping along under the upper crust of the ground, and consisteth of divers small round knobs set together; towards the top of the stalk there grow some single leaves, by each of which cometh a small cloven bulb, which when it is ripe, if it be set in the ground, it will grow to be a root.

As for the other Coralwort which groweth in this nation, it is more scarce than this, being a very small plant, much like coral-root, therefore some think it to be one of the sorts of crawfoot; I know not where to direct you to it, therefore I shall forbear the description.

Place.] The first groweth in Mayfield in Suffex, in a wood called Highread, and in another wood there also, called Foxholes.

Time.] They flower from the latter end of April to the middle of May, and before the middle of July they are gone, and not to be found.

Government and Virtues.] It is under the dominion of the Moon. It cleanseth the bladder, and provoketh urine, expel gravel and the stone, it easeth pains in the sides and bowels, is excellent good for inward wounds, especially such are held to be more effectual than the leaves, and the roots of little use. An ointment being made with them, taketh away spots and wrinkles of the skin, sun-burning and freckles, and adds beauty exceedingly; they remedy all infirmities of the head coming of heat and wind, as vertigo, evil altes, false apparitions, phrensies, falling sickness, palsies, convulsions, cramps, pains in the nerves; the roots ease pains in the back and bladder, and open the passages of urine. The leaves are good in wounds, and the flowers take away a burning. If the flowers be not well dried, and kept in a warm place, they will soon putrify and look green. Have a special eye over them. If you let them see the sun once a month, it will do neither the sun nor them harm.

Because they strengthen the brain and nerves, and remedy palsies, the Greeks give them the name Phal fir. The flowers preserved or conserved, and the quantity of a nutmeg eaten every morning, is a sufficient dose for inward diseases; but for wounds, spots, wrinkles, and sun burnings, an ointment is made of the leaves, and hog's grease.

Crabs Claws.

CALLED also Water Sengreen, Knights Pond Water, Water Houseleek, Pond Weed, and Fresh water Soldier.

Descript] It hath sundry long narrow leaves, with sharp prickles on the edges of them also, very sharp pointed; the stalks which bear the flowers seldom grow so high as the leaves, bearing a forked head, like a crab's claws, out of which comes a white flower, consisting of three leaves, with divers yellowish hairy threads in the middle; it taketh root in the mud in the bottom of the water.

Place] It groweth plentifully in the fens in Lincolnshire.

Time] It flowereth in June, and usually from thence till August.

Government and Virtues] It is a plant under the dominion of Venus, and thence a great strengthener of the reins. It is excellent good in that inflammation which is commonly called St. Anthony's fire; it assuageth all inflammations and swellings in wounds; and an ointment made of it, is excellent good to heal them; there is scarce a better remedy growing than this is for such as have bruised their kidneys, and upon that account pissing blood; a dram of the powder of the herb taken every morning, is a very good remedy to stop the terms.

Black Cresses.

Descript.] IT hath long leaves, deeply cut and jagged on both sides, not much unlike wild mustard; the stalks small, very limber, though very tough; you may twist them round as you may a willow, before they break. The flowers being very small and yellow, after which comes small cods, which contain the seed.

Place] It is a common herb, grows usually by the way-sides, and sometimes upon mud walls about London, but it delights most to grow among stones and rubbish.

Time.] It flowers in June and July, and the seed is ripe in August and September.

Government and Virtues] It is a plant of a hot and biting nature, under the dominion of Mars. The seed of Black Cresses strengthens the brain exceedingly, being in performing that office little inferior to mustard seed if at all; they are excellent good to stay those rheums which may fall down from the head upon the lungs; you may beat the seed into powder, if you please, and make it up into an electuary with honey; so you have an excellent remedy by you, not only for the premises, but also for the cough, yellow jaundice, and sciatica. The herb boiled into a poultice, is an excellent remedy for inflammations both in womens breasts and mens testicles.

Sciatica Cresses.

Descript] THESE are of two kinds. The first riseth up with a round stalk, about two feet high, spread into divers branches, whose lower leaves are somewhat larger than the upper, yet all of them cut or torn on the edges, somewhat like garden cresses, but smaller; the flowers are small and white, growing at the top of branches, where afterward grow husks, with small brownish seed therein, very strong and sharp in taste, more than the cresses of the garden; the root is long, white, and woody.

The other hath the lower leaves whole, somewhat long and broad, not torn at all, but only somewhat deeply dented about the edges towards the ends; but those that grow up higher

higher are lesser. The flowers and seeds are like the former, and so is the root likewise, and both root and seeds as sharp as it.

Place] They grow by the way sides in untilled places, and by the sides of old walls.

Time] They flower in the end of June, and their seed is ripe in July.

Government and Virtues] It is a Saturnine plant. The leaves, but especially the root, taken fresh in Summer-time, beaten or made into a poultice or salve with old hog's grease, and applied to the places pained with the sciatica, to continue thereon four hours, if it be on a man, and two hours on a woman; the place afterwards bathed with wine and oil mixed together, and then wrapped with wool or skins after they have sweat a little, will assuredly cure not only the same disease in hips, huckle bone, or other of the joints, as gout in the hands or feet, but all other old griefs in the head, (as inveterate rheums) and other parts of the body that are hard to be cured. And if of the former griefs any parts remain, the same medicine after twenty days is to be applied again. The same is also effectual in the diseases of the spleen, and applied to the skin, it taketh away the blemishes thereof, whether they be scars, leprosy, scabs, or scurf, which although it ulcerate the part, yet that is to be helped afterwards with a salve made of oil and wax. Esteem this as another secret.

Water Cresses.

Descript.] OUR ordinary Water Cresses spread forth with many, weak, hollow, sappy stalks, shooting out fibres at the joints, and upwards long winged leaves made of sundry broad sappy almost round leaves, of a brownish colour. The flowers are many and white, standing on long foot stalks, after which come small yellow seed contained in small long pods like horns. The whole plant abideth green in the Winter, and tasteth somewhat hot and sharp.

Place] They grow (for the most part) in small standing waters, yet sometimes in small rivulets of running water.

Time] They flower and seed in the beginning of Summer.

Government and Virtues.] It is an herb under the dominion of the Moon. They are more powerful against the scurvy,

scurvy, and to cleanse the blood and humours, than Brooklime is, and serve in all the other uses in which Brooklime is available, as to break the stone, and provoke urine and womens courses. The decoction thereof cleanseth ulcers, by washing them therewith. The leaves bruised, or the juice, is good to be applied to the face or other parts troubled with frecles, pimples, spots, or the like, at night, and washed away in the morning. The juice mixed with vinegar, and the forepart of the head bathed therewith, is very good for those that are dull and drousy, or have the lethargy.

Watercress pottage is a good remedy to cleanse the blood in the Spring, and help headachs, and consume the gross humours Winter hath left behind; those that would live in health, may use it if they please, if they will not, I cannot help it. If any fancy not pottage, they may eat the herb as a sallet.

Croswort.

Descript] COMMON Croswort groweth up with square hairy brown stalks a little above a foot high, having four small broad and pointed, hairy, yet smooth green leaves, growing at every joint, each against other crossway, which has caused the name. Towards the tops of the stalks at the joints, with the leaves in three or four rows downwards, stand small, pale, yellow flowers, after which come small blackish round seed, four for the most part set in every husk. The root is very small and full of fibres, or threads, taking good hold of the ground, and spreading with the branches a great deal of ground, which perish not in Winter, although the leaves die every year, and spring again new.

Place] It groweth in many moist grounds, as well meadows as untilled places about London, in Hampstead churchyard, at Wye in Kent, and sundry other places.

Time] It flowers from May all the Summer long, in one place or other, as they are open to the sun; the seed ripeneth soon after.

Government and Virtues] It is under the dominion of Saturn. This is a singular good wound herb, and is used inwardly, not only to stay bleeding of wounds, but to consolidate them, as it doth outwardly any green wound, which it quickly foldereth up, and healeth. The decoction of the herb in wine helpeth to expectorate phlegm out of the chest, and is good for obstructions in the breast, stomach or bowels and helpeth a decayed appetite. It is also good to wash any wound or sore with, to cleanse and heal it. The herb bruised, and then boiled applied outwardly for certain days together, renewing it often; and in the mean time the decoction of the herb in wine, taken inwardly every day, doth certainly cure the rupture in any, so as it be not too inveterate; but very speedily, if it be fresh and lately taken.

Crowfoot.

MANY are the names this furious biting herb hath obtained, almost enough to make up a Welshman's pedigree, if he fetch no farther than John of Gaunt, or William the Conqueror; for it is called Frogsfoot from the Greek name Barrakion; Crowfoot, Gold Knobs, Gold Cups, King's Knob, Baffners, Troilflowers, Polts, Locket Goulions, and Butterflowers.

Abundance are the sorts of this herb, that to describe them all would tire the patience of Socrates himself, but because I have not yet attained to the spirit of Socrates, I shall but describe the most usual.

Descript.] The most common Crowfoot hath many dark green leaves, cut into divers parts, in taste biting and sharp, biting and blistering the tongue. It bears many flowers, and those of a bright, resplendent, yellow colour. I do not remember, that I ever saw any thing yellower. Virgins in ancient time used to make powder of them to furrow bride beds; after which flowers come small heads, some spiked and rugged like a pine-apple.

Place] They grow very common every where; unless you turn your head into a hedge, you cannot but see them as you walk.

Time] They flower in May and June, even till September.

Government and Virtues] This fiery and hot spirited herb of Mars is no way fit to be given inwardly, but an ointment of the leaves or flowers will draw a blister, and may be so fitly applied to the nape of the neck to draw back rheum from the eye. The herb being bruised and mixed with a little mustard, draws a blister as well and as per-
fect-

fectly as Cantharides, and with far less danger to the vessels of urine, which Cantharides naturally delight to wrong: I knew the herb once applied to a pestilential rising that was fallen down, and it saved life even beyond hope; it were good to keep an ointment and plaister of it, if it were but for that.

Cuckow-point.

IT is called Atron, Janus, Barba aron, Calve-foot, Ramp, Starchwort, Cuckow pintle, Priests pintle, and Wake Robin.

Descript] This shooteth forth three, four, or five leaves at the most, from one root, every one whereof is somewhat large and long, broad at the bottom next the stalk, and forked, but ending in a point, without a cut on the edge, of a full green colour, each standing upon a thick round stalk of a hand-breadth long, or more, among which, after two or three months that they begin to wither, riseth up a bare, round, whitish green stalk, spotted and streaked with purple, somewhat higher than the leaves: At the top whereof standeth a long hollow husk, close at the bottom, but open from the middle upwards, ending in a point, in the middle whereof stand the small long pestle or clapper, smaller at the bottom than at the top, of a dark purple colour, as the husk is on the inside, though green without, which, after it hath so abided for some time, the husk with the clapper decayeth, and the foot or bottom thereof groweth to be a small long bunch of berries, green at the first, and of a yellowish red colour when they are ripe, of the bigness of a hazel nut kernel, which abideth thereon almost until Winter, the root is round, and somewhat long, for the most part lying along, the leaves shooting forth at the largest end, which, when it beareth his berries, are somewhat wrinkled and loose, another growing under it, which is solid and firm, with many small threads hanging thereat. The whole plant is of a very sharp biting taste, pricking the tongue as nettles do the hands, and so abideth for a great while without alteration. The root thereof was anciently used instead of starch to starch linen with.

There is another sort of Cuckow point with lesser leaves than the former, and sometimes harder, having blackish spots upon them, which for the most part abide longer

green

green in Summer than the former, and both leaves and roots are more sharp and fierce than it: In all things else it is like the former.

Place] These two sorts grow frequently almost under every hedge side in many places in this land.

Time] They shoot forth leaves in the Spring, and continue but until the middle of Summer, or somewhat later, their husks appearing before they fall away, and their fruit shewing in April.

Government and Virtues] It is under the dominion of Mars. Tragus reporteth, that a dram weight, or more if need be, of the spotted Wake Robin, either fresh and green, or dried, being beaten and taken, is a present and sure remedy for poison and the plague. The juice of the herb taken to the quantity of a spoonful hath the same effect. But if there be a little vinegar added thereto, as well as to the root aforesaid, it somewhat allayeth the sharp biting taste thereof upon the tongue. The green leaves bruised, and laid upon the boil or plague sore, doth wonderfully help to draw forth the poison. A dram of the powder of the dried root taken with twice so much sugar in the form of a licking electuary, or the green root, doth wonderfully help those that are pursy and shortwinded, as also those that have a cough; it breaketh, digesteth and riddeth away phlegm from the stomach, chest, and lungs. The milk wherein the root hath been boiled is effectual also for the same purpose. The said powder taken in wine or other drink, or the juice of the berries, or the powder of them, or the wine wherein they have been boiled, provoketh urine, and bringeth down womens courses, and purgeth them effectually after child bearing, to bring away the after birth. Taken with sheeps milk, it healeth the inward ulcers of the bowels. The distilled water thereof is effectual to all the purposes aforesaid. A spoonful taken at a time healeth the itch, and an ounce or more taken at a time for some days together doth help the rupture. The leaves, either green or dry, or the juice of them, doth cleanse all manner of rotten and filthy ulcers in what part of the body soever; and healeth the stinking sores in the nose, called Polypus. The water wherein the root hath been boiled, dropped into the eyes, cleanseth them from any film or skin, cloud or mists, which begin to hinder the

the sight, and helpeth the watering and redness of them, or when, by some chance, they become black and blue. The root mixed with bean flour, and applied to the throat or jaws that are inflamed, helpeth them. The juice of the berries boiled in oil of roses, or beaten into powder mixed with the oil, and dropped into the ears, easeth pains in them. The berries, or the roots beaten with hot ox dung and applied easeth the pains of the gout. The leaves and roots boiled in wine with a little oil, and applied to the piles, or the falling down of the fundament, easeth them, and so doth sitting over the hot fumes thereof. The fresh roots bruised and distilled with a little milk, yieldeth a most sovereign water to cleanse the skin from scurf, freckles, spots, or blemishes whatsoever therein.

Authors have left large commendations of this herb you see, but for my part, I have neither spoken with Dr Reason nor Dr Experience about it.

Cucumbers.

Government and Virtues] THERE is no dispute to be made, but that they are under the dominion of the Moon, tho' they are so much cried out against for their coldness, and if they were but one degree colder they would be poison. The best of Galenists hold them to be cold and moist in the second degree, and then not so hot as either lettuces or purslain; they are excellent good for a hot stomach, and hot liver; the unmeasurable use of them fills the body full of raw humours, and so indeed the unmeasurable use of any thing else doth harm. The face being washed with their juice cleanseth the skin, and is excellent good for hot rheum in the eyes; the seed is excellent good to provoke urine, and cleanseth the passages thereof when they are stopped; there is not a better remedy for ulcers in the bladder growing, than Cucumbers are. The usual course is, to use the seeds in emulsions, as they make almond milk, but a far better way (in my opinion) is this. When the season of the year is, take the Cucumbers and bruise them well, and distil the water from them, and let such as are troubled with ulcers in the bladder drink no other drink. The face being washed with the same water, cureth the reddest face that is; it is also excellent good for sun burning, freckles, and morphew.

Daisies.

Daisies.

THESE are so well known almost to every child, that I suppose it needless to write any description of them. Take therefore the virtues of them as followeth.

Government and Virtues] The herb is under the sign Cancer, and under the dominion of Venus, and therefore excellent good for wounds in the breast, and very fitting to be kept both in oils, ointments, and plaisters, as also in syrup. The greater wild Daisey is a wound herb of good respect, often used in those drinks or salves that are for wounds, either inward or outward. The juice or distilled water of these, or the small Daisey, doth much temper the heat and choler, and refresh the liver, and the other inward parts. A decoction made of them and drank, helpeth to cure the wounds made in the hollowness of the breast. The same cureth also all ulcers and pustules in the mouth or tongue, or in the secret parts. The leaves bruised and applied to the cods or to any other parts that are swoln and hot, doth dissolve it and temper the heat. A decoction made thereof, of wallwort and agrimony, and the places fomented or bathed therewith warm, giveth great ease to them that are troubled with the palsy, sciatica, or the gout. The same also dispereth and dissolveth the knots or kernels that grow in the flesh of any part of the body, and bruises and hurts that come of falls and blows; they are also used for ruptures and other inward burstings, with very good success. An ointment made thereof doth wonderfully help all wounds that have inflammations about them, or by reason of moist humours having access unto them, are kept long from healing, and such are these, for the most part, that happen to joints of the arms or legs. The juice of them dropped into the running eyes of any, doth much help them.

Dandelion, vulgarly called Piss-a-Beds.

Descript] It is well known to have many long and deep gashed leaves, lying on the ground round about the head of the roots, the ends of each gash or jag on both sides looking downwards towards the roots; the middle rib being white, which, being broken, yieldeth abundance of bitter milk, but the root much more; from among the leaves, which always abide green, arise many slender weak

weak, naked foot-stalks, every one of them bearing at the top one large yellow flower, consisting of many rows of yellow leaves, broad at the points, and nicked in with deep spots of yellow in the middle, which growing ripe, the green husk wherein the flowers stood turns itself down to the stalk, and the head of down becomes as round as a ball; with long reddish seed underneath, bearing a part of the down on the head of every one, which together is blown away with the wind, or may be at once blown away with one's mouth. The root growing downwards exceeding deep, which being broken off within the ground, will yet shoot forth again, and will hardly be destroyed where it hath once taken deep root in the ground.

Place.] It groweth frequently in all meadows and pasture grounds.

Time.] It flowereth in one place or other almost all the year long.

Government and Virtues.] It is under the dominion of Jupiter. It is of an opening and cleansing quality, and therefore very effectual for the obstructions of the liver, gall, and spleen, and the diseases that arise from them, as the jaundice and hypochondriac; it openeth the passages of the urine both in young and old; powerfully cleanseth imposthumes and inward ulcers in the urinary passage, and by its drying and temperate quality doth afterwards heal them, for which purpose the decoction of the roots or leaves in white wine, or the leaves chopped as pot herbs, with a few alisanders, and boiled in their broth, are very effectual. And whoever is drawing towards a consumption, or an evil disposition of the whole body, called Cachexia, by the use hereof for some time together, shall find a wonderful help. It helpeth also to procure rest and sleep to bodies distempered by the heat of ague fits, or otherwise. The distilled water is effectual to drink up pestilential fevers, and to wash the sores.

You see here what virtues this common herb hath, and that is the reason the French and Dutch so often eat them in the Spring; and now, if you look a little farther, you may see plainly, without a pair of spectacles, that foreign physicians are not so selfish as ours are, but more communicative of the virtues of plants to people.

Darnel.

Darnel.

IT is called Jum and Wray; in Sussex they call it Crop, it being a pestilent enemy among corn.

Descript.] This hath all the Winter long, sundry long, flat, and rough leaves, which, when the stalk riseth, which is slender and jointed, are narrower, but rough still; on the top groweth a long spike, composed of many heads set one above another, containing two or three husks, with sharp but short beards of awns at the end; the seed is easily shaked out of the ear, the husk itself being somewhat rough.

Place] The country husbandmen do know this too well to grow among their corn, or in the borders and pathways of the other fields that are fallow.

Government and Virtues] It is a malicious plant of sullen Saturn. As it is not without some vices, so hath it also many virtues. The meal of Darnel is very good to stay gangrenes and other such like fretting and eating cankers, and putrid sores. It also cleanseth the skin of all leprosies, morphew, ringworms, and the like, if it be used with salt and radish roots. And being used with quick brimstone and vinegar it dissolveth knots and kernels, and breaketh those that are hard to be dissolved, being boiled in wine with pigeons dung and linseed: A decoction thereof made with water and honey, and the places bathed therewith, is profitable for the sciatica. Darnel meal applied in a poultice draweth forth splinters and broken bones in the flesh: The red Darnel, boiled in red wine and taken, stayeth the lask and all other fluxes and women's bloody issues; and restraineth urine that passeth away too suddenly.

Dill.

Descript.] THE common Dill groweth up with seldom more than one stalk, neither so high nor so great usually as Fennel, being round and fewer joints thereon, whose leaves are sadder, and somewhat long, and so like Fennel that it deceiveth many, but harder in handling, and somewhat thicker, and of a stronger unpleasant scent. The tops of the stalks have four branches, and smaller umbels of yellow flowers, which turn into small seed, somewhat flatter and thinner than Fennel seed. The root is somewhat small and woolly, perisheth every year after it hath borne seed; and is also unprofitable, being never put to any use.

Place] It is most usually sown in gardens and grounds for the purpose, and is also found wild in many places.

Government and Virtues] Mercury hath the dominion of this plant, and therefore to be sure it strengthens the brain. The Dill being boiled and drank, is good to ease swellings and pains, it also stayeth the belly and stomach from casting. The decoction thereof helpeth women that are troubled with pains and windiness of the mother, if they sit therein. It stayeth the hiccough, being boiled in wine, and but smelled unto, being tied in a cloth. The seed is of more use than the leaves, and more effectual to digest raw and viscous humours, and is used in medicines that serve to expel wind, and the pains proceeding therefrom. The seed, being roasted or fried, and used in oils or plaisters, dissolve the imposthumes in the fundament; and drieth up all moist ulcers especially in the fundament; an oil made of Dill is effectual to warm or dissolve humours and imposthumes, to ease pains, and to produce rest. The decoction of Dill, be it herb or seed (only if you boil the seed you must bruise it) in white wine, being drank it is a gallant expeller of wind, and provoker of the terms.

Devil's-Bit.

Descript.] THIS rises up with a round green smooth stalk, about two feet high, set with divers long and somewhat narrow, smooth, dark green leaves, somewhat nipp'd about the edges, for the most part, being else all whole, and not divided at all, or but very seldom, even to the tops of the branches, which yet are smaller than those below, with one rib only in the middle. At the end of each branch standeth a round head of many flowers set together in the same manner, or more neatly than Scabious, and of a more bluish purple colour, which being past, there followeth seed that falleth away. The root somewhat thick but short and blackish, with many strings, abiding after seed time many years. This root was longer, until the devil (as the friars say) bit away the rest of it for spite, envying its usefulness to mankind, for sure he was not troubled with any disease for which it is proper.

There are two other sorts hereof, in nothing unlike the former, save that the one beareth white, and the other blush-coloured flowers.

Place]

Place] The first groweth as well in dry meadows and fields as moist, in many places of this land: But the other two are more rare, and hard to be met with, yet they are both found growing wild about Appledore, near Rye in Kent.

Time] They flower not usually until August.

Government and Virtues] The plant is venereal, pleasing and harmless. The herb or the root (all that the devil hath left of it) being boiled in wine, and drank, is very powerful against the plague and all pestilential diseases or fever poisons also, and the bitings of venomous beasts. It helpeth also those that are inwardly bruised by any casualty, or outwardly by fall or blows, dissolving the clotted blood, and the herb or root beaten and outwardly applied, taketh away the black and blue marks that remain in the skin. The decoction of the herb, with honey of roses put therein, is very effectual to help the inveterate tumours and swellings of the almonds and throat, by often gargling the mouth therewith. It helpeth also to procure womens courses, and easeth all pains of the mother, and to break and discuss wind therein, and in the bowels. The powder of the root taken in drink, driveth forth the worms in the body. The juice or distilled water of the herb, is effectual for green wounds, or old sores, and cleanseth the body inwardly, and the seed outwardly from sores, scurf, itch, pimples, freckles, morphew, or other deformities thereof, especially if a little vitriol be dissolved therein.

Dock.

MANY kinds of these are so well known, that I shall not trouble you with a description of them. My book grows big too fast.

Government and Virtues.] All Docks are under Jupiter, of which the Red Dock, which is commonly called Bloodwort, cleanseth the blood, and strengthens the liver, but the yellow Dock root is best to be taken when either the blood or liver is affected by choler. All of them leave a kind of cooling (but not all alike) drying quality, the Sorrel being most cold, and the bloody-worts most drying. Of the Burdock I have spoken already by itself. The seed of most of the other kinds, whether the gardens or fields, do stay laiks and fluxes of all sorts, the loathing of the stomach through choler, and is helpful for those that spit blood.

The root boiled in vinegar helpeth the itch, scabs, and breaking out of the skin, if it be bathed therewith. The distilled water of the herb and roots have the same virtue, and cleanseth the skin from freckles, morphews, and all other spots, and discolourings therein.

All Docks being boiled with meat, make it boil the sooner. Besides Blood wort is exceeding strengthening to the liver, and procures good blood, being as wholesome a pot herb as any grows in a garden; yet such is the nicety of our times (forsooth) that women will not put it into a pot because it makes the pottage black, pride and ignorance (a couple of monsters in the creation) preferring nicety before health.

Dodder of Thyme, Epithymum, and other Dodders.

Descript.] THIS first from seed giveth roots in the ground, which shooteth forth threads or strings, grosser or finer as the property of the plant wherein it groweth, and the climate doth suffer, creeping and spreading on that plant whereon it fasteneth, be it high or low. The strings have no leaves at all upon them, but wind and interlace themselves so thick upon a small plant, that it taketh away all comfort of the sun from it; and is ready to choak or strangle it. After these strings are risen up to that height, that they may draw nourishment from that plant, they seem to be broken off from the ground, either by the strength of their rising, or withered by the heat of the sun. Upon these strings are found clusters of small heads or husks, out of which shoot forth whitish flowers which afterwards give small pale-coloured seed, somewhat flat, and twice as big as a Poppy-seed. It generally participates of the nature of the plant which it climbeth upon; but the Dodder of Thyme is accounted the best, and is the only true Epithymum.

Government and Virtues.] All Dodders are under Saturn. Tell not me of physicians crying up Epithymum, or that Dodder which grows upon Thyme, (most of which comes from Hemetius in Greece, or Hybla in Sicily, because those mountains abound with Thyme) he is a physician indeed, that hath wit enough to choose his Dodder according to the nature of the disease and humour peccant. We see, Thyme is the hottest herb it usually grows upon, and there-

therefore that which grows upon Thyme is hotter than that which grows upon colder herbs; for it draws nourishment from what it grows upon, as well as from the earth where its root is, and thus you see old Saturn is wise enough to have two strings to his bow. This is accounted the most effectual for melancholy diseases, and to purge black or burnt choler, which is the cause of many diseases of the head and brain, as also for the trembling of the heart, faintings, and swoonings. It is helpful in all diseases and griefs of the spleen and melancholy, that arises from the windiness of the hypochondria. It purgeth also the reins or kidneys by urine, it openeth obstructions of the gall, whereby it profiteth them that have the jaundice; as also the leaves, the spleen, purging the veins of the choleric and phlegmatic humours, and helpeth children in agues, a little worm seed being put thereto.

The other Dodders do (as I said before) participate of the nature of those plants whereon they grow: as that which hath been found growing upon nettles in the west country, hath, by experience, been found very effectual to procure plenty of urine, where it hath been stopped or hindered. And so of the rest.

Sympathy and antipathy are two hinges upon which the whole mode of physic turns; and that physician which minds them not, is like a door off from the hooks, more like to do a man mischief than to secure him. Then all the diseases Saturn causeth, this helps by sympathy, and strengthens all the parts of the body he rules; such as be caused by Sol, it helps by antipathy. What those diseases are, see my judgment of diseases by astrology, and if you be pleased to look the herb Wormwood, you shall find a rational way for it.

Dog's-Grass, or Couch-grass.

Descript.] IT is well known, that the Grass creepeth far about under ground, with long white jointed roots, and small fibres almost at every joint, very sweet in taste, as the rest of the herb is, and interlacing one another, from whence shoot forth many fair grassy leaves, small at the ends, and cutting or sharp on the edges. The stalks are jointed like corn, with the like leaves on them, and a large spiked head, with a long husk in them, and hard
rough

rough seed in them. If you know it not by this description, watch the dogs when they are sick, and they will quickly lead you to it.

Place] It groweth commonly through this land in divers ploughed grounds, to the no small trouble of the husbandmen, as also of the gardeners, in gardens, to weed it out, if they can, for it is a constant customer to the place it gets footing in.

Government and Virtues.] 'Tis under the dominion of Jupiter, and is most medicineable of all the Quick Grasses. Being boiled and drank, it openeth the obstructions of the liver and gall, and the stopping of urine, and easeth the griping pains of the belly and inflammations; wasteth the matter of the stone in the bladder, and the ulcers thereof also. The roots bruised and applied do consolidate wounds. The seed doth more powerfully expel urine, and stayeth the lask and vomiting. The distilled water alone, or with a little wormseed, killeth the worms in children.

The way of use is to bruise the roots, and having well boiled them in white wine, drink the decoction. 'Tis opening, but not purging, very safe. 'Tis a remedy against all diseases coming of stopping, and such are half those that are incident to the body of man, and although a gardener be of another opinion, yet a physician holds half an acre of them to be worth five acres of Carrots twice told over.

Doves-Foot, or Cranes-Bill.

Descript] THIS hath divers small, round, pale green leaves, cut in about the edges, much like mallows, standing upon long, reddish, hairy stalks, lying in a round compass upon the ground; among which rise up two or three, or more reddish jointed, slender, weak hairy stalks, with such like leaves thereon, but smaller, and more cut in up to the tops, where grow many very small bright red flowers of five leaves a piece: after which follow small heads, with small short beaks pointed forth, as all other sorts of those herbs do.

Place.] It groweth in pasture grounds, and by the pathsides in many places, and will also be in gardens.

Time] It flowereth in June, July and August, some earlier and some later, and the seed is ripe quickly after.

Govern-

Government and Virtues.] It is a very gentle, though martial plant. It is found by experience to be singular good for the wind colic, as also to expel the stone and gravel in the kidneys. The decoction thereof in wine, is an excellent good cure for those that have inward wounds, hurts, or bruises, both to stay the bleeding, to dissolve and expel the congealed blood, and to heal the parts, as also to cleanse and heal outward sores, ulcers and fistulas; and for green wounds, many do only bruise the herb, and apply it to the place, and it healeth them quickly. The same decoction in wine some give to any place pained with the gout, or to joint aches, or pains of the sinews, giveth much ease. The powder or decoction of the herb taken for some time together, is found by experience to be singular good for ruptures and burstings in people, either young or old.

Ducks Meat.

THIS is so well known to swim on the top of standing waters, as ponds, pools, and ditches, that it is needless further to describe it.

Government and Virtues.] Cancer claims the herb and the Moon will be lady of it; a word is enough to a wise man. It is effectual to help inflammations and St. Anthony's fire, also the gout, either applied by itself, or in a poultice with barley meal. The distilled water by some is highly esteemed against all inward inflammations and pestilent fevers, also to help the redness of the eyes, and swelling of the cods, and of the breasts before they be grown too much. The fresh herb applied to the forehead, easeth the pains of the head coming of heat.

Down, or Cotton Thistle.

Descript.] THIS hath large leaves lying on the ground somewhat cut in, and as it were crumpled on the edges, of a green colour on the upper side, but covered with long hairy wool, or Cotton Down, set with most sharp and cruel pricks, from the middle of whose heads of flowers thrust forth many purplish crimson threads, and sometimes (though very seldom) white ones. The seed that followeth the heads, lying in a great deal of white down, is somewhat large, long and round, like the seed of Ladies thistle, but somewhat paler. The root is great and thick, spreading much, yet it usually dieth after seed time.

Place

Place.] It groweth in divers ditches, banks, and in corn fields and highways, generally every where throughout the land

Time.] It flowereth and beareth seed about the end of Summer, when other thistles do flower and seed.

Government and Virtues.] Mars owns the plant, and manifests to the world, that though it may hurt your finger, it will help your body; for I fancy it much for the ensuing virtues. Pliny and Dioscorides write, That the leaves and roots thereof taken in drink help those that have a crick in their neck, whereby they cannot turn their neck, but their whole body must turn also (sure they do not mean those that have got a crick in their neck by being under the hangman's hand). Galen saith, that the root and leaves hereof are of a heating quality, and good for such persons as have their bodies drawn together by some spasm or convulsions, as it is with children that have the rickets, or rather (as the college of physicians will have it) the Rachites, for which name of the disease they have (in a particular treatise lately set forth by them) learnedly disputed and put forth to public view, that the world may see they have taken much pains to little purpose.

Dragons.

THEY are so well known to every one that plants them in their gardens, that they need no description; if not, let them look down to the lower end of the stalks, and see how like a snake they look

Government and Virtues.] The Plant is under the dominion of Mars, and therefore it would be a wonder if it should want some obnoxious quality or other, in all herbs of that quality, the safest way is either to distil the herb in an alembic, in what vehicle you please, or else to press out the juice, and distil that in a glass still in sand. It scoureth and cleanseth the internal parts of the body mightily, and it cleareth the external parts also, being externally applied, from freckles, morphew, and sun burning. Your best way to use it externally, is to mix it with vinegar, an ointment of it is held to be good in wounds and ulcers, it consumes cankers, and that flesh growing in the nostrils, which they call Polypus: Also the distilled water being dropped into the eyes, taketh away spots there, or the pin and web and mends the dimness of sight; it is excellent good against pestilence and poison. Pliny and Dioscorides affirm, that no serpent will meddle with him that carries this herb about him.

The Elder Tree.

I HOLD it needless to write any description of this, since every boy that plays with a pot gun will not mistake another tree instead of Elder. I shall therefore in this place only describe the Dwarf Elder, called also Dead-wort, and Wall-wort.

The Dwarf Elder.

Descript.] THIS is but an herb every year, dying with his stalks to the ground, and rising fresh every Spring, and is like unto the Elder both in form and quality, rising up with a square rough hairy stalk, four feet high, or more sometimes. The winged leaves are somewhat narrower than the Elder, but else like them. The flowers are white with a dash of purple, standing in umbels, very like the Elder also, but more sweet in scent; after which come small blackish berries full of juice while they are fresh, wherein is small hard kernel or seed. The root doth creep under the upper crust of the ground, springing in divers places, being of the bigness of one's finger or thumb sometimes.

Place.] The Elder-tree groweth in hedges, being planted there to strengthen the fences and partitions of ground and to hold the banks by ditches and water courses.

The Dwarf Elder groweth wild in many places of England, where being once gotten into a ground, it is not easily gotten forth again.

Time.] Most of the Elder Trees flower in June, and their fruit is ripe for the most part in August. But the Dwarf Elder, or Wallwort, flowereth somewhat later, and his fruit is not ripe until September.

Government and Virtues.] Both Elder and Dwarf Tree are under the dominion of Venus. The first shoots of the common Elder boiled like asparagus, and the young leaves and stalks boiled in fat broth, doth mightily carry forth phlegm and choler. The middle or inward bark boiled in water, and given in drink, worketh much more violently, and the

berries

berries, either green or dry, expel the same humour, and are often given with good success to help the dropsy; the bark of the root boiled in wine or the juice thereof drank, worketh the same effects, but more powerfully than either the leaves or fruit. The juice of the root taken, doth mightily procure vomitings, and purgeth the watery humours of the dropsy. The decoction of the root taken, cureth the bite of an adder, and biting of mad dogs. It mollifieth the hardness of the mother, if a woman sit thereon, and openeth their veins, and bringeth down their courses. The berries boiled in wine performeth the same effect; and the hair of the head washed therewith, is made black. The juice of the green leaves applied to the hot inflammations of the eyes assuageth them; the juice of the leaves snuffed up into the nostrils purgeth the tunicles of the brain, the juice of the berries boiled with honey, and dropped into the ears, helpeth the pains of them; the decoction of the berries in wine being drank provoketh urine; the distilled water of the flowers is of much use to clean the skin from sun burning, freckles, morphew, or the like, and taketh away the head-ach, coming of a cold cause, the head being bathed therewith. The leaves or flowers distilled in the month of May, and the legs often washed with the said distilled water, it taketh away the ulcers and sores of them. The eyes washed therewith, it taketh away the redness and blood shot; and the hands washed morning and evening therewith, helpeth the palsy, and shaking of them.

The Dwarf Elder is more powerful than the common Elder in opening and purging choler, phlegm, and water; in helping the gout, piles, and womens diseases, coloureth the hair black, helpeth the inflammations of the eyes, and pains in the ears, the biting of serpents, or mad dogs, burnings and scaldings, the wind cholic, cholic and stone, the difficulty of urine, the cure of old sores, and fistulous ulcers. Either leaves or bark of Elder stripped upwards as you gather it, causeth vomiting. Also Dr Butler in a manuscript of his commends Dwarf Elder to the sky for dropsies, viz. to drink it, being boiled in white wine; to drink the decoction I mean, not the Elder.

The Elm Tree.

THIS tree is so well known, growing generally in all counties of this land, that it is needless to describe it.

Government

Government and Virtues.] It is a cold and Saturnine plant. The leaves thereof bruised and applied heal green wounds, being bound thereon with its own bark. The leaves, or the bark used with vinegar, cureth scurf and leprosy very effectually: The decoction of the leaves, bark or root, being bathed, heals broken bones. The water that is found in the bladders on the leaves, while it is fresh, is very effectual to cleanse the skin, and make it fair, and if cloths be often wet therein, and applied to the ruptures of children, it healeth them, if they be well bound up with a truss. The said water put into a glass, and set into the ground, or else in dung for twenty five days, the mouth thereof being close stopped, and the bottom set upon a lay of ordinary salt, that the fœces may settle and water become clear, is a singular and sovereign balm for green wounds, being used with soft tents. The decoction of the bark of the root fomented, mollifieth hard tumours, and the shrinking of the sinews. The roots of the Elm boiled for a long time in water, and the fat arising on the top thereof, being clean scummed off, and the place anointed therewith that is grown bald, and the hair fallen away, will quickly restore them again. The said bark ground with brine and pickle, until it come to the form of a poultice, and laid on the place pained with the gout, giveth great ease. The decoction of the bark in water, is excellent to bathe such places as have been burnt with fire.

Endive.

Descript.] COMMON garden Endive beareth a longer and larger leaf than succory, and abideth but one year, quickly running up to stalk and seed, and then perisheth; it hath blue flowers, and the seed of the ordinary Endive is so like succory seed, that it is hard to distinguish them.

Government and Virtues.] It is a fine cooling, cleansing, jovial plant. The decoction of the leaves, or the juice or the distilled water of Endive, serveth well to cool the excessive heat of the liver and stomach, and in the hot fits of agues and all other inflammations in any part of the body; it cooleth the heat and sharpness of the urine, and excoriations in the urinary parts. The seeds are of the same property, or rather more powerful, and besides are available for

fainting,

fainting, swoonings and passions of the heart. Outwardly applied, they serve to temper the sharp humours of fretting ulcers, hot tumours, swellings, and pestilential sores; and wonderfully help not only the redness and inflammations of the eyes, but the dimness of the sight also; they are also used to allay the pains of the gout. You cannot use it amiss, a syrup of it is a fine cooling medicine for fevers. See the end of this book, and the English Dispensatory.

Elecampane.

Descript.] IT shooteth forth many large leaves, long and broad, lying near the ground, small at both ends, somewhat soft in handling, of a whitish green on the upper side, and grey underneath, each set upon a short footstalk, from among which rise up divers great and strong hairy stalks, three or four feet high, with some leaves thereupon compassing them about at the lower end, and are branched towards the tops, bearing divers great and large flowers, like those of the corn marigold, both the border of leaves and the middle thrum being yellow, which turn into down, with long, small, brown seed among it, and is carried away with the wind. The root is great and thick, branched forth divers ways, blackish on the outside, and whitish within, of a very bitter taste, and strong but good scent, especially when they are dried; no part else of the plant having any smell.

Place.] It groweth in moist grounds and shadowy places, oftener than in the dry and open borders of fields and lanes, and in other waste places, almost in every county of this land.

Time.] It flowereth in the end of June and July, and the seed is ripe in August. The roots are gathered for use as well in the Spring before the leaves come forth, as in Autumn or Winter.

Government and Virtues.] It is a plant under the dominion of Mercury. The fresh roots of Elecampane preserved with sugar, or made into a syrup or conserve, are very effectual to warm a cold and windy stomach, or the pricking therein, and stitches in the sides caused by the spleen; and to help the cough, shortness of breath, and wheezing in the lungs. The dried root made into powder, and mixed with sugar and taken, serveth to the same purpose, and is also profitable for those who have their urine stopped, or the stopping of womens courses, the pains of the mother, and of the stone in the reins, kidneys, or bladder; it resisteth poison, and stayeth the spreading of the venom of serpents, as also putrid and pestilential fevers, and the plague itself. The roots and herb beaten and put into new ale or beer, and daily drank, cleareth, strengtheneth, and quickeneth the sight of the eyes wonderfully. The decoction of the roots in wine, or the juice taken therein, killeth and driveth forth all manner of worms in the belly, stomach, and maw, and gargled in the mouth, or the root chewed, fasteneth loose teeth, and helps to keep them from putrefaction; and being drank is good for those that spit blood, helpeth to remove cramps or convulsions, and the pains of the gout, the sciatica, the looseness and pains in the joints or those members that are out of joint by cold or moisture happening to them, applied outwardly as well as inwardly, and is also good for those that are bursten, or have any inward bruise. The root boiled well in vinegar, beaten afterwards, and made into an ointment with hog's suet, or oil of trotters, is an excellent remedy for scabs or itch in young or old; the places also bathed or washed with the decoction doth the same; it also helpeth all sorts of filthy old putrid sores or cankers whatsoever. In the roots of this herb lieth the chief effect for the remedies aforesaid. The distilled water of the leaves and roots together, is very profitable to cleanse the skin of the face, or other parts, from any morphew, spots, or blemishes therein, and make it clear.

Eringo, or Sea Holly.

Descript] THE first leaves of our ordinary Sea Holly, are nothing so hard and prickly as when they grow old, being almost round, and deeply dented about the edges, hard and sharp pointed, and a little crumpled, of a bluish green colour, every one upon a long foot stalk, but those that grow up higher with the stalk, do as it were compass it about. The stalk itself is round and strong, yet somewhat crested with joints, and leaves set thereat, but more divided, sharp and prickly; and branches rising from thence which have likewise other small branches, each of them bearing several bluish round prickly heads, with many small, jagged, prickly leaves under them, standing like a star and sometimes found greenish or whitish: The root groweth wonderful long, even to eight or ten feet in length, set with rings and circles toward the upper part, but smooth and without joints

joints downlower, brownish on the outside, and very white within, with a pith in the middle, of a pleasant taste, but much more, being artificially preserved, and candied with sugar.

Place] It is found about the sea coast in almost every county of this land which bordereth upon the sea.

Time] It flowereth in the end of Summer, and giveth ripe seed within a month after.

Government and Virtues] The plant is venereal, and breedeth seed exceedingly, and strengthens the spirit procreative; it is hot and moist, and under the celestial Balance. The decoction of the root hereof in wine is very effectual to open obstructions of the spleen and liver, and helpeth yellow jaundice, dropsy pains, of the loins, and wind colic, provoketh urine, and expelleth the stone, procureth womens courses. The continued use of the decoction for fifteen days, taken fasting, and next to bedward, doth help the stranguary, the pissing by drops, the stopping of urine, and stone, and all defects of the reins and kidneys, and if the said drink be continued longer, it is said that it cureth the stone; it is found good against the French pox. The roots bruised and applied outwardly, helpeth the kernels of the throat, commonly called the king's evil, or taken inwardly and applied to the place stung or bitten by any serpent, healeth it speedily. If the roots be bruised, and boiled in hog's grease, or salted lard, and applied to broken bones, thorns, &c remaining in the flesh, they do not only draw them forth, but heal up the place again, gathering new flesh where it was consumed. The juice of the leaves dropped into the ear, helpeth imposthumes therein. The distilled water of the whole herb, when the leaves and stalks are young, is profitably drank for all the purposes aforesaid, and helpeth the melancholy of the heart, and is available in quartan and quotidian agues, as also for them that have their necks drawn awry, and cannot turn them without turning their whole body.

Eyebright.

Descript.] COMMON Eyebright is a small low herb, rising up usually but with one blackish green stalk a span high, or not much more, spread from the bottom into sundry branches, whereon are small and almost round, yet pointed, dark green leaves, finely snipped about the edges, two always set together, and very thick. At the joints with the leaves, from the middle upward, come forth small white flowers, steeped with purple and yellow spots or stripes, after which follow small round heads, with very small seed therein. The root is long, small, and thready at the end.

Place.] It groweth in meadows, and grassy places in this land.

Government and Virtues.] It is under the sign of the Lion, and Sol claims dominion over it. If the herb was but as much used as it is neglected, it would half spoil the spectacle-makers trade; and a man would think that reason should teach people to prefer the preservation of their natural before artificial spectacles: which that they may be instructed how to do, take the virtues of Eyebright as followeth:

The juice or distilled water of Eyebright, taken inwardly in white wine or broth, or dropped into the eyes, for divers days together, helpeth all infirmities of the eyes that cause dimness of sight. Some make conserve of the flowers to the same effect. Being used any of the ways it also helpeth a weak brain or memory. This tunned up with strong beer, that it may work together, and drank, or the powder of the dried herb mixed with sugar, a little mace, and Fennel seed, and drank, or eaten in broth, or the said powder made into an electuary with sugar, and taken, hath the same powerful effect to help and restore the sight decayed through age, and Arnoldus de Villa Nova saith, it hath restored sight to them that have been blind a long time before.

Fern.

Descript.] Of this there are two kinds principally to be treated of, viz. the Male and Female. The Female groweth higher than the Male, but the leaves thereof are lesser, and more divided or dented, and of as strong a smell as the Male. The virtue of them are both alike, and therefore I shall not trouble you with any description or distinction of them.

Place.] They grow both in heaths and in shady places near the hedge-sides in all counties of this land.

Time.] They flower and give their seed at Midsummer.

The Female Fern is that plant which is in Sussex called Brake, the seed of which some authors hold to be so rare

Such

Such a thing there is I know, and may be easily had upon Midsummer Eve, and for ought I know, two or three days after it, if not more.

Government and Virtues.] It is under the dominion of Mercury, both Male and Female. The roots of both those sorts of Fern being bruised and boiled in mead, or honeyed water, and drank, killeth both the broad and long worms in the body, and abateth the swelling and hardness of the spleen. The green leaves eaten, purge the belly, and choleric and waterish humours that trouble the stomach. They are dangerous for women with child to meddle with, by reason they cause abortions. The roots bruised and boiled in oil, or hog's grease, make a very profitable ointment to heal wounds, or pricks gotten in the flesh. The powder of them used in foul ulcers, drieth up their malignant moisture, and causeth their speedier healing. Fern being burned, the smoke thereof driveth away serpents, gnats, and other noisome creatures which in fenny countries do, in the night-time, trouble and molest people lying on their beds with their faces uncovered; it causeth barrenness.

Osmond Royal or Water Fern.

Descript] THIS shooteth forth in Spring time (for in the Winter the leaves perish) divers rough hard stalks, half round and yellowish, or flat on the other side, two feet high, having divers branches of winged yellowish green leaves on all sides, set one against another, longer, narrower, and not nicked on the edges as the former. From the top of some of these stalks grow forth a long bush of small, and more yellow, green, scaly aglets, set in the same manner on the stalks as the leaves are, which are accounted the flowers and seeds. The root is rough, thick and scabby, with a white pith in the middle, which is called the heart thereof.

Place.] It groweth on moors, bogs, and watery places, in many parts of this land.

Time] It is green all the Summer, and the root only abideth in the Winter.

Government and Virtues] Saturn owns the plant. This hath all the virtues mentioned in the former Ferns, and is much more effectual than they, both for inward and outward griefs, and is accounted singular good in wounds, bruises, or the like. The decoction to be drank, or boiled into an ointment of oil, as a balsam or balm and so it is singular good against bruises, and bones broken, or out of joint, and giveth much ease to the colic and splenetic diseases; as also for ruptures or bursting. The decoction of the root in white wine provokes urine exceedingly, and cleanseth the bladder and the passages of the urine.

Feverfew, or Featherfew.

Descript.] COMMON Featherfew hath large, fresh, green leaves, much torn or cut on the edges. The stalks are hard and round, set with many such like leaves, but smaller, and at the tops stand many single flowers, upon small foot stalks, consisting of many small white leaves standing round about a yellow thrum in the middle. The root is somewhat hard and short, with many strong fibres about it. The scent of the whole plant is very strong and stuffing, and the taste is very bitter.

Place] This grows wild in many places of the land, but is for the most part nourished in gardens.

Time] It flowereth in the months of June and July.

Government and Virtues.] Venus commands this herb and hath commended it to succour her sisters (women) and to be a general strengthener of their wombs, and remedy such infirmities as a careless midwife hath there caused; if they will but be pleased to make use of her herb boiled in white wine, and drink the decoction; it cleanseth the womb, expels the after birth, and doth a woman all the good she can desire of an herb. And if any grumble because they cannot get the herb in Winter, tell them, if they please, they may make a syrup of it in Summer. It is chiefly used for the disease of the mother, whether it be the strangling or rising of the mother, or hardness, or inflammations of the same, applied outwardly thereunto. Or a decoction of the flowers in wine, with a little nutmeg or mace put therein, and drank often in a day, is an approved remedy to bring down women's courses speedily, and helpeth to expel the dead birth and after birth. For a woman to sit over the hot fumes of the decoction of the herb made in water or wine, is effectual for the same; and in some cases, to apply the herb warm to the privy parts. The decoction thereof made, with some sugar or honey put thereto, is used by many with good success to help the cough and stuffing of the chest, by colds, as also to cleanse the reins and bladder, and helps to expel the stone in them. The powder of the herb taken in wine, with some Oxymel, purgeth both choler and phlegm, and is available for those that are short winded, and are troubled with melancholy and heaviness, or sadness of spirits. It is very effectual for all pains in the head coming of a cold cause, the herb being bruised and applied to the crown of the head: As also for the vertigo, that is a running or swimming of the head. The decoction thereof drank warm, and the herb bruised with a few corns of Bay-salt, and applied to the wrists before the coming of the ague-fit, doth take them away. The distilled water taketh away freckles, and other spots and deformities in the face. The herb bruised and heated on a tile, with some wine to moisten it, or fried with a little wine and oil in a frying pan, and applied warm outwardly to the places, helpeth the wind and colic in the lower part of the belly. It is an especial remedy against opium taken too liberally.

Fennel.

EVERY garden affordeth this so plentifully, that it needs no description.

Government and Virtues] One good old fashion is not yet left off, viz. to boil Fennel with fish; for it consumes that phlegmatic humour, which fish most plentifully afford and annoy the body with, though few that use it know wherefore they do it; I suppose the reason of its benefit this way is because it is an herb of Mercury, and under Virgo, and therefore bears antipathy to Pisces. Fennel is good to break wind, to provoke urine, and ease the pains of the stone, and helps to break it. The leaves or seed boiled in barley water and drank are good for nurses, to increase their milk, and make it more wholesome for the child. The leaves, or rather the seeds, boiled in water, stayeth the hiccough, and taketh away the loathings which oftentimes happen to the stomachs of sick and feverish persons, and allayeth the heat thereof. The seed boiled in wine and drank, is good for those that are bitten with serpents, or have eaten poisonous herbs, or mushrooms. The seed and the roots much more help to open obstructions of the liver, spleen, and gall, and thereby help the painful and windy swellings of the spleen, and the yellow jaundice, as also the gout and cramps. The seed is of good use in medicines to help shortness of breath and wheezing by stopping of the lungs. It helpeth also to bring down the courses and to cleanse the parts after delivery. The roots are of most use in pottage, drinks and broths that are taken to cleanse the blood, to open obstructions of the liver, to provoke urine, and amend the ill colour in the face after sickness, and to cause a good habit through the body. Both leaves, seeds, and roots thereof are much used in drink or broth, to make people more lean that are too fat. The distilled water of the whole herb, or the condensate juice dissolved, but especially the natural juice, that in some counties issueth out hereof of its own accord, dropped into the eyes, cleanseth them from mists and films that hinder the sight. The sweet Fennel is much weaker in physical uses than the common Fennel. The wild Fennel is stronger and hotter than the tame, and therefore most powerful against the stone, but not so effectual to increase milk, because of its dryness.

Sow-Fennel, or Hog's-Fennel.

BESIDES the common name in English, Hog's Fennel, and the Latin name Peucidanum, it is called Hoar strange, and Hoar strong, Sulphur wort, and Brimstone wort.

Descript.] The common Sow Fennel hath divers branched stalks of thick and somewhat long leaves, three for the most part joined together at a place, among which ariseth a crested straight stalk less than Fennel, with some joints thereon, and leaves growing thereat, and towards the tops some branches issuing from thence; likewise on the tops of the stalks and branches stand divers tufts of yellow flowers, whereafter groweth somewhat flat, thin and yellowish seed, bigger than Fennel-seed. The roots grow great and deep, with many other parts and fibres about them of a strong scent like hot brimstone, and yield forth a yellowish milk, or clammy juice almost like a gum.

Place] It groweth plentifully in the salt low marshes near Feversham in Kent.

Time.] It flowereth plentifully in July and August.

Government and Virtues] This is also an herb of Mercury. The juice of Sow-fennel (saith Dioscorides, and Galen) used

used with vinegar and rose water, or the juice with a little euphorbium put to the nose, helpeth those that are troubled with the lethargy, frenzy, or giddiness of the head, the falling-sickness, long and inveterate head-ach, the palsy, sciatica, and the cramp, and generally all the diseases of the sinews, used with oil and vinegar. The juice dissolved in wine, or put into an egg, is good for a cough, or shortness of breath, and for those that are troubled with wind in the body. It purgeth the belly gently, expelleth the hardness of the spleen, giveth ease to women that have sore travel in child-birth, and easeth the pains of the reins and bladder, and also the womb. A little of the juice dissolved in wine, and dropped into the ears easeth the pains in them, and put into a hollow tooth, easeth the pains thereof. The root is less effectual to all the aforesaid disorders; yet the powder of the root cleanseth foul ulcers, being put into them, and taketh out splinters of broken bones, or other things in the flesh, and healeth them up perfectly, as also, drieth up old and inveterate running sores, and is of admirable virtue in all green wounds.

Fig-wort, or Throat-wort.

Descript] COMMON great Fig-wort sendeth out divers great, strong, hard, square brown stalks, three or four feet high, whereon grow large, hard, and dark green leaves, two at a joint, harder and larger than Nettle leaves, but not stinging; at the tops of the stalks stand many purple flowers set in husks, which are sometimes gaping and open, somewhat like those of Water Betony; after which come hard round heads, with a small point in the middle, wherein lie small brownish seed. The root is great, white, and thick, with many branches at it growing aslope under the upper crust of the ground, which abideth many years, but keepeth not his green leaves in Winter.

Place] It groweth frequently in moist and shadowy woods, and in the lower parts of the fields and meadows.

Time] It flowereth about July, and the seed will be ripe about a month after the flowers are fallen.

Government and Virtues] Some Latin authors call it Cervicaria, because it is appropriated to the neck; and the Throat-wort, because it is appropriated to the Throat. Venus owns the herb, and the Celestial Bull will not deny it; therefore a

better

better remedy, cannot be for the king's evil, because the Moon that rules the disease is exalted there. The decoction of the herb taken inwardly, and the bruised herb applied outwardly, dissolveth clotted and congealed blood within the body, coming by any wound, bruise or fall; and is no less effectual for the king's evil, or any other knobs, kernels, bunches, or wens growing in the flesh wheresoever; and for the hæmorrhoids, or piles. An ointment made hereof may be used at all times when the fresh herb is not to be had. The distilled water of the whole plant, roots and all, is used for the same purposes, and drieth up the superfluous, virulent moisture of hollow and corroding ulcers; it taketh away all redness, spots, and freckles in the face, as also the scurf, and any foul deformity therein, and the leprosy likewise.

Filipendula, or Drop-wort.

Descript.] THIS sendeth forth many leaves some bigger, some lesser, set on each side of a middle rib, and each of them cented about the edges, somewhat resembling wild Tansy or rather Agrimony, but harder in handling; among which rise up one or more stalks, two or three feet high, with the leaves growing thereon, and sometimes also divided into other branches spreading at the top into many white, sweet smelling flowers, consisting of five leaves a piece, with some threads in the middle of them standing together, in a pith or umbel, each upon a small foot stalk, which, after they have been blown upon a good while do fall away, and in their places appear small, round, chaffy heads like buttons, wherein are the chaffy seeds set and placed. The root consists of many small, black tuberous pieces fastened together by many small, long black strings, which run from one to another.

Place.] It groweth in many places of this land in the corners of dry fields and meadows, and the hedge sides.

Time.] They flower in June and July, and their seed is ripe in August.

Government and Virtues] It is under the dominion of Venus. It effectually opens the passages of the urine, helpeth the stranguary, the stone in the kidneys or bladder, the gravel, and all other pains of the bladder and reins, by taking the roots in powder, or a decoction of them in white wine, with

a little

a little honey. The roots made into powder, and mixed with honey in the form of an electuary, doth much help them whose stomachs are swollen, dissolving and breaking the wind which was the cause thereof; and is also very effectual for all the diseases of the lungs, as shortness of breath, wheezing, hoarseness of the throat, and the cough; and to expectorate tough phlegm, or any other parts thereabout. It is called Dropwort, because it helps such as piss by drops.

The Fig-tree.

FOR to give a description of a tree so well known to every body that keeps it in his garden, were needless. They prosper very well in our English gardens, yet are fitter for medicine, than for any other profit which is gotten by the fruit of them.

Government and Virtues.] The tree is under the dominion of Jupiter. The milk that issueth out from the leaves or branches where they are broken off, being dropped upon warts, taketh them away. The decoction of the leaves is excellent good to wash sore heads with; and there is scarcely a better remedy for the leprosy than it is. It clears the face also of morphew, and the body of white scurf, scabs, and running sores. If it be dropped into old fretting ulcers, it cleanseth out the moisture, and bringeth up the flesh, because you cannot have the leaves green all the year, you may make an ointment of them whilst you may. A decoction of the leaves being drank inwardly, or rather a syrup made of them, dissolves congealed blood caused by bruises or falls, and helps the bloody-flux. The ashes of the wood made into an ointment with hog's grease, helps kibes and chilblains. The juice being put into an hollow tooth, easeth pain, as also pain and noise in the ears, being dropped in them; and deafness. An ointment made of the juice and hog's grease is as excellent a remedy for the biting of mad dogs, or other venomous beasts, as most are. A syrup made of the leaves, or green fruit, is excellent good for coughs, hoarseness, or shortness of breath, and all diseases of the breast and lungs: it is also excellent good for the dropsy and falling sickness. They say that the Fig-tree, as well as the Bay-tree, is never hurt by lightning; as also if you tie a bull, be he ever so mad, to a Fig-tree, he will quickly become tame and gentle,

gentle. As for such figs as come from beyond sea, I have little to say, because I write not of exoticks; yet some authors say, the eating of them makes people lousy

The yellow Water Flag, or Flower-de-luce

Descript.] THIS groweth like the Flower-de-luce, but it hath much longer and narrower sad green leaves jointed together in that fashion; the stalk also growing oftentimes as high, bearing small yellow flowers shaped like the Flower-de-luce, with three falling leaves, and other three arched that cover their bottoms; but instead of the three upright leaves, as the Flower-de-luce hath, this hath only three short pieces standing in their places, after which succeed thick and long three-square heads, containing in each part somewhat big and flat seed, like those of the Flower-de-luce. The root is long and slender, of a pale brownish colour on the outside, and of a horse flesh colour on the inside, with many hard fibres thereat, and very harsh in taste.

Place] It usually grows in watery ditches, ponds, lakes, and moor sides, which are always overflowed with water.

Time] It flowereth in July and the seed is ripe in August.

Government and Virtues] It is under the dominion of the Moon. The root of this Water flag is very astringent, cooling, and drying; and thereby helps all lasks and fluxes, whether of blood and humours, as bleeding at the mouth, nose, or other parts, bloody flux, and the immoderate flux of womens courses. The distilled water of the whole herb, flowers and roots, is a sovereign good remedy for watering eyes, both to be dropped into them, and to have cloths or sponges wetted therein, and applied to the forehead. It also helpeth the spots and blemishes that happen in and about the eyes, or in any other parts. The said water fomented on swellings, and hot inflammations of womens breasts, upon cankers also, and those spreading ulcers called *Noli me tangere*, do much good. It helpeth also foul ulcers in the privities of man or woman; but an ointment made of the flowers is better for those external applications.

Flax-Weed, or Toad-Flax.

Descript] OUR common Flax-weed hath divers stalks full fraught with long and narrow ash-coloured leaves, and from the middle of them almost upward, stored with a number of pale yellow flowers, of a strong unpleasant scent, with deeper yellow mouths, and blackish flat seed in round heads. The root is somewhat woody and white especially the main downright one, with many fibres, abiding many years, shooting forth roots every way round about, and new branches every year.

Place] This groweth throughout this land, both by the way sides and in meadows as also by hedge sides, and upon the sides of banks, and borders of fields.

Time] It flowereth in Summer, and the seed is ripe usually before the end of August.

Government and Virtues] Mars owns the herb: In Sussex we call it Gallwort, and lay it in our chickens water to cure them of the gall, it relieves them when they are drooping. This is frequently used to spend the abundance of those watery humours by urine, which cause the dropsy. The decoction of the herb, both leaves and flowers in wine taken and drank, doth somewhat move the belly downwards, openeth obstructions of the liver, and helpeth the yellow jaundice; expelleth poison, provoketh womens courses, driveth forth the dead child, and after birth. The distilled water of the herb and flower, is effectual for all the same purposes; being drank with a dram of the powder of the seeds of bark, or the roots of Wall wort, and a little cinnamon, for certain days together, it is held a singular remedy for the dropsy. The juice of the herb or the distilled water dropped into the eyes, is a certain remedy for all heat, inflammation and redness in them. The juice or water put into foul ulcers, whether they be cancerous or fistulous, with tents put therein, or parts washed and injected therewith, cleanseth them thoroughly from the bottom, and healeth them up safely. The same juice or water also cleanseth the skin wonderfully of all sorts of deformity, as leprosy, morphew, scurf, wheals, pimples, or spots, applied of itself, or used with some powder of Lupines.

Flea-

Flea-Wort.

Descript] ORDINARY Flea-wort riseth up with a stalk two feet high or more, full of joints and branches on every side up to the top, and at every joint two small, long, and narrow whitish green leaves somewhat hairy. At the top of every branch stand divers small, short, scaly, or chaffy heads, out of which come forth small whitish yellow threads, like to those of the plantain herbs, which are the bloomings of flowers. The seed inclosed in these heads is small and shining while it is fresh, very like unto fleas both for colour and bigness, but turning black when it groweth old. The root is not long, but white, hard and woody, perishing every year, and rising again of it's own seed for divers years, if it be suffered to shed. The whole plant is somewhat whitish and hairy, smelling somewhat like rosin.

There is another sort hereof, differing not from the former in the manner of growing, but only that this stalk and branches being somewhat greater, do a little more bow down to the ground. The leaves are somewhat greater, the heads somewhat lesser, the seed alike and the root and leaves abide all Winter and perisheth not as the former.

Place] The first groweth only in gardens, the second plentifully in fields that are near the sea.

Time] They flower in July, or thereabouts.

Government and Virtues] The herb is cold, dry, and Saturnine. I suppose it obtained the name of Flea-wort, because the seeds are like Fleas. The seed fried, and taken, stayeth the flux or lask of the belly, and the corrosions that come by reason of hot choleric, or sharp and malignant humours, or by too much purging of any violent medicine, as Scammony, or the like. The mucilage of the seed made with Rose-water, and a little sugar candy put thereto, is very good in all hot agues and burning fevers, and other inflammations, to cool the thirst, and lenity the dryness and roughness of the tongue and throat. It helpeth hoarseness of the voice, and diseases of the breast and lungs, caused by heat, or sharp salt humours, and the pleurisy also. The mucilage of the seed made with plantain water, whereunto the yolk of an egg or two, and a little populeon are put, is a most safe and sure remedy to ease the sharpness, pricking, and pains of the hæmorrhoids or piles, ples, if it be laid on a cloth, and bound thereto. It helpeth all inflammations in any part of the body, and the pains that come thereby, as the head-ach and megrims, and all hot impoithumes, swellings or breaking out of the skin, as blains, wheals, pushes, purples, and the like; as also the joints of those that are out of joint, the pains of the gout and sciatica, the bursting of young children, and the swelling of the navel, applied with oil of roses and vinegar. It is also good to heal the nipples and sore breasts of women, being often applied thereunto. The juice of the herb with a little honey put into the ears helpeth the running of them, and the worms breeding in them: The same also mixed with hog's grease, and applied to corrupt and filthy ulcers, cleanseth and healeth them.

Fluxweed.

Descript] It riseth up with a round upright hard stalk, four or five feet high, spread into sundry branches, whereon grow many greyish green leaves, very finely cut and severed into a number of short and almost round parts. The flowers are very small and yellow, growing spike fashion, after which come small long pods, with small yellowish seed in them. The root is long and woody, perishing every year.

There is another sort, differing in nothing, save only it hath somewhat broader leaves; they have a strong evil savour, being smelled unto, and are of a drying taste.

Place] They flower wild in the fields by hedge sides and high ways, and among rubbish and other places.

Time.] They flower and seed quickly after, namely in June and July.

Government and Virtues.] This herb is Saturnine also. Both the herb and seed of Fluxweed are of excellent use to stay the flux or lask of the belly, being drank in water wherein gads of steel heated have been often quenched; and it is no less effectual for the same purpose than plantain or comfrey, and to restrain any other flux of blood in man or woman, as also to consolidate bones broken or out of joint. The juice thereof drank in wine, or the decoction of the herb drank, doth kill the worms in the stomach or belly, or the worms that grow in putrid and filthy ulcers; and made into a salve doth quickly heal all old sores, how foul, or malignant soever they be.

The

The distilled water of the herb worketh the same effects, although somewhat weaker, yet it is a fair medicine, and more acceptable to be taken. It is called Fluxweed because it cures the flux, and for its uniting broken bones, &c. Paracelsus extols it to the skies. It is fitting that syrup, ointment, and plaisters of it were kept in your houses.

Flower-de-luce.

IT is so well known, being now shed up in most gardens, that I shall not need to spend time in writing a description thereof.

Time.] The flaggy kinds thereof have the most physical uses; the dwarf kinds thereof flower in April, the greater sorts in May.

Government and Virtues] The herb is Lunar. The juice or decoction of the green root of the flaggy kind of Flower-de-luce with a little honey drank, doth purge and cleanse the stomach of gross and tough phlegm, and choler therein; it helpeth the jaundice and the dropsy, evacuating those humours both upwards and downwards, and because it somewhat hurts the stomach, is not to be taken without honey and spikenard. The same being drank, doth ease the pains and torments of the belly and sides, the shaking of agues, the diseases of the liver and spleen, the worms of the belly, the force in the reins, convulsions and cramps that come of old humours; it also helps those whose seed passeth from them unawares. It is a remedy against the bitings and stingings of venomous creatures, being boiled in water and vinegar and drank. Boiled in water and drank, it provoketh urine, helpeth the colic, bringeth down womens courses, and made up into a pessary with honey, and put up into the body, draweth forth the dead child. It is much commended against the cough, to expectorate tough phlegm; it much easeth pains in the head, and procureth sleep, being put into the nostril it procureth sneezing, and thereby purgeth the head of phlegm. The juice of the root applied to the piles or hæmorrhoids giveth much ease. The decoction of the roots gargled in the mouth, easeth the tooth-ach, and helpeth a stinking breath. Oil called Oleum Irinum, if it be rightly made of the great broad flag Flower-de-luce (and not of the green bulbed Flower-de-luce as is used by some apothecaries) and roots of the same of the flaggy kind, is

very

very effectual to warm and comfort all cold joints and sinews, as also the gout and sciatica, and mollifieth, dissolveth, and consumeth tumours and swellings in any part of the body, as also of the matrix; it helpeth the cramp, or convulsions of the sinews. The head and temples anointed therewith, helpeth the catarrh, or thin rheum distilled from thence; and used upon the breast or stomach, helpeth to extenuate the cold tough phlegm, it helpeth also pains and noise in the ears, and the stench of the nostrils. The root itself, either green or in powder, helpeth to cleanse, heal, and incarnate wounds, and to cover the naked bones with flesh again, that ulcers have made bare, and is also very good to cleanse and heal up fistulas and cankers that are hard to be cured.

Fluellin, or Lluellin.

Descript] IT shooteth forth many long branches partly lying upon the ground, and partly standing upright, set with almost red leaves, yet a little pointed, and sometimes more long and round, without order thereon, somewhat hairy, and of an evil greenish white colour, at the joints all along the stalks, and with the leaves come forth small flowers, one at a place, upon a very small short footstalk, gaping somewhat like snap dragons, or rather like toad flax, with the upper jaw of a yellow colour, and the lower of a purplish, with a small heel or spur behind; after which come forth small round heads, containing small black seed. The root is small and thready, dying every year, and raiseth itself again of its own sowing.

There is another sort of Lluellin which hath longer branches wholly trailing upon the ground, two or three feet long, and somewhat more thin, set with leaves thereon, upon small foot stalks. The leaves are a little larger, and somewhat round, and cornered sometimes in some places on the edges; but the lower part of them being the broadest, hath on each side a small point, making it seem as if they were ears, sometimes hairy, but not hoary, and a better green colour than the former. The flowers come forth like the former, but the colours therein are more white than yellow and the purple not so fair. It is a large flower, and so are the seed and seed vessels. The root is like the other, and perisheth every year.

Place] They grow in divers corn fields, and in borders
about

about them, and in other fertile grounds about Southfleet in Kent abundant; at Bechrite, Hamerton, and Richmanworth in Huntingdonshire, and in divers other places.

Time.] They are in flower about June and July, and the whole plant is dry and withered before August be done.

Government and Virtues.] It is a Lunar herb. The leaves bruised and applied with barley meal to watering eyes that are hot and inflamed by defluctions from the head, do very much help them; as also the fluxes of blood or humours, as the lask, bloody flux, women's courses, and stayeth all manner of bleeding at the nose, mouth, or any other place, or that cometh by any bruise or hurt, or bursting of a vein, it wonderfully helpeth all these inward parts that need consolidating or strengthening, and is no less effectual both to heal and close green wounds, than to cleanse and heal all foul or old ulcers, fretting or spreading cankers, or the like. Bees are industrious, and go abroad to gather honey from each plant and flower; but drones lie at home, and eat up what the bees have taken pains for. Just so do the college of physicians lie at home and domineer, and suck out the sweetness of other men's labour and studies, themselves being as ignorant in the knowledge of herbs as a child of four years old, as I can make appear to any rational man by their last dispensatory. Now then to hide their ignorance, there is no readier way in the world than to hide knowledge from their countrymen, that so no body might be able so much as to smell out their ignorance. When simples were in use, mens bodies were better in health by far than now they are, or shall be, if the college can help it. The truth is, this herb is of a fine cooling, drying quality, and an ointment or plaister of it might do a man a courtesy that hath any hot virulent sores: 'tis admirable for the ulcers of the French pox; if taken inwardly, may cure the disease. It was first called Female Speedwell, but a gentleman of Wales, whose nose was almost eaten off with the pox, and so near the matter, that the doctors commanded it to be cut off, being cured only by the use of this herb, and to honour the herb, for saving his nose whole, gave it one of her country names, Fluellin.

Fox-Gloves.

Descript.] It hath many long and broad leaves lying upon the ground dented upon the edges, a little soft or woolly, and of a hoary green colour, among which riseth up sometimes sundry stalks, but one very often, bearing such leaves thereon from the bottom to the middle, from whence to the top it is stored with large and long hollow reddish purple flowers, a little more long and imminent at the lower edge, with some white spots with them, one above another, with small green leaves at every one, but all of them turning their heads one way, and hanging downwards, having some threads also in the middle, from whence rise round heads, pointed sharp at the ends, wherein small brown seed lieth. The roots are so many small fibres, and some greater things among them: the flowers have no scent, but the leaves have a bitter hot taste.

Place] It groweth on dry sandy ground for the most part, and as well on the higher as the lower places under hedge sides in almost every county of this land.

Time] It seldom flowereth before July, and the seed is ripe in August.

Government and Virtues] The plant is under the dominion of Venus, being of a gentle cleansing nature, and withal very friendly to nature. The herb is familiarly and frequently used by the Italians to heal any fresh or green wound, the leaves being but bruised and bound thereon, and the juice thereof is also used in old sores, to cleanse, dry, and heal them. The decoction hereof made up with some sugar or honey, is available to cleanse and purge the body both upwards and downwards, sometimes of tough phlegm and clammy humours, and to open obstructions of the liver and spleen. It hath been found by experience to be available for the king's evil, the herb bruised and applied, or an ointment made with the juice thereof, and so used; and a decoction of two handfuls thereof, with four ounces of Polypody in ale, hath been found by late experience to cure divers of the falling sickness that have been troubled with it above twenty years. I am confident that an ointment of it is one of the best remedies for a scabby head that is.

Fumitory.

Descript] OUR common Fumitory is a tender sappy herb, sendeth forth from one square, a slender weak stalk, and leaning downwards on all sides, many branches two or three feet long, with finely cut and jagged leaves

leaves of whitish, or rather bluish sea green colour. At the tops of the branches stand many small flowers, as it were in a long spike one above another, made like little birds, of a reddish purple colour, with whitish bellies, after which come small round husks, containing small black seeds. The root is yellow, small, and not very long, full of juice while it is green, but quickly perishes with the ripe seed. In the corn field in Cornwall, it beareth white flowers.

Place.] It groweth in corn fields almost everywhere, as well as in gardens.

Time.] It flowereth in May, for the most part, and the seed ripeneth shortly after.

Government and Virtues.] Saturn owns the herb, and presents it to the world as a cure for his own disease, and strengthener of the parts of the body he rules. If by my astrological judgment of diseases from the decumbiture you find Saturn author of the disease, or it by direction from a nativity you fear a Saturnine disease approaching, you may by this herb prevent it in the one, and cure it in the other, and therefore it is fit to keep a syrup of it always by you. The juice or syrup made thereof, or the decoction made in whey by itself, with some other purging or opening herbs and roots to cause it to work the better (itself being but weak) is very effectual for the liver and spleen, opening the obstructions thereof, and clarifying the blood from saltish, choleric, and adult humours, which cause leprosy, scabs, tetters, and itches, and such like breakings out of the skin, and after the purgings doth strengthen all the inward parts. It is also good against the yellow jaundice, and spendeth it by urine, which it procureth in abundance. The powder of the dried herb given for some time together cureth melancholy, but the seed is strongest in operation for all the former diseases. The distilled water of the herb is also of good effect in the former diseases, and conduceth much against the plague and pestilence, being taken with good treacle. The distilled water also, with a little water and honey of roses, helpeth all the sores of the mouth or throat, being gargled often therewith. The juice dropped into the eyes cleareth the sight, and taketh away redness and other defects in them, although it procureth some pain for the present, and causes tears. Dioscorides saith it hindereth any fresh springing of hairs on the eye lids (after they are pulled away) if the eye-lids be anointed ed with juice hereof, with Gum Arabick diffolved therein. The juice of the Fumitory and Docks mixed with vinegar, and the places gently wafhed or wet therewith cureth all forts of fcabs, pimples, blotches, wheals, and pufhes which arife on the face or hands, or any other parts of the body.

The Furz Bufh.

IT is as well known by this name, as it is in fome counties by the name of Gorz or Whins, that I fhall not need to write any defcription thereof, my intent being to each my countrymen what they know not, rather than to tell them again of that which is generally known before.

Place.] They are known to grow on dry barren heaths, and other wafte, gravelly, or fandy grounds, in all counties of this land.

Time.] They alfo flower in the Summer months.

Government and Virtues.] Mars owns the herb. They are hot and dry, and open obftructions of the liver and fpleen. A decoction made with the flowers thereof hath been found effectual againft the jaundice, as alfo to provoke urine, and cleanfe the kidneys from gravel or ftone ingendered in them. Mars doth alfo this by fympathy.

Garlick.

THE offenfivenefs of the breath of him that hath eaten Garlick, will lead you by the nofe to the knowledge hereof, and (inftead of a defcription) direct you to the place where it groweth in gardens, which kinds are the beft and moft phyfical.

Government and Virtues.] Mars owns this herb. This was anciently accounted the poor man's treacle, it being a remedy for all difeafes, and hurts (except thofe which itfelf breed.) It provoketh urine and womens courfes, helpeth the biting of mad dogs, and other venomous creatures; killeth worms in children, cutteth and voideth tough phlegm, purgeth the head, helpeth the lethargy, is a good prefervative againft, and a remedy for any plague, fore, or foul ulcer; taketh away fpots and blemifhes in the fkin, eafeth pain in the ears, ripeneth and breaketh impofthumes, or other fwellings. And for all thefe difeafes the onions are as effectual. But the

Garlick hath some more peculiar virtues besides the former, viz. It hath a special quality to discuss inconveniences coming by corrupt agues or mineral vapours, or by drinking corrupt and stinking waters; as also by taking wolf bane, hen-bane, hemlock or other poisonous and dangerous herbs. It is also held good in hydropic diseases the jaundice, falling sickness, cramps, convulsions, the piles or hæmorrhoids, or other cold diseases. Many authors quote many diseases this is good for: but conceal its vices. Its heat is very vehement, and all vehement hot things send up but ill favoured vapours to the brain. In choleric men it will add fuel to the fire, in men oppressed by melancholy, it will attenuate the humour, and send up strong fancies, and as many strange visions to the head: therefore let it be taken inwardly with great moderation; outwardly you may make more bold with it.

Gentian, Felwort, or Baldmony.

IT is confessed that Gentian, which is most used amongst us, is brought over from beyond sea, yet we have two sorts of it growing frequently in our nation, which, besides the reasons so frequently alledged why English herbs should be fittest for English bodies, hath been proved by the experience of divers physicians, to be not a whit inferior in virtue to that which cometh from beyond sea, therefore be pleased to take the description of them as followeth.

Descript.] The greater of the two hath many small long roots thrust down deep into the ground, and abiding all the Winter. The stalks are sometimes more, sometimes fewer, of a brownish green colour, which is sometimes two feet high, if the ground be fruitful, having many long, narrow, dark green leaves, set by couples up to the top; the flowers are long and hollow, of a purple colour, ending in fine corners. The smaller sort which is to be found in our land, groweth up with sundry stalks, not a foot high, parted into several small branches, whereon grow divers small leaves together, very like those of the lesser Centaury, of a whitish green colour; on the tops of these stalks grow divers perfect blue flowers standing in long husks, but not so big as the other; the root is very small, and full of threads.

Place] The first groweth in divers places of both the East and West countries and as well in wet as in dry grounds, as near Longfield by Gravesend, near Cobham in Kent, near
Lillingstone

Lillinstone in Kent, also in a chalk pit hard by a paper mill not far from Dartford in Kent. The second groweth also in divers places in Kent, as about Southfleet and Longfield; upon Barton's Hills in Bedfordshire; also not far from St Albans, upon a piece of waste chalky ground, as you go out of Dunstable way towards Gorhambury.

Time.] They flower in August.

Government and Virtues] They are under the dominion of Mars, and of them the most principal herbs he is ruler of. They resist putrefactions, poison, and a more sure remedy cannot be found to prevent the pestilence than it is; it strengthens the stomach exceedingly, helps digestion, comforts the heart, and preserves it against faintings and swoonings. The power of the dry roots help the biting of mad dogs and venomous beasts, opens obstructions of the liver, and restoreth an appetite of their meat to such as have lost it. The herb steeped in wine, and the wine drank, refresheth such as be over weary with travel, and grow lame in their joints, either by cold or evil lodgings; it helps stitches, and griping pains in the sides; is an excellent remedy for such as are bruised by falls; it provokes urine and the terms exceedingly, therefore let it not be given to women with child. The same is very profitable for such as are troubled with cramps and convulsions, to drink the decoction: Also they say it breaks the stone, and helps ruptures most certainly, it is excellent in all cold diseases, and such as are troubled with tough phlegm, scabs, itch, or any fretting sores and ulcers; it is an admirable remedy to kill the worms, by taking half a dram of the powder in a morning in any convenient liquor; the same is excellent good to be taken inwardly for the king's evil. It helps agues of all sorts, and the yellow jaundice, as also the bots in cattle: when kine are bitten on the udder by any venomous beast, do but stroke the place with the decoction of any of these, and it will instantly heal them.

Clove Gilliflowers.

IT is vain to describe an herb so well known.

Government and Virtues.] They are gallant, fine, temperate flowers, of the nature and under the dominion of Jupiter; yea, so temperate, that no excess, neither in heat, cold

cold, dryness, nor moisture, can be perceived in them; they are great strengtheners both of the brain and heart, and will therefore serve either for cordials or cephalicks, as your occasion will serve. There is both a syrup and a conserve made of them alone, commonly to be had at every apothecary's. To take now and then a little of either, strengthens nature much in such as are in consumptions. They are also excellent good in hot pestilent fevers, and expel poison.

Germander.

Descript] COMMON Germander shooteth forth sundry stalks, with small and somewhat round leaves, dented about the edges. The flowers stand at the tops, of a deep purple colour. The root is composed of divers sprigs, which shoot forth a great way round about, quickly over spreading a garden.

Place] It groweth usually with us in gardens.

Time.] And flowereth in June and July.

Government and Virtues] It is a most prevalent herb of Mercury, and strengthens the brain and apprehension exceedingly; (you may see what human virtues are under Mercury, in the latter end of my Ephemeris for 1652) strengthens them when weak, and relieves them when drooping. This taken with honey (saith Dioscorides) is a remedy for coughs, hardness of the spleen, and difficulty of urine, and helpeth those that are fallen into a dropsy, especially at the beginning of the disease, a decoction being made thereof when it is green, and drank. It also bringeth down women courses and expelleth the dead child. It is most effectual against the poison of all serpents, being drank in wine, and the bruised herb outwardly applied, used with honey, it cleanseth old and foul ulcers, and made into an oil, and the eyes anointed therewith, taketh away the dimness and moistness. It is likewise good for the pains in the sides and cramps. The decoction thereof taken for four days together, driveth away and cureth both tertian and quartan agues. It is also good against all diseases of the brain, as continual head-ach, falling sickness, melancholy, drowsiness and dullness of the spirits, convulsions and palsies. A dram of the seed taken in powder purgeth by urine and is good against the yellow jaundice. The juice of the leaves dropped into the ears kill eth the worms in them. The tops thereof, when they are in flowers, steeped twenty-four hours in a draught of white wine, and drank, killeth the worms in the belly.

Stinking Gladwin.

Descript] THIS is one of the kinds of Flower de-luce, having divers leaves arising from the roots, very like a Flower de luce, but that they are sharp edged on both sides, and thicker in the middle, of a deeper green colour, narrower and sharper pointed, and a strong ill scent, if they be bruised between the fingers. In the middle riseth up a reasonable strong stalk, a yard high at the least, bearing three or four flowers at the top, made somewhat like the flowers of the Flower de luce, with three upright leaves, of a dead purplish ash colour, with some veins discoloured in them; the other three do not fall down, nor are the three other small ones so arched, nor cover the lower leaves as the Flower de luce doth, but stand loose or asunder from them. After they are past, there come up three square hard husks opening wide into three parts when they are ripe, wherein lie reddish seed turning back when it hath abiden long. The root is like that of the Flower-de-luce, but reddish on the outside and whitish within, very sharp and hot in the taste, of as evil scent as the leaves.

Place] This groweth as well in upland grounds as in moist places, woods, and shadowy places by the sea-side in many places of this land, and is usually nursed up in gardens.

Time] It flowereth not until July, and the seed is ripe in August or September; yet the husks after they are ripe, opening themselves, will hold their seed with them for two or three months, and not shed them.

Government and Virtues] It is supposed to be under the dominion of Saturn. It is used by many country people to purge corrupt phlegm and choler, which they do by drinking the decoction of the roots; and some, to make it more gentle, do but infuse the sliced roots in ale; and some take the leaves, which serve well for the weaker stomachs: The juice hereof put up, or snuffed up the nose, causeth sneezing, and draweth from the head much corruption; and the powder thereof doth the same. The powder thereof drank in wine helpeth those that are troubled with cramps and convulsions, or with the gout and sciatica, and giveth ease to those that have griping pains in their body and belly, and helpeth those that have the stranguary. It is given with much profit to those that have had long fluxes by the sharp and evil quality of humours, which it stayeth, having first cleansed and purged them by the drying and binding property therein. The root boiled in wine and drank doth effectually procure womens courses, and used as a pessary worketh the same effect, but causeth abortion in women with child. Half a dram of the seed beaten to powder and taken in wine, doth speedily cause one to piss, which otherwise cannot. The same taken with vinegar, dissolveth the hardness and swellings of the spleen. The root is effectual in all wounds, especially of the head; as also to draw forth any splinters, thorns, or broken bones, or any other thing sticking in the flesh without causing pains, being used with a little verdigrease and honey, and the great Centaury root. The same boiled in vinegar, and laid upon any tumour or swelling, doth very effectually dissolve and consume them; yea even the swellings of the throat called the king's evil, the juice of the leaves or roots healeth the itch, and all running or spreading scabs, sores, blemishes, or scars in the skin, wheresoever they be.

Golden Rod.

Descript.] THIS ariseth up with brownish small round stalks, two feet high, and sometimes more, having thereon many narrow and long dark green leaves, very seldom with any dents about the edges, or any stalks or white spots therein, yet they are sometimes so found divided at the tops into many small branches, with divers small yellow flowers on every one of them, all which are turned one way, and being ripe do turn into down, and are carried away by the wind. The root consists of many small fibres, which grow not deep in the ground, but abideth all the Winter therein, shooting forth new branches every year, the old one lying down to the ground.

Place.] It groweth in the open places of woods and copses, both moist and dry ground, in many places of this land.

Time.] It flowereth about the month of July.

Government and Virtues.] Venus claims the herb, and therefore to be sure it respects beauty lost. Arnoldus de Villa Nova commends

commends it much against the stone in the [ ] and kidneys, and to provoke urine in abundance whereby also all the gravel and stone may be voided. The decoction of the herb, green or dry, or the distilled water thereof, is very effectual for inward bruises, as also to be outwardly applied, it stayeth bleeding in any part in the body, and of wounds, also the fluxes of humours, the bloody flux, and womens courses; and is no less prevalent in all ruptures or burstings, being drank inwardly, and outwardly applied. It is a sovereign wound herb, inferior to none, both for inward and outward hurts; green wounds, old sores and ulcers, are quickly cured therewith. It also is of especial use in all lotions for sores or ulcers in the mouth, throat, or privy parts of man or woman. The decoction also helpeth to fasten the teeth that are loose in the gums.

Goutwort, or Herb Gerrard.

Descript.] IT is a low herb, seldom rising half a yard high, having sundry leaves standing on brownish green stalks by three, snipped about, and of a strong unpleasant favour: The umbels of the flowers are white, and the seed blackish, the root runneth in the ground, quickly taking a great deal of room.

Place] It groweth by hedge and wall sides, and often in the boarder and corners of fields, and in gardens also

Time] It flowereth and seedeth about the end of July.

Government and Virtues] Saturn rules it. Neither is it to be supposed Goutwort hath its name for nothing, but upon experiment to heal the gout and sciatica; as also joint-achs, and other cold griefs. The very bearing of it about one easeth the pains of the gout, and defends him that bears it from the disease.

Gromel.

OF this I shall briefly describe their kinds, which are principally used in physic, the virtues whereof are alike, though somewhat different in their manner and form of growing.

Descript.] The greater Gromel groweth up with slender hard and hairy stalks, trailing and taking root in the ground, as it lieth thereon, and parted into many other small branches with hairy dark green leaves thereon. At the joints with the leaves come forth very small blue flowers, and after them hard stoney roundish seed. The root is long and woody, abiding the Winter, and shooteth forth fresh stalks in the Spring.

The smaller wild Gromel sendeth forth divers upright hard branched stalks, two or three feet high, full of joints, at every of which groweth small, long, hard, and rough leaves like the former, but lesser, among which leaves come forth small white flowers, and after them greyish round seed like the former; the root is not very big, but with many strings thereat.

The garden Gromel hath divers upright, slender, woody, hairy stalks, blown and cressed, very little branched, with leaves like the former, and white flowers; after which, in rough brown husks, is contained a white, hard, round seed, shining like pearl, and greater than either of the former; the root is like the first described, with divers branches and sprigs thereat, which continueth (as the first doth) all the Winter.

Place.] The two first grow wild in barren or untilled places, and by the way sides in many places of this land. The last as a nursling in the gardens of the curious.

Time.] They all flower from Midsummer until September sometimes, and in the mean time the seed ripeneth.

Government and Virtues.] The herb belongs to Dame Venus, and therefore if Mars cause the colic or stone, as usually he doth, if in Virgo, this is your cure. These are accounted to be of as singular force as any herb or seed whatsoever, to break the stone and to void it, and the gravel either in the reins or bladder, as also to provoke urine being stopped, and to help the stranguary. The seed is of greatest use when bruised and boiled in white wine or in broth, or the like, or the powder of the seed taken therein. Two drams of the seed in powder taken with women's breast milk, is very effectual to procure a very speedy delivery to such women as have sore pains in their travail, and cannot be delivered. The herb itself, (when the seed is not to be had) either boiled, or the juice thereof drank, is effectual to all the purposes aforesaid, but not so powerful and speedy in operation.

Gooseberry-Bush.

CALLED also Feaberry, and in Sussex Dewberry-Bush, and in some counties Wineberry.

Government and Virtues] They are under the dominion of Venus. The berries while they are unripe, being scalded, or baked, are good to stir up a fainting or decayed appetite, especially such whose stomachs are afflicted by choleric humours. They are excellent good to stay longings of women with child. You may keep them preserved with sugar all the year long. The decoction of the leaves of the tree cools hot swellings and inflammations, as also St Anthony's fire. The ripe Gooseberries being eaten, are an excellent remedy to allay the violent heat both of the stomach and liver. The young tender leaves break the stone, and expel gravel both from the kidneys and bladder. All the evils they do to the body of man is, they are supposed to breed crudities, and by crudities, worms.

Winter-Green.

Descript.] THIS sends forth seven, eight, or nine leaves from a small brown creeping root, every one standing upon a long foot stalk, which are almost as broad as long, round pointed, of a sad green colour, and hard in handling, and like the leaf of a Pear tree, from whence ariseth a slender weak stalk, yet standing upright, bearing at the top many small white sweet smelling flowers, laid open like a star, consisting of five round pointed leaves, with many yellowish threads standing in the middle about a green head, and a long stalk with them, which being ripe is found five square with a small point at it, wherein is contained seed as small as dust.

Place] It groweth seldom in fields, but frequent in the woods northwards, viz. in Yorkshire, Lancashire, and Scotland.

Time] It flowereth about June and July.

Government and Virtues] Winter-green is under the dominion of Saturn, and is a singular good wound herb, and an especial remedy for to heal green wounds speedily, the green leaves being used and applied, or the juice of them. A salve made of the green herb stamped, or the juice boiled with hog's lard, or with sallad oil and wax, and some turpentine added unto it, is a sovereign salve, and highly extolled by the Germans, who use it to heal all manner of wounds and sores. The herb boiled in wine and water, and given to drink to them that have any inward ulcers in their kidneys, or neck of the bladder, doth wonderfully help them. It stayeth all fluxes, as the lask, bloody flux, womens courses, and bleeding of wounds, and taketh away any inflammations rising upon pains of the heart; it is no less helpful for foul ulcers hard to be cured; as also for cankers or fistulas. The distilled water of the herb doth effectually perform the same things.

Groundsel.

Descript.] OUR common Groundsel hath a round green and somewhat brownish stalk, spreading toward the top into branches, set with long and somewhat narrow green leaves, cut in on the edges, somewhat like the oak-leaves, but lesser, and round at the end. At the tops of the branches stand many small green heads, out of which grow small yellow threads or thrumbs, which are the flowers, and continue many days blown in that manner, before it pass away into Down, and with the seed is carried away in the wind. The root is small and thready, and soon perisheth, and as soon riseth again of its own sowing, so that it may be seen many months in the year, both green and in flowers and seed, for it will spring and seed twice in a year at least, if it be suffered in a garden.

Place.] This groweth almost every where, as well on tops of walls, as at the foot, amongst rubbish and untilled grounds, but especially in gardens.

Time.] It flowereth, as is said before, almost in every month throughout the year.

Government and Virtues.] This herb is Venus's mistress piece, and is a gallant and universal medicine for all diseases coming of heat, in what part of the body soever they be, as the sun shines upon; it is very safe and friendly to the body of man; yet causeth vomiting if the stomach be afflicted, if not, purging, and it doth it with more gentleness than can be expected; it is moist, and something cold withal, thereby causing expulsion, and repressing the heat caused by the motion of the internal parts in purges and vomits. Lay by our

learned

learned receipts; take so much Sena, so much Scammony, so much Colocynthis, so much infusion of Crocus Metallorum, &c. this herb alone preserved in a syrup, in a distilled water, or in an ointment, shall do the deed for you in all hot diseases, and shall do it, 1. Safely, 2. Speedily.

The decoction of the herb (saith Dioscorides) made with wine and drank, helpeth the pains of the stomach, proceeding of choler, (which it may well do by a vomit) as daily experience sheweth. The juice thereof taken in drink, or the decoction of it in ale, gently performeth the same. It is good against the jaundice and falling sickness, being taken in wine; as also against difficulty of making water. It provoketh urine, expelleth gravel in the reins or kidneys; a dram thereof given in oxymel after some walking or stirring of the body. It helpeth also the sciatica, griping of the belly, the colic; defects of the liver, and provoketh womens courses. The fresh herb boiled, and made into a poultice, applied to the breasts of women that are swollen with pain and heat, as also the privy parts of man or woman, the seat or fundament, or the arteries, joints and sinews, when they are inflamed and swollen, doth much ease them; and used with some salt, helpeth to dissolve knots or kernels in any part of the body. The juice of the herb, or (as Dioscorides saith) the leaves and flowers, with some fine frankincense in powder, used in wounds of the body, nerves, or sinews, do singularly help to heal them. The distilled water of the herb performeth well all the aforesaid cures, but especially for inflammations or watering of the eyes, by reason of the defluction of rheum unto them.

Heart's-Ease.

THIS is that herb which such physicians as are licensed to blaspheme by authority, without danger of having their tongues burned through with an hot iron, called an herb of the Trinity. It is also called by those that are more moderate, Three Faces in a hood, Live in Idleness, Cull me to you, and in Sussex we call them Pancies.

Place] Besides those which are brought up in gardens, they grow commonly wild in the fields, especially in such as are very barren; sometimes you may find it on the tops of the high hills.

Time] **They** flower all the Spring and Summer long.

Government

Government and Virtues] The herb is really Saturnine, something cold, viscous and slimy. A strong decoction of the herbs and flowers (if you will, you may make into syrup) is an excellent cure for the French pox, the herb being a gallant antivenerean, and that antivenereans are the best cure for that disease, far better and safer than to torment them with the flux, divers foreign physicians have confessed. The spirit of it is excellent good for the convulsions in children, as also for the falling sickness, and a gallant remedy for the inflammation of the lungs and breasts, pleurisy, scabs, itch, &c. It is under the celestial sign Cancer.

Artichokes.

THE Latins call them Cinera, only our college calls them Artichocus.

Government and Virtues] They are under the dominion of Venus, and therefore it is no marvel if they provoke lust as indeed they do, being something windy meat; and yet they stay the involuntary course of natural seed in man, which is commonly called nocturnal pollutions. And here I care not greatly if I quote a little of Galen's nonsense in his treatise of the faculties of nourishment. He saith, they contain plenty of choleric juice (which notwithstanding I can scarcely believe) of which he faith is engendered melancholy juice, and of that melancholy juice then choleric blood. But to proceed; this is certain, that the decoction of the root boiled in wine, or the root bruised and distilled in wine in an alembic, and being drank, purgeth by urine exceedingly.

Harts-Tongue.

Descript] THIS hath divers leaves arising from the root, every one severally, which fold themselves in their first springing and spreading when they are full grown are about a foot long, smooth and green above, but hard and with little sap in them, and streaked on the back, thwart on both sides of the middle rib with small and somewhat long brownish marks; the bottoms of the leaves are a little bowed on each side of the middle rib, somewhat narrow with the length, and somewhat small at the end. The root is of many black threads, folded or interlaced together.

Time] It is green all the Winter; but new leaves spring every year.

Govern

Government and Virtues] Jupiter claims dominion over this herb, therefore it is a singular remedy for the liver, both to strengthen it when weak, and ease it when afflicted, you shall do well to keep it in a syrup all the year: For though authors say it is green all the year, I scarce believe it. Harts Tongue is much commended against the hardness and stoppings of the spleen and liver, and against the heat of the liver and stomach, and against lasks, and the bloody flux. The distilled water thereof is also very good against the passions of the heart, and to stay the hiccough, to help the falling of the palate, and to stay the bleeding of the gums, being gargled in the mouth. Dioscorides saith, it is good against the stinging or biting of serpents. As for the use of it, my direction at the latter end will be sufficient, and enough for those that are studious in physic, to whet their brains upon for one year or two.

Hazel-Nut.

HAZEL Nuts are so well known to every body, that they need no description.

Government and Virtues.] They are under the dominion of Mercury. The parted kernels made into an electuary, or the milk drawn from the kernels with mead or honeyed water, is very good to help an old cough; and being parched, and a little pepper put to them and drank, digesteth the distillations of rheum from the head. The dried husks and shells, to the weight of two drams, taken in red wine, stayeth lasks and womens courses, and so doth the red skin that covers the kernels, which is more effectual to stay womens courses.

And if this be true, as it is, then why should the vulgar so familiarly affirm, that eating Nuts causeth shortness of breath? than which nothing is falser. For, how can that which strengthens the lungs cause shortness of breath? I confess, the opinion is far older than I am; I knew tradition was friend to error before, but never that he was the father of slander: Or are mens tongues so given to slandering one another, that they must slander Nuts too, to keep their tongues in use? If any thing of the Hazel-Nut be stopping, it is the husks and shells, and no body is so mad to eat them, unless physically; and the red skin which covers the kernel, you may easily pull off. And so thus have I made apology for Nuts, which cannot speak for themselves.

Hawk

Hawk-weed.

Descript.] It hath many large leaves lying upon the ground, much rent or torn on the sides into gashes like Dandelion, but with greater parts, more like the smooth Sow Thistle, from among which riseth a hollow, rough stalk, two or three feet high, branched from the middle upward, whereon are set at every joint longer leaves, little or nothing rent or cut, bearing on their top sundry pale, yellow flowers, consisting of many small narrow leaves, broad pointed, and nicked in at the ends, set in a double row or more, the outermost being larger than the inner, which from most of the Hawk-weeds (for there are many kinds of them) do hold, which turn into down, and with the small brownish seed is blown away with the wind. The root is long, and somewhat greater, with many small fibres thereat. The whole plant is full of bitter milk.

Place] It groweth in divers places about the field sides, and the path ways in dry grounds.

Time] It flowereth and flies away in Summer months.

Government and Virtues.] Saturn owns it. Hawk-weed (saith Dioscorides) is cooling, somewhat drying and binding, and therefore good for the heat of the stomach, and gnawings therein; for inflammations, and the hot fits of agues. The juice thereof in wine, helpeth digestion, discusseth wind, hindereth crudities abiding in the stomach, and helpeth the difficulty of making water, the biting of venomous serpents, and stinging of the scorpion, if the herb be also outwardly applied to the place, and is very good against all other poisons. A scruple of the dried root given in wine and vinegar, is profitable for those that have the dropsy. The decoction of the herb taken with honey, digesteth the phlegm in the chest or lungs, and with hyssop helpeth the cough. The decoction thereof, and of wild succory, made with wine, and taken, helpeth the wind colic, and hardness of the spleen; it procureth rest and sleep, hindereth venery and venerous dreams, cooling heats, purgeth the stomach, increaseth blood, and helpeth the diseases of reins and bladder. Outwardly applied, it is singularly good for all the defects and diseases of the eyes, used with some womens milk; and used with good success in fretting or creeping ulcers, especially in the beginning. The green leaves bruised, and with a little salt applied to any place

place burnt with fire, before blisters do arise, helpeth them; as also inflammations, St Anthony's fire, and all pushes and eruptions, hot and salt phlegm. The same applied with meal and fair water in manner of a poultice, to any place affected with convulsions and the cramp, such as are out of joint, doth give help and ease. The distilled water cleanseth the skin, and taketh away freckles, spots, morphew, or wrinkles in the face.

Hawthorn.

IT is not my intent to trouble you with a description of this tree, which is so well known that it needeth none. It is ordinarily but a hedge bush, although being pruned and dressed, it groweth to a tree of a reasonable height.

As for the Hawthorn Tree at Glastenbury, which is said to flower yearly on Christmas-day, it rather sheweth the superstition of those that observe it for the time of its flowering, than any great wonder, since the like may be found in divers other places of this land; as in Whey street in Romney-Marsh, and near unto Nantwich in Cheshire, by a place called White Green, where it flowereth about Christmas and May. If the weather be frosty, it flowereth not until January, or that the hard weather be over.

Government and Virtues] It is a tree of Mars. The seeds in the berries beaten to powder, being drank in wine, are held singular good against the stone, and are good for the dropsy. The distilled water of the flowers stayeth the lask. The seed cleared from the down, bruised and boiled in wine, and drank, is good for inward tormenting pains. If cloths and spunges be wet in the distilled water, and applied to any place wherein thorns and splinters, or the like, do abide in the flesh, it will notably draw them forth.

And thus you see the thorn gives a medicine for his own pricking, and so doth almost every thing else.

Hemlock.

Descript] THE common great Hemlock groweth up with a green stalk, four or five feet high, or more, full of red spots sometimes, and at the joints very large winged leaves set at them, which are divided into many other winged leaves one set against the other, dented about the edges,

edges, of a sad green colour, branched towards the top, where it is full of umbels of white flowers, and afterwards with whitish flat seed. The root is long, white, and sometimes crooked, and hollow within. The whole plant, and every part, hath a strong, heady, and ill-favoured scent, much offending the senses.

Place] It groweth in all counties of this land, by walls and hedge sides, in waste grounds and untilled places.

Time.] It flowereth and feedeth in July, or thereabouts.

Government and Virtues] Saturn claims dominion over this herb, yet I wonder why it may not be applied to the privities in a *Priapism*, or continual standing of the yard; it being very beneficial to that disease. I suppose, my author's judgment was first upon the opposite disposition of Saturn to Venus in those faculties, and therefore he forbade the applying of it to those parts, that it might not cause barrenness, or spoil the spirit procreative; which if it do, yet applied to the privities, it stops its lustful thoughts. Hemlock is exceedingly cold, and very dangerous, especially to be taken inwardly. It may safely be applied to inflammations, tumours, and swellings in any part of the body (save the privy parts) as also to St Anthony's fire, wheals, pushes, and creeping ulcers that arise of hot sharp humours, by cooling and repelling the heat; the leaves bruised and laid to the brow or forehead are good for the eyes that are red and swollen, as also to take away a pin and web growing in the eye, this is a tried medicine: Take a small handful of this herb, and half so much Bay salt, beaten together, and applied to the contrary wrist of the hand, for 24 hours, doth remove it in thrice dressing. If the root thereof be roasted under the embers, wrapped in double wet paper, until it be soft and tender, and then applied to the gout in the hands or fingers, it will quickly help this evil. If any through mistake eat the herb Hemlock instead of Parsley, or the roots instead of a Parsnip (both of which it is very like) whereby happeneth a kind of frenzy, or perturbation of the senses, as if they were stupid and drunk, the remedy is (as Pliny saith) to drink of the best and strongest pure wine, before it strikes to the heart, or gentian put in wine, or a draught of vinegar, wherewith Tragus doth affirm that he cured a woman that had eaten the root.

Hemp.

Hemp.

THIS is so well known to every good housewife in the country, that I do not need to write any description of it.

Time.] It is sown in the end of March, or beginning of April, and is ripe in August or September.

Government and Virtues] It is a plant of Saturn, and good for something else, you see, than to make halters only. The seed of Hemp consumeth wind, and by too much use thereof disperseth it so much, that it drieth up the natural seed for procreation; yet, being boiled in milk, and taken, helpeth such as have a hot dry cough. The Dutch make an emulsion out of the seed, and give it with good success to those that have the jaundice, especially in the beginning of the disease, if there be no ague accompanying it, for it openeth obstructions of the gall, and causeth digestion of choler. The emulsion or decoction of the seed stayeth lasks and continual fluxes, easeth the colic, and allayeth the troublesome humours in the bowels, and stayeth bleeding at the mouth, nose, or other places, some of the leaves being fried with the blood of them that bleed, and so given them to eat. It is held very good to kill the worms in men or beasts; and the juice dropped into the ears killeth worms in them; and draweth forth earwigs, or other living creatures gotten in them. The decoction of the root allayeth inflammations of the head, or any other parts; the herb itself, or the distilled water thereof, doth the like. The decoction of the roots easeth pains of the gout, the hard humours of knots in the joints, the pain and shrinking of the sinews, and the pains of the hips. The fresh juice mixed with a little oil and butter, is good for any place that hath been burnt with fire, being thereto applied.

Henbane.

Descript.] OUR common Henbane hath very large, thick, soft, woolly leaves, lying on the ground, much cut in, or torn on the edges, of a dark, ill greyish green colour; among which rise up divers thick and short stalks, two or three feet high, spread into divers small branches, with lesser leaves on them, and many hollow flowers, scarce appearing above the husk, and usually torn on one side,

side, ending in five round points, growing one above another of a deadish yellowish colour, somewhat paler towards the edge, with many purplish veins therein, and a dark yellowish purple in the bottom of the flower, with a small point of the same colour in the middle, each of them standing in a hard close husk, which after the flowers are past, groweth very like the husk of Harabacca and somewhat sharp at the top points wherein is contained much small seed very like Poppy seed, but of a dusky, greyish colour. The root is great, white and thick, branching forth divers ways under ground, so like a Parsnip root (but that it is not so white) that it hath deceived others. The whole plant, more than the root, hath a very heavy, ill, soporiferous smell, somewhat offensive.

Place] It commonly groweth by the way sides, and under hedge sides and walls.

Time] It flowereth in July, and springeth again yearly of its own seed. I doubt my authors mistook July for June, if not for May.

Government and Virtues] I wonder how astrologers could take on them to make this an herb of Jupiter; and yet Mezaldus, a man of a penetrating brain, was of that opinion as well as the rest; the herb is indeed under the dominion of Saturn, and I prove it by this argument: All the herbs which delight most to grow in Saturnine places, are Saturnine herbs. But Henbane delights most to grow in Saturnine places and whole cart loads of it may be found near the places where they empty the common Jacks, and scarce a ditch to be found without it growing by it. Ergo, it is an herb of Saturn. The leaves of Henbane do cool all hot inflammations in the eyes, or any other part of the body; and are good to assuage all manner of swellings of the cods, or womens breasts, or elsewhere, if they be boiled in wine, and either applied themselves, or the fomentation warm; it also assuageth the pain of the gout, the sciatica, and other pains in the joints which arise from a hot cause. And applied with vinegar to the forehead and temples, helpeth the head-ach and want of sleep in hot fevers. The juice of the herb or seed, or the oil drawn from the seed, do the like. The oil of the seed is helpful for deafness, noise, and worms in the ears, being dropped therein. The juice of the herb or root doth the same. The decoction of the herb or seed, or both, killeth lice in man

man or beast. The fume of the dried herb, stalks and seed burned, quickly healeth swellings, chilblains or kibes in the hands or feet, by holding them in the fume thereof. The remedy to help those that have taken Henbane is to drink goat's milk, honeyed water, or pine kernels, with sweet wine; or, in the absence of these, Fennel-seed, Nettle seed, the seed of Cresses, Mustard, or Radish; as also Onions or Garlick taken in wine, do all help to free them from danger, and restore them to their due temper again.

Take notice, that this herb must never be taken inwardly; outwardly, an oil, ointment, or plaister of it, is most admirable for the gout, to cool the venereal heat of the reins in the French pox; to stop the tooth ach, being applied to the aching side. to allay all inflammations, and to help the diseases before premised.

Hedge Hyssop.

Descript] DIVERS sorts there are of this plant; the first of which is an Italian by birth, and only nursed up here in the gardens of the curious. Two or three sorts are found commonly growing wild here, the description of two of which I shall give you. The first is a smooth, low plant, not a foot high, very bitter in taste, with many square stalks, diversely branched from the bottom to the top, with divers joints, and two small leaves at each joint, broader at the bottom than they are at the end, and full of veins. The flowers stand at the joints, being of a fair purple colour, with some white spots in them, in fashion like those of dead nettles. The seed is small and yellow and the roots spread much under ground.

The second seldom groweth half a foot high, sending up many small branches, whereon grow many small leaves, set one against the other somewhat broad but very short. The flowers are like the flowers of the other in fashion, but of a pale reddish colour. The seeds are small and yellowish. The root spreadeth like the other. neither will it yield to its fellow one ace of bitterness.

Place] They grow in wet low grounds, and by the water-sides; the last may be found among the bogs on Hamstead Heath.

Time]

Time.] They flower in June and July, and the seed is ripe presently after.

Government and Virtues.] They are herbs of Mars, and as cholerick and churlish as he is, being most violent purges, especially of choler and phlegm. It is not safe taking them inwardly, unless they be well rectified by the art of the alchymist, and only the purity of them given, so used they may be very helpful both for the dropsy, gout, and sciatica; outwardly used in ointments they kill worms, the belly being anointed with it, and are excellent good to cleanse old and filthy ulcers.

Black Hellebore.

IT is also called Setter-wort, Setter-grass, Bear's foot, Christmas herb, and Christmas flower.

Descript.] It hath sundry fair green leaves rising from the root, each of them standing about an handful high from the earth; each leaf is divided into seven, eight, or nine parts, dented from the middle of the leaf to the point on both sides, abiding green all the Winter; about Christmas time, if the weather be any thing temperate the flowers appear upon foot stalks, also consisting of five large, round, white leaves a piece, which sometimes are purple towards the edges, with many pale yellow thumbs in the middle; the seeds are divided into several cells, like those of Columbines, save only that they are greater; the seeds are in colour black, and in form long and round. The root consisteth of numberless blackish strings all united into one head. There is another Black Hellebore which grows up and down in the woods very like this, but only that the leaves are smaller and narrower, and perish in the Winter, which this doth not.

Place.] The first is maintained in gardens. The second is commonly found in the woods in Northamptonshire.

Time.] The first flowereth in December or January, the second in February or March.

Government and Virtues.] It is an herb of Saturn, and therefore no marvel if it hath some sullen conditions with it, and would be far safer, being purified by the art of the alchymist than given raw. If any have taken any harm by taking it, the common cure is to take goat's milk: If you cannot get goat's milk, you must make a shift with such as you can get. The roots are very effectual against all melancholy diseases, especially such as are of long standing, as quartian agues and madness; it helps the falling sickness, the leprosy, both the yellow and black jaundice, the gout, sciatica, and convulsions, and this was found out by experience, that the root of that which groweth wild in our country, works not so churlishly as those do which are brought from beyond sea, as being maintained by a more temperate air. The root, used as a pessary, provokes the terms exceedingly; also being beaten into powder, and strewed upon foul ulcers, it consumes the dead flesh, and instantly heals them; nay, it will help grangrenes in the beginning. Twenty grains taken inwardly is a sufficient dose for one time, and let that be corrected with half so much cinnamon, country people used to rowel their cattle with it. If a beast be troubled with a cough, or have taken any poison, they bore a hole through his ear, and put a piece of the root in it, this will help him in 24 hours time. Many other uses farriers put it to which I shall forbear.

Herb Robert.

Descript] IT riseth up with a reddish stalk two feet high, having divers leaves thereon, upon very long and reddish foot stalks, divided at the ends into three or five divisions, each of them cut in on the edges, some deeper than others, and all dented likewise about the edges, which sometimes turn reddish. At the tops of the stalks come forth divers flowers made of five leaves, much larger than the dove's-foot, and a more reddish colour, after which come black heads as in others. The root is small and thready, and smelleth as the whole plant, very strong, almost stinking.

Place] This groweth frequently every where by the way-sides, upon ditch banks and waste grounds wheresoever one goeth.

Time.] It flowereth in June and July chiefly, and the seed is ripe shortly after.

Government and Virtues] It is under the dominion of Venus. Herb Robert is commended not only against the stone, but to stay blood, where or howsoever flowing; it speedily healeth all green wounds, and is effectual in old ulcers in the privy parts, or elsewhere. You may persuade yourself this is true, and also conceive a good reason for it do but consider it is an herb of Venus, for all it hath a man's name.

Herb True-love, or One-berry.

Descript] ORDINARY Herb True-love, hath a small creeping root running under the uppermost crust of the ground, somewhat like couch grass root, but not so white, shooting forth stalks with leaves, some whereof carry no berries, the others do; every stalk smooth without joints, and blackish green, rising about half a foot high, if it bear berries, otherwise seldom so high, bearing at the top four leaves set directly one against another, in manner of a cross or ribband tied (as it is called) in a true-loves knot, which are each of them apart somewhat like unto a nightshade leaf, but somewhat broader, having sometimes three leaves, sometime five, sometimes six, and those sometimes greater than others. In the middle of the four leaves riseth up one small slender stalk, about an inch high, bearing at the tops thereof one flower spread like a star, consisting of four small and long narrow-pointed leaves of a yellowish green colour, and four others lying between them lesser than they, in the middle whereof stands a round dark purplish button or head, compassed about with eight small yellow mealy threads with three colours, making it the more conspicuous, and lovely to behold. This button or head in the middle, when the other leaves are withered, becometh a blackish purple berry, full of juice, of the bigness of a reasonable grape, having within it many white seeds. The whole plant is without any manifest taste.

Place] It groweth in woods and copses, and sometimes in the corners or borders of fields, and waste ground in very many places of this land, and abundantly in the woods, copses, and other places about Chiselhurst, and Maidstone in Kent.

Time] They spring up in the middle of April or May, and are in flower soon after. The berries are ripe in the end of May, and in some places in June.

Government and Virtues.] Venus owns it. The leaves or berries hereof are effectual to expel poison of all sorts, especially that of the aconites, as also, the plague and other pestilential disorders. Matthiolus saith, that some that have lain long in a lingering sickness, and others that by witchcraft (as it was thought) were become half foolish by taking a dram of the seeds or berries hereof in powder every day for 20 days together, were restored to their former health. The roots in powder taken in wine easeth the pains of the colic speedily. The leaves are very effectual as well for green wounds as to cleanse and heal up filthy old sores and ulcers; and is very powerful to discuss all tumours and swellings in the cods, privy parts, the groin, or in any part of the body, and speedily to allay all inflammations. The juice of the leaves applied to felons, or those nails of the hands or toes that have imposthumes or sores gathered together at the roots of them, healeth them in a short space. The herb is not to be described for the premises, but is fit to be nourished in every good woman's garden.

Hyssop.

HYSSOP is so well known to be an inhabitant in every garden that it will save me labour in writing a description thereof. The virtues are as follow.

Temperature and Virtues] The herb is Jupiter's, and the sign Cancer. It strengthens all the parts of the body under Cancer and Jupiter; which what they may be, is found amply discoursed in my astrological judgment of diseases. Dioscorides saith, that Hyssop boiled with rue and honey, and drank, helpeth those that are troubled with coughs, shortness of breath, wheezing and rheumatic distillations upon the lungs; taken also with oxymel, it purgeth gross humours by stool, and with honey killeth worms in the belly; and with fresh and new figs bruised, helpeth to loosen the belly, and more forcibly if the root of Flower de luce and cresses be added thereto. It amendeth and cherisheth the native colour of the body, spoiled by the yellow jaundice; and being taken with figs and nitre, helpeth the dropsy and spleen, being boiled with wine, it is good to wash inflammation, and taketh away the black and blue spots and marks that come by strokes, bruises, or falls, being applied with warm water. It is an excellent medicine for the quinsy, or swelling in the throat, to wash and gargle it, being boiled in figs, it helpeth the toothach, being boiled in vinegar and gargled therewith. The hot vapours of the decoction taken by a funnel in at the ears, easeth the inflammations and singing noise of them. Being bruised, and salt, honey, and cummin seed put to it, helpeth those that are stung by serpents. The oil thereof (the head being anointed) killeth lice, and taketh away itching of the head. It helpeth those that have the falling sickness, which way soever it be applied. It helpeth to expectorate tough phlegm, and is effectual in all cold griefs or diseases of the chests or lungs, being taken either in syrup or licking medicine. The green herb bruised and a little sugar put thereto, doth quickly heal any cut or green wounds being thereunto applied.

Hops.

THESE are so well known that they need no description; I mean the manured kind, which every good husband or housewife is acquainted with.

Descript.] This wild hop groweth up as the other doth, ramping upon trees or hedges, that stand next to them, with rough branches and leaves like the former, but it giveth smaller heads, and in far less plenty than it, so that there is scarce a head or two seen in a year on divers of this wild kind, wherein consisteth the chief difference.

Place] They delight to grow in low moist grounds, and are found in all parts of this land.

Time.] They spring not up until April, and flower not until the latter end of June; the heads are not gathered until the middle or latter end of September.

Government and Virtues] It is under the dominion of Mars. This, in physical operations, is to open obstructions of the liver and spleen, to cleanse the blood, to loosen the belly, to cleanse the reins from gravel, and provoke urine. The decoction of the tops of Hops, as well of the tame as the wild, worketh the same effects. In cleansing the blood they help to cure the French disease, and all manner of scabs, itch and other breakings-out of the body; as also all tetters, ringworms, and spreading sores, the morphew, and all discolouring of the skin. The decoction of the flowers and tops do help to expel poison that any one hath drank. Half a dram of the seed in powder taken in drink, killeth worms in the body, bringeth down womens courses, and expelleth urine. A syrup made of the juice and sugar cureth the yellow jaundice, easeth the head ach that comes of heat, and tempereth

the

the heat of the liver and stomach, and is profitably given in long and hot agues that rise in choler and blood. Both the wild and the manured are of one property, and like effectual in all the aforesaid diseases. By all these testimonies beer appears to be better than ale.

Mars owns the plant, and then Dr Reason will tell you how it performs these actions.

Horehound.

Descript.] COMMON Horehound groweth up with square hairy stalks, half a yard or two feet high, set at the joints with two round crumpled rough leaves of a sullen hoary green colour, of a reasonable good scent, but a very bitter taste. The flowers are small, white, and gaping, set in a rough, hard prickly husk round about the joints, with the leaves in the middle of the stalk upward, wherein afterward is found small round blackish seed. The root is blackish, hard and woody, with many strings, and abideth many years.

Place.] It is found in many parts of this land, in dry grounds, and waste green places.

Time.] It flowereth in July, and the seed is ripe in August.

Government and Virtues.] It is an herb of Mercury. A decoction of the dried herb, with the seed, or the juice of the green herb taken with honey, is a remedy for those that are short-winded, have a cough, or are fallen into a consumption, either through long sickness, or thin distillations of rheum upon the lungs. It helpeth to expectorate tough phlegm from the chest, being taken from the roots of Iris or Orris. It is given to women to bring down their courses, to expel their after birth, and to them that have sore and long travails; as also to those that have taken poison, or are stung or bitten by venomous serpents. The leaves used with honey purge foul ulcers, stay running or creeping sores and the growing of the flesh over the nails. It also helpeth pains of the sides. The juice thereof with wine and honey helpeth to clear the eye sight, and snuffed up into the nostrils purgeth away the yellow jaundice, and with a little oil of roses dropped into the ears easeth the pains of them. Galen saith, it openeth obstructions both of the liver and spleen, and purgeth the breast and lungs of phlegm; and used outwardly it both cleanseth and digesteth. A decoction of Horehound (saith Matthiolus)

Matthiolus) is available for those that have hard livers, and for such as have itches and running tetters. The powder hereof taken, or the decoction, killeth worms. The green leaves bruised and boiled in old hog's grease into an ointment, healeth the bitings of dogs, abateth the swellings and pains that come by any pricking of thorns, or such like means, and used with vinegar, cleanseth and healeth tetters. There is a syrup made of Harehound to be had at the apothecaries, very good for old coughs, to rid phlegm; as also to void cold rheums from the lungs of old folks, and for those that are asthmatic or short-winded.

Horsetail.

OF that there are many kinds, but I shall not trouble you nor myself with any large description of them, which to do, were but as the proverb is, To find a knot in a rush, all the kinds thereof being nothing else but knotted rushes, some with leaves, and some without. Take the description of the most eminent sort as followeth:

Descript] The great Horsetail at the first springing hath heads somewhat like those of asparagus, and after grow to be hard, rough, hollow stalks, jointed at sundry places up to the top, a foot high, so made as if the lower parts were put into the upper, where grow on each side a bush of small long rush-like hard leaves, each part resembling a horsetail, from whence it is so called. At the tops of the stalks come forth small catkins, like those of trees. The root creepeth under ground, having joints at sundry places.

Place.] This, (as most of the other sorts hereof) groweth in wet grounds.

Time] They spring up in April, and their blooming catkins in July, seeding for the most part in August, and then perish down to the ground, rising afresh in the Spring.

Government and Virtues] The herb belongs to Saturn, yet is very harmless, and excellent good for the things following. Horsetail, the smoother rather than the rough, and the leaved rather than the bare, is most physical. It is very powerful to staunch bleeding either inward or outward, the juice or the decoction thereof being drank, or the juice, decoction, or distilled water applied outwardly. It also stayeth all sorts of lasks and fluxes in man or woman, and the pissing of blood; and healeth also not only the inward ulcers, and the excoriation

tion of the entrails, bladder, &c. but all other sorts of foul, moist and running ulcers, and soon sodereth together the tops of green wounds. It cureth all ruptures in children. The decoction thereof in wine being drank provoketh urine, and helpeth the stone and stranguary; and the distilled water thereof drank two or three times in a day, and a small quantity at a time, also easeth the entrails or guts, and is effectual against a cough that comes by distillation from the head. The juice or distilled water being warmed, and hot inflammations, pustles or red wheals, and other breakings-out in the skin, being bathed therewith, doth help them, and doth no less ease the swelling heat and inflammations of the fundament, or privy parts in men and women.

Houseleek, or Sengreen.

BOTH these are so well known to my countrymen, that I shall not need to write any description of them

Place] It groweth commonly upon walls and house sides, and flowereth in July

Government and Virtues.] It is an herb of Jupiter, and it is reported by Mezaldus, to preserve what it grows upon from fire and lightning. Our ordinary Houseleek is good for all inward heats as well as outward, and in the eyes or other parts of the body; a posset made with the juice of Houseleek, is singular good in all hot agues, for it cooleth and tempereth the blood and spirits, and quencheth the thirst; and also good to stay all hot defluctions or sharp and salt rheums in the eyes, the juice being dropped into them, or into the ears, helpeth them. It helpeth also other fluxes of humours in the bowels, and the immoderate courses of women. It cooleth and restraineth all other hot inflammations, St Anthony's fire, scaldings and burnings, the shingles, fretting ulcers cankers, tetters, ringworms, and the like; and much easeth the pain of the gout proceeding from a hot cause. The juice also taketh away warts and corns in the hands or feet, being often bathed therewith, and the skin and leaves being laid on them afterwards. It easeth also the head-ach, and distempered heat of the brain in frenzies, or through want of sleep being applied to the temples and forehead The leaves bruised and laid upon the crown or seam of the head, stayeth bleeding at the nose very quickly. The distilled water of the herb is profitable for all the purposes aforesaid. The leaves being gently rubbed on any place stung with nettles or bees, doth quickly take away the pain.

Hound's Tongue.

Descript.] THE great ordinary Hound's Tongue hath many long and somewhat narrow, soft, hairy, darkish green leaves, lying on the ground, somewhat like unto Buglofs leaves, from amongst which riseth up a rough hairy stalk about two feet high, with some smaller leaves thereon, and branched at the tops into divers parts, with a small leaf at the foot of every branch, which is somewhat long, with many flowers set along the same, which branch is crooked or turneth inwards before it flowereth, and openeth by degrees as the flowers do blow, which consist of small purplish red leaves of a dead colour, rising out of the husks wherein they stand with some threads in the middle. It hath sometimes a white flower. After the flowers are past, there cometh rough flat seed, with a small pointle in the middle, easily cleaving to any garment that it toucheth, and not so easily pulled off again. The root is black, thick, and long, hard to break, and full of clammy juice, smelling somewhat strong, of an evil scent, as the leaves also do.

Place.] It groweth in moist places of this land, in waste grounds, and untilled places, by highway-sides, lanes, and hedge-sides.

Time.] It flowereth about May or June, and the seed is ripe shortly after.

Government and Virtues.] It is a plant under the dominion of Mercury. The root is very effectually used in pills, as well as the decoction, or otherwise, to stay all sharp and thin defluctions of rheum from the head into the eyes or nose, or upon the stomach or lungs, as also for coughs and shortness of breath. The leaves boiled in wine (saith Dioscorides, but others do rather appoint it to be made with water, and do add thereto oil and salt) mollifieth or openeth the belly downwards. It also helpeth to cure the biting of a mad dog, some of the leaves being also applied to the wound: The leaves bruised, or the juice of them boiled in hog's-lard, and applied, helpeth falling away of the hair, which cometh of hot and sharp humours; as also for any place that is scalded or burnt,

the

the leaves bruised and laid to any green wound doth heal it quickly; the root baked under the embers, wrapped in paste or wet paper, or in a wet double cloth, and thereof a suppository made, and put up into or applied to the fundament, doth very effectually help the painful piles or hæmorrhoids. The distilled water of the herbs and roots is very good to all the purposes aforesaid, to be used as well inwardly to drink, as outwardly to wash any sore place, for it healeth all manner of wounds and punctures, and those foul ulcers that arise by the French pox. Mizaldus adds, that the leaves laid under the feet will keep the dogs from barking at you. It is called Hound's tongue, because it ties the tongues of hounds; whether true, or not, I never tried, yet I cured the biting of a mad dog with this only medicine.

Holy Holm, or Hulver Bush.

FOR to describe a tree so well known is needless.

Government and Virtues] The tree is Saturnine. The berries expel wind, and therefore are held to be profitable in the colic. The berries have a strong faculty with them; for if you eat a dozen of them in the morning fasting when they are ripe and not dried, they purge the body of gross and clammy phlegm, but if you dry the berries, and beat them into powder, they bind the body, and stop fluxes, bloody-fluxes, and the terms in women. The bark of the tree, and also the leaves, are excellent good, being used in fomentations for broken bones, and such members as are out of joint. Pliny saith, the branches of the tree defend houses from lightning, and men from witchcraft.

St John's Wort.

Descript.] COMMON St John's Wort shooteth forth brownish, upright, hard, round stalks, two feet high, spreading branches from the sides up to the tops of them, with two small leaves set one against another at every place, which are of a deep green colour, somewhat like the leaves of the lesser centaury, but narrow, and full of small holes in every leaf, which cannot be so well perceived, as when they are held up to the light, at the tops of the stalks and branches stand yellow flowers of five leaves a-piece, with many yellow threads in the middle, which being bruised do yield a reddish juice like blood; after which come small round heads wherein is contained small blackish seed smelling like rosin. The root is hard and woody, with divers strings and fibres at it, of a brownish colour, which abideth in the ground many years, shooting anew every Spring.

Place] This groweth in woods and copses as well those that are shady, as open to the sun.

Time] They flower about Midsummer and July, and their seed is ripe about the latter end of July or August.

Government and Virtues] It is under the celestial sign Leo, and the dominion of the Sun. It may be, if you meet a Papist, he will tell you especially if he be a lawyer, that St John made it over to him by a letter of attorney. It is a singular wound herb, boiled in wine and drank, it healeth inward hurts or bruises; made into an ointment, it opens obstructions, dissolves swellings, and closes up the lips of wounds. The decoction of the herb and flowers, especially of the seed, being drank in wine, with the juice of knot-grass, helpeth all manner of vomiting and spitting of blood, is good for those that are bitten or stung by any venomous creature, and for those that cannot make water. Two drams of the seed of St John's Wort made into powder, and drank in a little broth, doth gently expel choler or congealed blood in the stomach. The decoction of the leaves and seeds drank somewhat warm before the fits of agues, whether they be tertians or quartians, alters the fits, and, by often using, doth take them quite away. The seed is much commended, being drank for forty days together, to help the sciatica, the falling-sickness, and the palsy.

Ivy.

IT is well known, to every child almost, to grow in woods upon the trees, and upon the stone walls of churches, houses, &c. and sometimes to grow alone of itself, though but seldom.

Time] It floweth not until July, and the berries are not ripe till Christmas, when they have felt Winter frosts.

Government and Virtues] It is under the dominion of Saturn. A purgel of the flowers, which may be about a dram, (saith Dioscorides,) drank twice a day in red wine, helpeth the lask, and bloody-flux. It is an enemy to the nerves and sinews,

sinews, being much taken inwardly, but very helpful unto them being outwardly applied. Pliny saith, the yellow berries are good against the jaundice; and taken before one be set to drink hard, preserveth from drunkenness, and helpeth those that spit blood; and that the white berries being taken inwardly, or applied outwardly, killeth the worms in the belly. The berries are a singular remedy to prevent the plague, as also to free them from it that have got it, by drinking the berries thereof made into powder, for two or three days together. They being taken in wine, do certainly help to break the stone, provoke urine, and womens courses. The fresh leaves of Ivy boiled in vinegar, and applied warm to the sides of those that are troubled with the spleen, ach, or stitch in the sides, do give much ease. The same applied with some Rosewater, and oil of Roses, to the temples and forehead, easeth the head-ach, though it be of long continuance. The fresh leaves boiled in wine, and old filthy ulcer hard to be cured washed therewith, do wonderfully help to cleanse them. It also quickly healeth green wounds, and is effectual to heal all burnings and scaldings, and all kinds of exulcerations coming thereby, or by salt phlegm or humours in other parts of the body. The juice of the berries or leaves snuffed up into the nose, purgeth the head and brain of rheum that maketh defluxions into the eyes and nose, and curing the ulcers and stench therein; the same dropped into the ears, helpeth the old and running sores of them; those that are troubled with the spleen shall find much ease by continual drinking out of a cup made of Ivy, so as the drink may stand some small time therein before it be drank. Cato saith, That wine put into the cup will soak through it, by reason of the antipathy that is between them.

There seems to be a very great antipathy between wine and Ivy; for if one hath got a surfeit by drinking of wine, his speediest cure is to drink a draught of the same wine wherein a handful of Ivy leaves, being first bruised, have been boiled.

Juniper Bush.

FOR to give a description of a bush so commonly known is needless.

Place.] They grow plentifully in divers woods in Kent, Warney Common near Brentwood in Essex, upon Finchely Common without Highgate;-hard by the New-found Wells near Dulwich, upon a Common between Mitcham and Croydon, in the Highgate near Amersham in Buckinghamshire, and many other places.

Time] The berries are not ripe the first year, but continue green two Summers and one Winter before they are ripe; at which time they are all of a black colour, and therefore you shall always find upon the bush green berries, the berries are ripe about the fall of the leaf.

Government and Virtues.] This admirable solar shrub is scarce to be paralleled for its virtues. The berries are hot in the third degree, and dry but in the first, being a most admirable counter poison, and as great a resister of the pestilence as any grows; they are excellent good against the bitings of venomous beasts, they provoke urine exceedingly, and therefore are very available to dysuries and stranguaries. It is so powerful a remedy against the dropsy, that the very lee made of the ashes of the herb being drank, cures the disease. It provokes the terms, helps the fits of the mother, strengthens the stomach exceedingly, and expels the wind. Indeed there is scarce a better remedy for wind in any part of the body, or the colic, than the chymical oil drawn from the berries; such country people as know not how to draw the chymical oil may content themselves by eating ten or a dozen of the ripe berries every morning fasting. They are admirable good for a cough, shortness of breath and consumption, pains in the belly, ruptures, cramps, and convulsions. They give safe and speedy delivery to women with child, they strengthen the brain exceedingly, help the memory, and fortify the sight by strengthening the optic nerves, are excellent good in all sorts of agues; help the gout and sciatica and strengthen all the limbs of the body. The ashes of the wood is a speedy remedy to such as have the scurvy, to rub their gums with. The berries stay all fluxes, help the hæmorrhoids or piles, and kill worms in children. A lee made of the ashes of the wood, and the body bathed with it cures the itch, scabs and leprosy. The berries break the stone, procure appetite when it is lost, and are excellent good for all palsies, and falling sickness.

Kidney-

Kidneywort, or Wall Pennyroyal, or Wall Pennywort.

Descript.] It hath many thick, flat, and round leaves growing from the root, every one having a long footstalk, fastened underneath, about the middle of it, and a little unevenly weaved sometimes about the edges, of a pale green colour, and somewhat yellow on the upper side like a saucer; from among which arise one or more tender, smooth, hollow stalks half a foot high, with two or three small leaves thereon, usually not round as those below, but somewhat long, and divided at the edges; the tops are somewhat divided into long branches, bearing a number of flowers, set round about a long spike one above another, which are hollow like a little bell of a whitish green colour, after which come small heads, containing very small brownish seed, which falling on the ground will plentifully spring up before Winter, if it have moisture. The root is round and most usually smooth, greyish without, and white within, having small fibres at the head of the root, and bottom of the stalk.

Place] It groweth very plentifully in many places in this land, but especially in all the west parts thereof, upon stone and mud walls, upon rocks also, and in stony places upon the ground, at the bottom of old trees, and sometimes on the bodies of them that are decayed and rotten.

Time] It usually flowereth in the beginning of May, and the seed ripening quickly after, sheddeth itself; so that about the end of May, usually the leaves and stalks are withered, dry, and gone until September, and the leaves spring up again, and so abide all Winter.

Government and Virtues] Venus challengeth the herb under Libra. The juice or the distilled water being drank, is very effectual for all inflammations and unnatural heats, to cool a fainting hot stomach, a hot liver, or the bowels; the herb, juice, or distilled water thereof, outwardly applied, healeth pimples, St. Anthony's fire, and other outward heats. The said juice or water helpeth to heal sore kidneys, torn or fretted by the stone, or exulcerated within; it also provoketh urine, is available for the dropsy and helpeth to break the stone. Being used as a bath, or made an ointment, it cooleth the painful piles or hæmorrhoidal veins. It is no less effectual to give ease to pains of the gout, the sciatica, and the inflammations and swellings in the cods, it helpeth the kernels or knots in the neck or throat, called the king's evil; healing kibes and chilblains if they be bathed with the juice, or anointed with ointment made thereof, and some of the skin of the leaf upon them, it is also used in green wounds to stay the blood, and to heal them quickly.

Knapweed.

Descript.] THE common sort hereof hath many long and somewhat broad dark green leaves, rising from the root, dented about the edges, and sometimes a little rent or torn on both sides in two or three places, and somewhat hairy withal; amongst which ariseth a long round stalk, four or five feet high, divided into many branches, at the tops whereof stand great scaly green heads, and from the middle of them thrust forth a number of dark purplish red thrumbs or threads, which after they are withered and past, there are found divers black seeds, lying in a great deal of down, somewhat like unto Thistle seed, but smaller; the root is white, hard and woody, and divers fibres annexed thereunto, which perisheth not, but abideth with leaves thereon all the Winter, shooting out fresh every Spring.

Place] It groweth in most fields and meadows, and about their borders and hedges, and in many waste grounds also every where.

Time] It usually flowereth in June or July, and the seed is ripe shortly after.

Government and Virtues] Saturn challengeth the herb for his own. This knapweed helpeth to stay fluxes, both of blood at the mouth or nose, or other outward parts, and those veins that are inwardly broken, or inward wounds, as also the fluxes of the belly; it stayeth distillations of thin and sharp humours from the head upon the stomach and lungs; it is good for those that are bruised by any fall, blows, or otherwise, and is profitable for those that are bursten, and have ruptures, by drinking the decoction of the herb and root in wine, and applying the same outwardly to the place. It is singularly good in all running sores, cancerous and fistulous, drying up of the moisture, and healing them up gently, without sharpness; it doth the like to running sores or scabs of the

the head or other parts. It is of special use for the soreness of the throat, swelling of the uvula and jaws, and excellent good to stay bleeding, and heal up all green wounds.

Knotgrass.

IT is generally known so well, that it needeth no description.

Place] It groweth in every county of this land, by the highway sides, and by foot paths in fields; as also by the sides of old walls.

Time.] It springeth up late in the Spring, and abideth until the Winter, when all the branches perish

Temperature and Virtues.] Saturn seems to me to own the herb, and yet some hold the sun, out of all doubt 'tis Saturn. The juice of the common kind of Knotgrass is most effectual to stay bleeding of the mouth, being drank in steeled or red wine; and the bleeding at the nose, to be applied to the forehead or temples, or to be squirted up into the nostrils. It is no less effectual to cool and temper the heat of the blood and stomach, and to stay any flux of the blood and humours, as lask, bloody flux, womens courses, and running of the reins. It is singular good to provoke urine, help the stranguary, and allayeth the heat that cometh thereby; and is powerful by urine to expel the gravel or stone in the kidneys and bladder, a dram of the powder of the herb being taken in wine for many days together Being boiled in wine and drank, it is profitable to those that are stung or bitten by venomous creatures, and very effectual to stay all defluxions of rheumatic humours upon the stomach, and killeth worms in the belly or stomach, quieteth inward pains that arise from the heat, sharpness and corruption of blood and choler The distilled water hereof taken by itself, or with the powder of the herb or seed, is very effectual to all the purposes aforesaid, and is accounted one of the most sovereign remedies to cool all manner of inflammations, breaking out through heat hot swellings and imposthumes, gangrene and fistulous cankers, or foul filthy ulcers, being applied or put into them; but especially for all sorts of ulcers and sores happening in the privy parts of men and women It helpeth all fresh and green wounds, and speedily healeth them The juice dropped into the ears cleanseth them, being foul, and having running matter in them.

It is very prevalent for the premises; as also for broken joints and ruptures.

Ladies-Mantle.

Descript] IT hath many leaves rising from the root standing upon long hairy foot stalks, being almost round, and a little cut on the edges, into eight or ten parts, making it seem like a star, with so many corners and points, and dented round about, of a light colour, somewhat hard in handling, and as it were folded or plaited at first, and then crumpled in divers places, and a little hairy, as the stalk is also, which riseth up among them to the height of two or three feet; and being weak, is not able to stand upright, but bendeth to the ground, divided at the top into two or three branches, with small yellowish green heads, and flowers of a whitish colour breaking out of them: which being past, there cometh a small yellowish seed like a poppy seed. The root is somewhat long and black, with many strings and fibres thereat.

Place] It groweth naturally in many pastures and wood sides in Hertfordshire, Wiltshire, and Kent, and other places of this land.

Time] It flowereth in May and June, abideth after seed time green all the Winter.

Government and Virtues.] Venus claims the herb as her own. Ladies Mantle is very proper for those wounds that have inflammations, and is very effectual to stay bleeding, vomitings, fluxes of all sorts, bruises by falls or otherwise, and helpeth ruptures; and such women or maids as have over great flagging breasts, causing them to grow less and hard, being both drank, and outwardly applied for 20 days together helpeth conception, and to retain the birth, if the woman do sometimes also sit in a bath made of the decoction of the herb. It is one of the most singular wound herbs that is, and therefore highly prized and praised by the Germans, who use it in all wounds inward and outward, to drink a decoction thereof, and wash the wounds therewith, or dip tents therein, and put them into the wounds which wonderfully drieth up all humidity of the sores, and abateth inflammations therein. It quickly healeth all green wounds, not suffering any

corruptions

corruptions to remain behind, and cureth all old sores, though fistulous and hollow.

Lavender.

BEING an inhabitant almost in every garden, it is so well known, that it needeth no description.

Time.] It flowereth about the end of June, and beginning of July.

Government and Virtues.] Mercury owns the herb, and it carries his effects very potently. Lavender is of a special good use for all the griefs and pains of the head and brain that proceed of a cold cause, as the apoplexy, falling sickness, the dropsy, or sluggish malady, cramps, convulsions, palsies, and often faintings. It strengthens the stomach, and freeth the liver and spleen from obstructions, provoketh womens courses, and expelleth the dead child and after-birth. The flowers of Lavender steeped in wine, helpeth them to make water that are stopped, or are troubled with the wind or colick, if the place be bathed therewith. A decoction made with the flowers of Lavender, Hore hound, Fennel, and Asparagus root, and a little Cinnamon, is very profitably used to help the falling sickness, and the giddiness or turning of the brain; to gargle the mouth with the decoction thereof is good against the tooth ach. Two spoonfuls of the distilled water of the flowers taken, helpeth them that have lost their voice, as also the tremblings and passions of the heart, and faintings and swooning, not only being drank, but applied to the temples, or nostrils to be smelt unto; but it is not safe to use it where the body is replete with blood and humours, because of the hot and subtile spirits wherewith it is possessed. The chymical oil drawn from Lavender, usually called Oil of Spike, is of so fierce and piercing a quality, that it is cautiously to be used, some few drops being sufficient, to be given with other things, either for inward or outward griefs.

Lavender-Cotton.

IT being a common garden herb, I shall forbear the description, only take notice, that it flowereth in June and July.

Government and Virtues] It is under the dominion of Mercury. It resisteth poison, putrefaction, and heals the biting of venomous beasts: A dram of the powder of the dried leaves taken every morning fasting stops the running of the reins in men, and whites in women. The seed beaten into powder, and taken as worm seed, kills the worms, not only in children, but also in people of riper years; the like doth the herb itself, being steeped in milk, and the milk drank the body bathed with the decoction of it, helps scabs and itch.

Ladies Smock, or Cuckow-Flowers.

Descript.] THE root is composed of many small white threads, from whence spring divers long stalks of winged leaves, consisting of round, tender, dark, green leaves, set one against another upon a middle rib the greatest being at the end, amongst which arise up divers tender, weak, round, green stalks, somewhat streaked, with longer and smaller leaves upon them: on the tops of which stand flowers, almost like the Stock Gilliflowers, but rounder, and not so long, of a blushing white colour; the seed is reddish, and groweth to small bunches, being of a sharp biting taste, and so hath the herb.

Place] They grow in moist places, and near to brooksides.

Time.] They flower in April and May, and the lower leaves continue green all the Winter.

Government and Virtues] They are under the dominion of the Moon, and very little inferior to Water Cresses in all their operations; they are excellent good for the scurvy; they provoke urine, and break the stone, and excellently warm a cold and weak stomach, restoring lost appetite, and help digestion.

Lettuce.

IT is so well known, being generally used as a Sallet herb, that it is altogether needless to write any description thereof

Government and Virtues.] The Moon owns them, and that is the reason they cool and moisten what heat and dryness Mars causeth, because Mars hath his fall in Cancer; and they cool the heat because the Sun rules it, between whom and
the

the Moon is a reception in the generation of man, as you may see in my guide for women. The juice of Lettuce mixed or boiled with Oil of Roses, applied to the forehead and temples procureth sleep, and easeth the head-ach proceeding of an hot cause: Being eaten boiled, it helpeth to loosen the belly. It helpeth digestion, quencheth thirst, increaseth milk in nurses, easeth griping pains in the stomach and bowels, that come of choler. It abateth bodily lust, represseth venerous dreams, being outwardly applied to the cods with a little Camphire. Applied in the same manner to the region of the heart, liver or reins, or by bathing the said place with the juice of distilled water, wherein some white Sanders, or red Roses are put; also it not only represseth the heat and inflammations therein, but comforts and strengthens those parts, and also tempereth the heat of urine. Galen adviseth old men to use it with spice, and where spices are wanting, to add mints, rochet, and such like hot herbs, or else citron, lemon or orange seeds, to abate the cold of one and heat of the other. The seed and distilled water of the Lettuce work the same effects in all things; but the use of Lettuce is chiefly forbidden to those that are short-winded, or have any imperfection in the lungs, or spit blood.

Water Lily.

OF these there are two principally noted kinds, viz. the White, and the Yellow

Descript] The White Lily hath very large and thick dark green leaves lying on the water, sustained by long and thick foot-stalks, that arise from a great, thick, round, and long tuberous black root, spongy or loose, with many knobs thereon, like eye, and whitish within from amidst which rise other the like thick green stalks, sustaining one large great flower thereon, green on the outside, but as white as snow within, consisting of divers rows of long and somewhat thick and narrow leaves, smaller and thinner the more inward they be, encompassing a head with many yellow threads or thrumbs in the middle, where, after they are past, stand round Poppy like heads, full of broad oily and bitter seed

The Yellow kind is little different from the former, save only that it hath fewer leaves on the flowers, greater and more shining seed, and a whitish root, both within and without. The root of both is somewhat sweet in taste.

Place.

Place.] They are found growing in great pools, and standing waters, and sometimes in slow running rivers, and less ditches of water, in sundry places of this land.

Time.] They flower most commonly about the end of May, and their seed is ripe in August.

Government and Virtues.] The herb is under the dominion of the Moon, and therefore cools and moistens like the former. The leaves and flowers of the Lilies are cold and moist, but the roots and seeds are cold and dry; the leaves do cool all inflammations, both outward and inward heat of agues, and so doth the flowers also, either by the syrup or conserve; the syrup helpeth much to procure rest, and to settle the brain of frantick persons, by cooling the hot distemperature of the head. The seed as well as the root is effectual to stay fluxes of blood or humours, either of wounds or of the belly; but the roots are most used, and more effectual to cool, bind, and restrain all fluxes in men and women; also running of the reins, and passing away of the seed when one is asleep, but the frequent use hereof extinguisheth venerous action. The root is likewise very good for those whose urine is hot and sharp, to be boiled in wine and water, and the decoction drank. The distilled water of the flowers is very effectual for all the diseases aforesaid, both inwardly taken, and outwardly applied; and is much commended to take away freckles, spots, sunburn, and morphew from the face, or other parts of the body. The oil made of the flowers, as Oil of Roses is made, is profitably used to cool hot tumours, and to ease the pains, and help the sores.

Lily of the Valley.

CALLED also Conval Lily, Male Lily, and Lily Constancy.

Descript.] The root is small, and creepeth far in the ground, as grass roots do. The leaves are many, against which riseth up a stalk half a foot high, with many white flowers, like little bells with turned edges, of a strong, though pleasing smell; the berries are red, not much unlike those of Asparagus.

Place.] They grow plentifully upon Hampstead Heath, and many other places in this nation.

Time.] They flower in May, and the seed is ripe in September.

Tempe-

Temperature and Virtues.] It is under the dominion of Mercury, and therefore it strengthens the brain, recruits a weak memory, and makes it strong again: The distilled water dropped into the eyes helps inflammations there; as also that infirmity which they call a pin and web. The spirit of the flowers distilled in wine restoreth lost speech, helps the palsy, and is exceeding good in the apoplexy, comforteth the heart and vital spirits. Gerrard sayeth, that the flowers being close stopped up in a glass, put into an ant hill, and taken away again a month after, ye shall find a liquor in the glass, which, being outwardly applied, helps the gout.

White Lilies.

IT were in vain to describe a plant so commonly known in every one's garden: therefore I shall not tell you what they are, but what they are good for.

Government and Virtues] They are under the dominion of the Moon, and by antipathy to Mars expel poison; they are excellent good in pestilential fevers, the roots being bruised and boiled in wine, and the decoction drank; for it expels the venom to the exterior parts of the body: The juice of it being tempered with barley meal, baked, and so eaten for ordinary bread, is an excellent cure for the dropsy. An ointment made of the root, and hog's grease, is excellent good for scald heads, unites the sinews when they are cut, and cleanses ulcers. The root boiled in any convenient decoction, give speedy delivery to women in travail, and expels the after birth. The root roasted, and mixed with a little hog's grease, makes a gallant poultice to ripen and break plague-sores. The ointment is excellent good for swellings in the privities, and will cure burnings and scaldings without a scar, and trimly deck a black place with hair.

Liquorice.

Descript] OUR English Liquorice riseth up with divers woody stalks, wherein are set at several distances many narrow, long, green leaves, set together on both sides of the stalk, and an odd one at the end, very well resembling a young ash tree sprung up from the seed. This by many years continuance in a place without removing, and not else, will bring forth flowers, many standing together
spike

spike fashion, one above another upon the stalk, of the form of pease blossoms, but of a very pale blue colour, which turn into long, somewhat flat and smooth cods, wherein is contained a small, round, hard seed: The roots run down exceeding deep into the ground with divers other small roots and fibres growing with them, and shoot out suckers from the main roots all about, whereby it is much increased, of a brownish colour on the outside, and yellow within.

Place] It is planted in fields and gardens, in divers places of this land, and thereof good profit is made.

Government and Virtues.] It is under the dominion of Mercury. Liquorice boiled in fair water, with some Maidenhair and figs, maketh a good drink for those that have a dry cough or hoarseness, wheezing or shortness of breath, and for all the griefs of the breast and lungs, pthysic, or consumptions caused by the distillation of salt humours on them. It is also good in all pains of the reins, the stranguary, and heat of urine: The fine powder of Liquorice blown through a quill into the eyes that have a pin and web (as they call it) or rheumatic distillations in them, doth cleanse and help them. The juice of Liquorice is as effectual in all the diseases of the breast and lungs, the reins and the bladder, as the decoction. The juice distilled in Rose-water, with some gum tragacanth, is a fine licking medicine for hoarseness, wheezing, &c.

Liverwort.

Descript] COMMON Liverwort groweth close, and spreadeth much upon the ground in moist and shady places, with many small green leaves, or rather (as it were) sticking flat to one another, very unevenly cut in on the edges and crumpled; from among which arise small slender stalks an inch or two high at most, bearing small star-like flowers at the top; the roots are very fine and small.

Government and Virtues] It is under the dominion of Jupiter, and under the sign Cancer. It is a singular good herb for all the diseases of the liver, both to cool and cleanse it, and helpeth the inflammations in any part, and the yellow jaundice likewise: Being bruised and boiled in small beer, and drank, it cooleth the heat of the liver and kidneys, and helpeth the running of the reins in men, and the whites in women;

women; it is a singular remedy to stay the spreading of tetters, ringworms, and other fretting and running sores and scabs, and is an excellent remedy for such whose livers are corrupted by surfeits, which cause their bodies to break out, for it fortifieth the liver exceedingly, and makes it impregnable.

Loosestrife, or Willowherb.

Descript] COMMON yellow Loosestrife groweth to be four or five feet high, or more, with great round stalks a little crested, diversely branched from the middle of them to the tops into great and long branches, on all which at the joints grow long and narrow leaves, but broader below, and usually two at a joint, yet sometimes three or four, somewhat like willow leaves, smooth on the edges, and a fair green colour from the upper joints of the branches, and at the tops of them also stand many yellow flowers of five leaves a piece, with divers yellow threads in the middle, which turn into small round heads, containing small cornered seeds; the root creepeth under ground, almost like couch-grass, but greater, and shooteth up every Spring brownish heads, which afterwards grow up into stalks. It hath no scent or taste, but only astringent.

Place] It groweth in many places of this land in moist meadows, and by water sides.

Time.] It flowereth from June to August.

Government and Virtues] This herb is good for all manner of bleeding at the mouth, nose, or wounds, and all fluxes of the belly, and the bloody flux given either to drink or taken by clyster, it stayeth also the abundance of womens courses; it is a singular good wound herb for green wounds, to stay the bleeding, and quickly close together the lips of the wound, if the herb be bruised, and the juice only applied. It is often used in gargling for sore mouths, as also for the secret parts. The smoke hereof being burned, driveth away flies and gnats, which in the night-time molest people inhabiting near marshes, and in the fenny countries.

Loosestrife, with spiked Heads of Flowers.

Descript] THIS groweth with many woody square stalks, full of joints, about three feet high at least;

at

at every one whereof stand two long leaves, shorter, narrower, and a larger green colour than the former, and some brownish. The stalks are branched into many long stems of spiked flowers half a foot long, growing in bundles one above another, out of small husks, very like the spiked heads of lavender, each of which flowers have five round pointed leaves of a purple violet colour, or somewhat inclining to redness, in which husks stand small round heads after the flowers are fallen, wherein is contained small seed. The root creepeth under ground like unto the yellow, but is greater than it, and so are the heads of the leaves when they first appear out of the ground, and more brown than the other.

Place] It groweth usually by rivers, and ditch sides in wet grounds, as about the ditches at and near Lambeth, and in many other places of this land.

Time] It flowereth in the months of June and July.

Government and Virtues.] It is an herb of the Moon, and under the sign Cancer, neither do I know a better preserver of the sight when 'tis well, nor a better cure for sore eyes than Eyebright, taken inwardly, and this used outwardly; 'tis cold in quality. This herb is no whit inferior unto the former, it having not only all the virtues which the former hath, but some peculiar virtues of its own, found out by experience, as namely, That distilled water is a present remedy for hurts and blows on the eyes, and for blindness so as the Crystalline humour be not perished or hurt; and this hath been sufficiently proved true by the experience of a man of judgment, who kept it long to himself as a great secret. It cleareth the eyes of dust, or any thing gotten into them, and preserveth the sight. It is also very available against wounds and thrusts, being made into an ointment in this manner. To every ounce of the water, add two drams of May butter without salt, and of sugar and wax, of each as much also; let them boil gently together. Let tents dipped into that liquor that remaineth after it is cold be put into the wounds, and the place covered with a linen cloth doubled and anointed with the ointment, and this is also an approved medicine. It likewise cleanseth and healeth all foul ulcers, and sores whatsoever, and stayeth their inflammations by washing them with the water, and laying on them a green leaf or two in the Summer, or dry leaves in the Winter.

his water gargled warm in the mouth, and sometimes drank so, doth cure the quinsy, or king's evil in the throat. The said water applied warm, taketh away all spots, marks and scabs in the skin; and a little of it drank, quencheth thirst when it is extraordinary.

Lovage.

Descript.] It hath many long and great stalks of large winged leaves, divided into many parts, like smallage, but cut much larger and greater, every leaf being cut about the edges, broadest forward, and smallest at the stalk, of a sad green colour, smooth and shining: from among which rise up sundry strong, hollow green stalks, five or six, sometimes seven or eight feet high, full of joints, but lesser leaves set on them than grow below; and with them towards the tops come forth large branches, bearing at their tops large umbels of yellow flowers, and after them flat brownish seed. The root groweth thick, great and deep, spreading much, and enduring long, of a brownish colour on the outside, and whitish within. The whole plant and every part of it smelling strong, and aromatically, and is of a hot, sharp, biting taste.

Place] It is usually planted in gardens, where, if it be suffered, it groweth huge and great.

Time.] It flowereth in the end of July, and seedeth in August.

Government and Virtues.] It is an herb of the Sun, under the sign Taurus. If Saturn offend the throat (as he always doth if he be occasioner of the malady, and in Taurus is the Genesis) this is your cure. It openeth, cureth, and digesteth humours, and mightily provoketh womens courses and urine. Half a dram at a time of the dried root in powder taken in wine doth wonderfully warm a cold stomach, helpeth digestion, and consumeth all raw and superfluous moisture therein, easeth all inward gripings and pains, dissolveth wind and resisteth poison and infection. It is a known and much praised remedy to drink the decoction of the herb for any sort of ague, and to help the pains and torments of the body and bowels coming of cold. The seed is effectual to all the purposes aforesaid (except the last) and worketh more powerfully. The distilled water of the herb helpeth the quinsy in the throat, if the mouth and throat be gargled and washed therewith, and helpeth the pleurisy, being drank three or four times. Being dropped into the eyes, it taketh away the redness or dimness of them; it likewise taketh away spots or freckles in the face. The leaves bruised and fried with a little hog's lard, and laid hot to any blotch or boil will quickly break it.

Lungwort.

Descript.] THIS is a kind of moss that groweth on sundry sorts of trees, especially oaks and beeches, with broad, greyish, tough leaves diversely folded, crumpled, and gashed in on the edges, and some spotted also with many small spots on the upper side. It was never seen to bear any stalk or flower at any time.

Government and Virtues] Jupiter seems to own this herb. It is of great use to physicians to help the diseases of the lungs, and for coughs, wheezings, and shortness of breath, which it cureth both in man and beast. It is very profitable to put into lotions that are taken to stay the moist humours that flow to ulcers, and hinder their healing, as also to wash all other ulcers in the privy parts of a man or woman. It is an excellent remedy boiled in beer for broken-winded horses.

Madder.

Descript.] GARDEN Madder shooteth forth many very long, weak, four-square, reddish stalks, trailing on the ground a great way, very rough and hairy, and full of joints: At every one of these joints come forth divers long and narrow leaves, standing like a star about the stalks, rough also and hairy, towards the tops whereof come forth many small pale yellow flowers, after which come small round heads, green at first, and reddish afterwards, but black when they are ripe, wherein is contained the seed. The root is not very great, but exceeding long, running down half a man's length into the ground, red and very clear while it is fresh, spreading divers ways.

Place.] It is only manured in gardens, or larger fields, for the profit that is made thereof.

Time] It flowereth towards the end of Summer, and the seed is ripe quickly after.

Government and Virtues.] It is an herb of Mars. It hath

opening quality, and afterward to bind and strengthen. is a sure remedy for the yellow jaundice, by opening the obstructions of the liver and gall, and cleansing those parts; openeth also the obstructions of the spleen, and diminisheth the melancholy humour: It is available for the palsy and sciatica, and effectual for bruises inward and outward, and is therefore much used in vulnerary drinks. The root for all those aforesaid purposes is to be boiled in wine or water, as the cause requireth, and some honey and sugar put thereunto afterwards. The seed hereof taken in vinegar and honey helpeth the swelling and hardness of the spleen. The decoction of the leaves and branches is a good fomentation for women to sit over that have not their courses. The leaves and roots beaten and applied to any part that is discoloured with freckles, morphew, the white scurf, or any such deformity of the skin, cleanseth thoroughly, and taketh them away.

Maiden-Hair.

Descript.] OUR common Maiden Hair doth, from a number of hard black fibres, send forth a great many blackish shining brittle stalks, hardly a span long, many not half so long, on each side set very thick with small, round, dark green leaves, and spitted on the back of them like a fern.

Place.] It groweth upon old stone walls, in the West parts of Kent, and divers other places of this land; it delighteth likewise to grow by springs, wells, and rocky moist and shady places, and is always green.

Wall Rue, or White Maiden-Hair.

Descript.] THIS hath very fine pale green stalks, almost as fine as hairs, set confusedly with divers pale green leaves on very short foot-stalks, somewhat in form, but more diversely cut in on the edges, and thicker, smooth in the upper part, and spotted finely underneath.

Place.] It groweth in many places of this land, at Dartford, and the bridge at Ashford in Kent, at Beaconsfield in Buckinghamshire, at Wolly in Huntingdonshire, on Framingham Castle in Suffolk, on the church walls at Mayfield in Sussex, in Somersetshire, and divers other places of this land, and is green in Winter as well as Summer.

Government and Virtues.] Both this and the former are
under

under the dominion of Mercury, and so is that also which followeth after, and the virtue of both these are so near alike, that though I have described them and their places of growing severally, yet I shall, in writing the virtues of them, join them both together as followeth:

The decoction of the herb Maiden-Hair being dark, helpeth those that are troubled with the cough, shortness of breath, yellow jaundice, diseases of the spleen, stopping of urine, and helpeth exceedingly to break the stone in the kidneys, (in all which diseases the Wall Rue is also very effectual.) It provoketh women's courses, and stays both bleedings and fluxes of the stomach and belly, especially when the herb is dry; for being green, it looseneth the belly, and voideth choler and phlegm from the stomach and liver; it cleanseth the lungs, and by rectifying the blood causeth a good colour to the whole body. The herb boiled in oil of camomile dissolveth knots, allayeth swellings, and drieth up moist ulcers. The lee made thereof is singular good to cleanse the head from scurf, and from dry and running sores, stayeth the falling or shedding of the hair, and causeth it to grow thick, fair, and well coloured: for which purpose some boil it in wine, putting some Smallage thereto, and afterwards some oil. The Wall Rue is as effectual as Maiden Hair in all diseases of the head, or falling and recovering of the hair again, and generally for all the aforementioned diseases And besides, the powder of it taken in drink for forty days together, helpeth the burstings in children.

Golden Maiden Hair.

TO the former give me leave to add this, and I shall no more but only describe it unto you, and for the virtue refer you to the former, since whatsoever is said of them, may be also said of this.

Descript.] It hath many small, brownish, red hairs to make up the form of leaves growing about the ground from the root, and in the middle of them, in Summer, the small stalks of the same colour set with very fine yellowish green hairs on them, and bearing a small gold, yellow head, lesser than a wheat corn, standing in a great husk. The root is very small and thready.

Time.] It groweth in bogs and moorish places, and also on dry shady places, as Hampstead Heath, and elsewhere.

Mallows

Mallows and Marshmallows.

COMMON Mallows are generally so well known that they need no description.

Our common Marshmallows have divers soft hairy white stalks, rising to be three or four feet high, spreading forth many branches, the leaves whereof are soft and hairy, somewhat lesser than the other Mallow leaves, but longer pointed, out (for the most part) into some few divisions, but deep. The flowers are many, but smaller also than the other Mallows, and white, or tending to a bluish colour. After which come such long, round cases and seeds, as in the other mallows. The roots are many and long, shooting from one head, of the bigness of a thumb or finger, very pliant, tough, and being like liquorice, of a whitish yellow colour on the outside, and more white within, full of a slimy juice, which being laid in water, will thicken, as if it were a jelly.

Place.] The common Mallows grow in every county of this land. The common Marshmallows in most of the salt marshes, from Woolwich down to the sea, both on the Kentish and Essex shore, and in divers other places of this land.

Time.] They flower all the Summer months, even until the Winter do pull them down.

Government and Virtues.] Venus owns them both. The leaves of either of the sorts before specified, and the roots also boiled in wine and water, or in broth with parsley or fennel roots do help to open the body, and are very convenient in hot agues or other distempers of the body, to apply the leaves so boiled warm to the belly. It not only voideth hot, choleric, and other offensive humours, but easeth the pains and torments of the belly coming thereby; and are therefore used in all clysters conducing to those purposes. The same used by nurses, procureth them store of milk. The decoction of the seed of any of the common Mallows made in milk or wine, doth marvellously help excoriation, the phthisic, pleurisy, and other diseases of the chest and lungs, that proceed of hot causes, if it be continued taking for some time together. The leaves and roots work the same effects. They help much also in the excoriations of the guts and bowels, and hardness of the mother, and in all hot and sharp diseases thereof.

thereof. The juice drank in wine, or the decoction of them therein, doth help women to a speedy and easy delivery. Pliny saith, that whosoever shall take a spoonful of any of the Mallows, shall that day be free from all diseases that may come unto him; and that it is special good for the falling sickness. The syrup also and conserve made of the flowers, are very effectual for the same diseases, and to open the body, being costive. The leaves bruised, and laid to the eyes with a little honey, take away the imposthumes of them. The leaves bruised or rubbed upon the place stung with bees, wasps, or the like, presently take away the pains, redness, and swellings that arise thereupon. And Dioscorides saith, The decoction of the roots and leaves helpeth all sorts of poison, so as the poison be presently voided by vomit. A poultice made of the leaves, boiled and bruised, with some bean or barley flower, and oil of roses added, is an especial remedy against all hard tumours and inflammations, or imposthumes, or swellings of the cods, and other parts, and easeth the pains of them; as also against the hardness of the liver or spleen, being applied to the places. The juice of Mallows boiled in old oil and applied, taketh away all roughness of the skin, as also the scurf, dandriff, or dry scabs in the head, or other parts, if they be anointed therewith, or washed with the decoction, and preserveth the hair from falling off. It is also effectual against scaldings and burnings, St Anthony's fire, and all other hot, red and painful swellings in any part of the body. The flowers boiled in oil or water (as every one is disposed) whereunto a little honey and allum is put, is an excellent gargle to wash, cleanse or heal any sore mouth or throat in a short space. If the feet be bathed or washed with the decoction of the leaves, roots and flowers, it helpeth much the defluctions of rheum from the head; if the head be washed therewith, it stayeth the falling and shedding of the hair. The green leaves (saith Pliny) beaten with nitre, and applied, draw out thorns or prickles in the flesh.

The Marshmallows are more effectual in all the diseases before-mentioned: The leaves are likewise used to loosen the belly gently, and in decoctions for clysters to ease all pains of the body, opening the strait passages, and making them slippery, whereby the stone may descend the more easily,

and

and without pain, out of the reins, kidneys and bladder, and to ease the torturing pains thereof. But the roots are of more special use for those purposes, as well for coughs, hoarseness, shortness of breath and wheezings, being boiled in wine, or honeyed water, and drank. The roots and seeds hereof, boiled in wine and water, are with good success used by them that have excoriations in the guts, or the bloody-flux, by qualifying the violence of sharp fretting humours, easing pains, and healing the soreness. It is profitably taken of them that are troubled with ruptures, cramps, or convulsions of the sinews, and boiled in white wine, for the imposthumes of the throat, commonly called the king's evil, and of those kernels that rise behind the ears, and inflammations or swellings in womens breasts. The dried roots boiled in milk and drank, is special good for the chincough. Hippocrates used to give the decoction of the roots, or the juice thereof, to drink, to those that are wounded, and ready to faint through loss of blood, and applied the same mixed with honey and rosin to the wounds. As also, the roots boiled in wine to those that have received any hurt by bruises, falls, or blows, or had any bone or member out of joint, or any swelling pain, or ach in the muscles, sinews or arteries. The mucillage of the roots, and of linseed and fenugreek put together, is much used in poultices, ointments, and plasters, to mollify and digest all hard swellings, and the inflammation of them, and to ease pains in any part of the body. The seed either green or dry, mixed with vinegar, cleanseth the skin of Morphew, and all other discolourings, being boiled therewith in the sun.

You may remember, that not long since there was a raging disease called the bloody-flux; the college of physicians not knowing what to make of it, called it the plague of the guts, for their wits were at *ne plus ultra* about it. My son was taken with the same disease, and the excoriation of his bowels was exceeding great; myself being in the country, was sent for up; the only thing I gave him was Mallows bruised and boiled both in milk and drink, in two days (the blessing of God being upon it) it cured him. And I here, to shew my thankfulness to God, in communicating it to his creatures, leave it to posterity.

Maple Tree.

Government and Virtues.] IT is under the dominion of Jupiter. The decoction either of the leaves or bark must needs strengthen the liver much, and so you shall find it to do, if you use it. It is excellent good to open obstructions both in the liver and spleen, and easeth pains of the sides thence proceeding.

Wild Marjoram.

CALLED also Origane, Origanum, Eastward Marjoram, Wild Marjoram, and Grove Marjoram.

Descript] Wild or field Marjoram hath a root which creepeth much under ground, and continueth a long time, sending up sundry brownish, hard, square stalks, with small dark green leaves, very like those of Sweet Marjoram, but harder and somewhat broader; at the top of the stalks stand tufts of flowers, of a deep purplish red colour. The seed is small and something blacker than that of sweet Marjoram.

Place.] It groweth plentifully in the borders of corn fields, and in some copses.

Time] It flowereth towards the latter end of Summer.

Government and Virtues] This is also under the dominion of Mercury. It strengthens the stomach and head much, there being scarce a better remedy growing for such as are troubled with a sour humour in the stomach; it restores the appetite being lost; helps the cough, and consumption of the lungs; it cleanseth the body of choler, expelleth poison, and remedieth the infirmities of the spleen; helps the bitings of venomous beasts, and helps such as have poisoned themselves by eating hemlock, henbane, or opium. It provoketh urine, and the terms in women, helps the dropsy, and the scurvy, scabs, itch and yellow jaundice. The juice being dropped into the ears, helps deafness, pain and noise in the ears. And thus much for this herb, between which and adders, there is a deadly antipathy.

Sweet Marjoram.

SWEET Marjoram is so well known, being an inhabitant in every garden, that it is needless to write any description thereof, neither of the Winter Sweet Marjoram, or Pot Marjoram.

Place.] They grow commonly in gardens, some sort there are

are that grow wild in the borders of corn fields and pastures, in sundry places of this land; but it is not my purpose to insist upon them. The garden kinds being most used and useful.

Time.] They flower in the end of Summer.

Government and Virtues] It is an herb of Mercury, and under Aries, and therefore is an excellent remedy for the brain and other parts of the body and mind, under the dominion of the same planet. Our common Sweet Marjoram is warming and comfortable in the cold diseases of the head, stomach, sinews, and other parts, taken inwardly or outwardly applied. The decoction thereof being drank, helpeth all diseases of the chest which hinder the freeness of breathing, and is also profitable for the obstructions of the liver and spleen. It helpeth the cold griefs of the womb, and the windiness thereof, and the loss of speech, by resolution of the tongue. The decoction thereof made with some pellitory of Spain, and long pepper, or with a little acorns or origanum, being drank, is good for those that are beginning to fall into a dropsy, for those that cannot make water, and against pains and torments in the belly; it provoketh womens courses, if it be put as a pessary. Being made into powder, and mixed with honey, it taketh away the black marks of blows, and bruises, being thereunto applied; it is good for the inflammations and watering of the eyes, being mixed with fine flour, and laid upon them. The juice dropped into the ears, easeth the pains and singing noise in them. It is profitably put into those ointments and salves that are warm and comfort the outward parts, as the joints and sinews, for swellings also, and places out of joint. The powder thereof, snuffed up into the nose provoketh sneezing, and thereby purgeth the brain, and chewed in the mouth, draweth forth much phlegm. The oil made thereof, is very warm and comfortable to the joints that are stiff, and the sinews that are hard, to mollify and supple them. Marjoram is much used in all odoriferous waters, powders, &c. that are for ornament or delight.

Marigolds.

THESE being so plentiful in every garden, are so well known that they need no description.

Time.] They flower all the Summer long, and sometimes in Winter, if it be mild.

Government and Virtues.] It is an herb of the Sun, and under Leo. They strengthen the heart exceedingly, and are very expulsive, and little less effectual in the small pox and measles than saffron. The juice of Marigold leaves mixed with vinegar, and any hot swellings bathed with it, instantly giveth ease and assuageth it. The flowers, either green or dried, are much used in possets, broths, and drink, as a comforter of the heart and spirits, and to expel any malignant or pestilential quality which might annoy them. A plaister made with the dry flowers in powder, hogs-grease, turpentine, and rosin, applied to the breast, strengthens and succours the heart infinitely in fevers, whether pestilential or not pestilential.

Masterwort.

Descript.] COMMON Masterwort hath divers stalks of winged leaves divided into sundry parts, three for the most part standing together at a small foot stalk on both sides of the greater, and three likewise at the end of the stalk, somewhat broad, and cut in on the edges into three or more divisions, all of them dented about the brims, of a dark green colour, somewhat resembling the leaves of Angelica, but that these grow lower to the ground, and on lesser stalks; among which rise up two or three short stalks about two feet high, and slender, with such like leaves at the joints which grow below, but with lesser and fewer divisions, bearing umbels of white flowers, and after them thin, flat blackish seeds, bigger than Dill-seeds. The root is somewhat greater, and growing rather sideways than down deep in the ground, shooting forth sundry heads, which taste sharp, biting on the tongue, and is the hottest and sharpest part of the plant, and the seed next unto it being somewhat blackish on the outside, and smelling well.

Place.] It is usually kept in gardens with us in England.

Time.] It flowereth and seedeth about the end of August.

Government and Virtues.] It is an herb of Mars. The root of Masterwort is hotter than pepper, and very available in cold griefs and diseases both of the stomach and body, dissolving very powerfully upwards and downwards. It is also used in a decoction with wine against all cold rheums, distillation upon the lungs, or shortness of breath, to be taken morning and evening. It also provoketh urine and

helpeth

helpeth to break the stone, and expel the gravel from the kidneys; provoketh womens courses, and expelleth the dead birth. Is singular good for strangling of the mother, and other such like feminine diseases. It is effectual also against the dropsy, cramps, and falling sickness; for the decoction in wine being gargled in the mouth, draweth down much water and phlegm, from the brain, purging and easing it of what oppresseth it. It is of a rare quality against all sorts of cold poison to be taken as there is cause; it provoketh sweat. But lest the taste hereof, or of the seed (which worketh to the like effect, tho' not so powerfully) should be too offensive, the best way is to take the water distilled both from the herb and root. The juice hereof dropped, or tents dipped therein, and applied either to green wounds or filthy rotten ulcers, and hose that come by envenomed weapons, doth soon cleanse and heal them. The same is also very good to help the gout coming of a cold cause.

Sweet Maudlin.

Descript.] COMMON Maudlin hath somewhat long and narrow leaves, snipped about the edges. The stalks are two feet high, bearing at the tops many yellow flowers set round together, and all of an equal height, in umbels or tufts, like unto Tansy; after which followeth small whitish seed, almost as big as wormseed.

Place and Time] It groweth in gardens, and flowereth in June and July.

Government and Virtues.] The virtues hereof being the same with Costmary or Alecost, I shall not make any repetition thereof, lest my book grow too big; but rather refer you unto Costmary for satisfaction.

The Medlar.

Descript.] THE Tree groweth near the bigness of the Quince Tree, spreading branches reasonably large, with longer and narrower leaves than either the apple or quince, and not dented about the edges. At the end of the sprigs stand the flowers, made of five white, great, broad pointed leaves, nicked in the middle with some white threads also; after which cometh the fruit, of a brownish green colour being ripe, bearing a crown as it were on the top, which were the five green leaves; and being rubbed off,

off, or fallen away, the head of the fruit is seen to be somewhat hollow. The fruit is very harsh before it is mellowed, and hath usually five hard kernels within it. There is another kind hereof nothing differing from the former, but that it hath some thorns on it in several places, which the other hath not; and usually the fruit is small, and not so pleasant.

Time and Place.] They grow in this land, and flower in May for the most part, and bear fruit in September and October.

Government and Virtues.] The fruit is old Saturn's, and sure a better medicine he hardly hath to strengthen the retentive faculty; therefore it stays womens longings. The good old man cannot endure womens minds should run a gadding. Also a plaister made of the fruit dried before they are rotten, and other convenient things, and applied to the reins of the back, stops miscarriage in women with child. They are very powerful to stay any fluxes of blood or humours in men and women; the leaves also have this quality. The fruit eaten by women with child, stayeth their longing after unusual meats, and is very effectual for them that are apt to miscarry and may be delivered before their time, to help that malady, and make them joyful mothers. The decoction of them is good to gargle and wash the mouth, throat and teeth, when there is any defluxions of blood to stay it, or of humours, which causeth the pains and swellings. It is a good bath for women to sit over, that have their courses flow too abundant; or for the piles when they bleed too much. If a poultice or plaister be made with dried Medlars, beaten and mixed with the juice of red roses, whereunto a few cloves and nutmegs may be added, and a little red coral also, and applied to the stomach, that is given to casting or loathing of meat, it effectually helpeth it. The dried leaves in powder strewed on fresh bleeding wounds restraineth the blood, and healeth up the wound quickly. The Medlar stones made into powder, and drank in wine, wherein some Parsley roots have lain infused all night, or a little boiled, do break the stone in the kidneys, helping to expel it.

Mellilot, or King's Claver.

Descript.] THIS hath many green stalks, two or three feet high, rising from a tough, long, white root

root, which dieth not every year, set round about at the joints with small and somewhat long, well smelling leaves, set three together unevenly dented about the edges. The flowers are yellow, and well-smelling also, made like other trefoil, but small standing in long spikes one above another, for an hand-breadth long or better, which afterwards turn into long crooked cods, wherein is contained flat seed, somewhat brown.

Place] It groweth plentifully in many places of this land, as in the edge of Suffolk, and in Essex, as also in Huntingdonshire and in other places, but most usually in corn fields, in corners of meadows.

Time] It flowereth in June and July, and is ripe quickly after.

Government and Virtues] Melilot boiled in wine, and applied, mollifieth all hard tumours and inflammations that happen in the eyes, or other parts of the body, as the fundament, or privy parts of men and women, and sometimes the yolk of a roasted egg, or fine flour, or poppy-seed, or endive, is added unto it. It helpeth the spreading ulcers in the head, it being washed with a lee made thereof. It helpeth the pains of the stomach, being applied fresh; or boiled with any of the aforenamed things. Also, the pains of the ears, being dropped into them, and steeped in vinegar, or rose-water, it mitigateth the head-ach. The flowers of Melilot or camomile are much used to be put together in clysters to expel wind, and ease pains; and also in poultices for the same purpose, and to assuage swelling tumours in the spleen or other parts, and helpeth inflammations in any part of the body. The juice dropped into the eyes, is a singular good medicine to take away the film or skin that cloudeth or dimneth the eye sight. The head often washed with the distilled water of the herb and flower, or a lee made therewith, is effectual for those that suddenly lose their senses, as also to strengthen the memory, to comfort the head and brain, and to preserve them from pain, and the apoplexy.

French and Dogs Mercury.

Descript] THIS riseth up with a square green stalk full of joints, two feet high, or thereabouts, with two leaves at every joint, and the branches likewise from both sides of the stalk, set with fresh green leaves, somewhat broad and long, about the bigness of the leaves of Basil, finely dented about the edges; towards the tops of the stalks and branches, come forth at every joint in the male mercury two small round green heads, standing together upon a short foot-stalk, which growing ripe, are seeds not having flowers. The female stalk is longer, spike fashion, set round about with small green husks, which are the flowers, made like small bunches of grapes, which give no seed, but abide long upon the stalks without shedding. The root is composed of many small fibres, which perisheth every year at the first approach of Winter, and riseth again of its own sowing, and if once it is suffered to sow itself, the ground will never want afterwards, even both sorts of it.

Dog Mercury.

HAVING described unto you that which is called French Mercury, I come now to shew you a description of this kind also.

Descript] This is likewise of two kinds, male and female, having many stalks slender and lower than Mercury, without any branches at all upon them, the root is set with two leaves at every joint, somewhat greater than the female, but more pointed and full of veins, and somewhat harder in handling, of a dark green colour, and less dented or snipp'd about the edges. At the joints with the leaves come forth longer stalks than the former, with two hairy round seeds upon them, twice as big as those of the former Mercury. The taste hereof is herby, and the smell somewhat strong and virulent. The female has much harder leaves standing upon longer foot-stalks, and the stalks are also longer, from the joints come forth spikes of flowers like the French Female Mercury. The roots of them both are many, and full of small fibres which run under ground, and mat themselves very much, not perishing as the former Mercuries do, but abiding the Winter, and shoot forth new branches every year, for the old lie down to the ground.

Place] The male and female French Mercury are found wild in divers places in this land, as by a village called Brookland in Rumney Marsh in Kent.

The Dog Mercury in sundry places of Kent also, and elsewhere; but the female more seldom than the male.

Time.]

Time] They flower in the Summer months, and therein give their seed.

Government and Virtues] Mercury, they say, owns the herb, but I rather think it is Venus's, and I am partly confident of it too, for I never heard that Mercury ever minded womens businefs so much: I believe he minds his study more. The decoction of the leaves of Mercury, or the juice thereof in broth, or drank with a little fugar put to it, purgeth choleric and waterifh humours. Hippocrates commended it wonderfully for womens difeafes, and applied to the fecret parts, to eafe the pains of the mother; and ufed the decoction of it, both to procure womens courfes, and to expel the after birth; and gave the decoction thereof with myrrh or pepper, or ufed to apply the leaves outwardly againft the ftranguary and difeafes of the reins and bladder. He ufed it alfo for fore and watering eyes, and for the deafnefs and pains in the ears, by dropping the juice thereof into them, and bathing them afterwards in white wine. The decoction thereof made with water and a cock chicken, is a moft fafe medicine againft the hot fits of agues. It alfo cleanfeth the breaft and lungs of phlegm, but a little offendeth the ftomach. The juice or diftilled water fnuffed up into the noftrils, purgeth the head and eyes of catarrhs and rheums. Some ufe to drink two or three ounces of the diftilled water, with a little fugar put to it, in the morning fafting, to open and purge the body of grofs, vifcous, and melancholy humours. It is wonderful (if it be not fabulous) which Diofcorides and Theophraftus do relate of it, viz. That if women ufe thefe herbs either inwardly or outwardly, for three days together after conception, and their courfes be paft, they fhall bring forth male or female children, according to that kind of herb they ufe. Matthiolus faith, that the feed both of the male and female Mercury boiled with wormwood and drank cureth the yellow jaundice in a fpeedy manner. The leaves or the juice rubbed upon warts, taketh them away. The juice mingled with fome vinegar, helpeth all running fcabs, tetters, ringworms, and the itch. Galen faith, that being applied in manner of a poultice to any fwelling or inflammation, it digefteth the fwelling, and allayeth the inflammation, and is therefore given in clyfters to evacuate from the belly offenfive humours. The Dog Mercury, although it be lefs ufed, yet may ferve in the fame manner to the same purpose, to purge waterish and melancholy humours.

Mint.

OF all the kinds of Mint, the Spear Mint, or Heart Mint, being most useful, I shall only describe as follows:

Descript.] Spear Mint hath divers round stalks, and long but narrowish leaves set thereon, of a dark green colour. The flowers stand in spiked heads at the tops of the branches, being of a pale blue colour. The smell or scent thereof is somewhat near unto Basil; it increaseth by the root under ground, as all others do.

Place] It is an usual inhabitant in gardens: And because it seldom giveth any good seed, the effects is recompensed by the plentiful increase of the root, which being once planted in a garden, will hardly be rid out again.

Time] It flowereth not until the beginning of August, for the most part.

Government and Virtues] It is an herb of Venus. Dioscorides saith it hath a heating, binding and drying quality, and therefore the juice taken in vinegar stayeth bleeding. It stirreth up venery, or bodily lust, two or three branches thereof taken in the juice of four pomegranates, stayeth the hiccough, vomiting, and allayeth the choler. It dissolveth imposthumes, being laid to with barley meal. It is good to repress the milk in womens breasts, and for such as have swollen, flagging, or great breasts. Applied with salt, it helpeth the biting of a mad dog; with mead and honeyed water, it easeth the pains of the ears, and taketh away the roughness of the tongue, being rubbed thereupon. It suffereth not milk to curdle in the stomach, if the leaves thereof be steeped or boiled in it before you drink it: Briefly, it is very profitable to the stomach. The often use hereof is a very powerful medicine to stay womens courses and the whites. Applied to the forehead and temples, it easeth the pains in the head, and is good to wash the heads of young children therewith, against all manner of breakings-out, sores or scabs therein, and healeth the chops of the fundament. It is also profitable against the poison of venomous creatures. The distilled water of mint is available to all the purposes aforesaid, yet more weakly. But if a spirit thereof be rightly and chymically

mically drawn, it is much more powerful than the herb itself. Simeon Sethi saith, it helpeth a cold liver, strengtheneth the belly, causeth digestion, stayeth vomits and the hiccough; it is good against the gnawing of the heart, provoketh appetite, taketh away obstructions of the liver, and stirreth up bodily lust; but therefore too much must not be taken because it maketh the blood thin and wheyish and turneth it into choler, and therefore choleric persons must abstain from it. It is a safe medicine for the biting of a mad dog, being bruised with salt, and laid thereon. The powder of it being dried and taken after meat, helpeth digestion, and those that are splenetic. Taken with wine, it helpeth women in their sore travail in child bearing. It is good against the gravel and stone in the kidneys, and the stranguary. Being smelled unto, it is comfortable for the head and memory. The decoction thereof gargled in the mouth, cureth the gums and mouth that is sore, and mendeth an ill favoured breath; as also the rue and coriander, causeth the palate of the mouth to turn to its place, the decoction being gargled and held in the mouth.

The virtues of the Wild or Horse Mint, such as grow in ditches (whose description I purposely omitted, in regard they are well enough known) are especially to dissolve wind in the stomach, to help the colic, and those that are shortwinded, and are an especial remedy for those that have venereal dreams and pollutions in the night, being outwardly applied to the testicles or cods. The juice dropped into the ears easeth the pains of them, and destroyeth the worms that breed therein. They are good against the venomous biting of serpents. The juice laid on warm, helpeth the king's evil, or kernels in the throat. The decoction or distilled water helpeth a stinking breath proceeding from corruption of the teeth, and snuffed up the nose purgeth the head. Pliny saith, that eating of the leaves hath been found by experience to cure the leprosy, applying some of them to the face, and to help the scurf or dandriff of the head used with vinegar. They are extreme bad for wounded people; and they say a wounded man that eats Mint, his wound will never be cured, and that is a long day.

Misselto.

Misselto.

Descript] THIS riseth up from the branch or arm of the tree whereon it groweth, with a woody stem, putting itself into sundry branches, and they again divided into many other smaller twigs, interlacing themselves one within another, very much covered with a greyish green bark, having two leaves set at every joint, and at the end likewise, which are somewhat long and narrow, small at the bottom, but broader towards the end. At the knots or joints of the boughs and branches grow small yellow flowers, which run into small, round, white, transparent berries, three or four together, full of a glutinous moisture, with a blackish seed in each of them, which was never yet known to spring, being put into the ground, or any where else to grow.

Place] It groweth very rarely on oaks with us, but upon sundry other, as well timber as fruit-trees, plentifully in woody groves, and the like, through all this land.

Time] It flowereth in the Spring time, but the berries are not ripe until October, and abideth on the branches all the Winter, unless the black birds, and other birds, do devour them.

Government and Virtues] This is under the dominion of the Sun, I do not question, and can also take for granted, that that which grows upon oaks, participates something of the nature of Jupiter, because an oak is one of his trees, as also that which grows upon pear trees, and apple trees, participates something of his nature, because he rules the tree it grows upon, having no root of its own. But why that should have most virtues that grows upon oaks I know not, unless because it is rarest and hardest to come by, and our college opinion is in this contrary to scripture, which saith, *God's tender mercies are over all his works*, and so it is, let the college of physicians walk as contrary to him as they please, and that is as contrary as the east to the west. Clusius affirm, that which grows upon pear trees to be as prevalent, and gives order, that it should not touch the ground after it is gathered, and also saith, that, being hung about the neck, it remedies witchcraft. Both the leaves and berries of Misselto do heat and dry, and are of subtile parts; the bir lime doth mollify hard knots, tumour, and imposthumes; ripeneth and discusseth them, and draweth forth thick as well as thin

thin humours from the remote parts of the body, digesting and separating them. And being mixed with equal parts of rosin and wax, doth mollify the hardness of the spleen, and helpeth old ulcers and sores. Being mixed with sandaric and orpiment, it helpeth to draw off foul nails; and if quick-lime, and wine lees be added thereunto, it worketh the stronger. The Misselto itself of the oak (as the best) made into powder, and given in drink to those that have the falling-sickness, doth assuredly heal them, as Matthiolus saith; but it is fit to use it for forty days together. Some have so highly esteemed it for the virtues thereof, that they have called it *Lignum Sanctæ Crucis*, Wood of the Holy Cross, believing it helps the falling sickness, apoplexy and palsy very speedily, not only to be inwardly taken, but to be hung at their neck. Tragus saith, that the fresh wood of any Misselto bruised, and the juice drawn forth and dropped in the ears that have imposthumes in them, doth help and ease them within a few days.

Moneywort, or Herb Twopence.

Descript.] THE common Moneywort sendeth forth from a small thready root, divers long, weak, and slender branches, lying and running upon the ground two or three feet long or more, set with leaves two at a joint one against another at equal distances, which are almost round, but pointed at the ends, smooth, and of a good green colour. At the joints with the leaves from the middle forward come forth at every point sometimes one yellow flower, and sometimes two, standing each on a small foot stalk, and made of five leaves, narrow pointed at the end, with some yellow threads in the middle, which being past, there stand in their places small round heads of seed.

Place.] It groweth plentifully in almost all places of this land, commonly in moist grounds by hedge sides, and in the middle of grass fields.

Time.] They flower in June and July, and their seed is ripe quickly after.

Government and Virtues] Venus owns it. Moneywort is singular good to stay all fluxes in man or woman, whether they be lasks, bloody fluxes, the flowing of womens courses, bleeding inwardly or outwardly, and the weakness of the

stomach

stomach that is given to casting. It is very good also for the ulcers or excoriations of the lungs, or other inward parts. It is exceeding good for all wounds, either fresh or green to heal them speedily, and for all old ulcers that are of a spreading nature. For all which purposes the juice of the herb, or the powder drank in water wherein hot steel hath been often quenched, or the decoction of the green herb in wine or water drank, or used to the outward place, to wash or bathe them, or to have tents dipped therein and put into them, are effectual.

Moonwort.

Descript.] It riseth up usually but with one dark, green, thick and flat leaf, standing upon a short foot stalk, not above two fingers breadth; but when it flowers it may be said to bear a small slender stalk about four or five inches high, having but one leaf in the middle thereof, which is much divided on both sides, into sometimes five or seven parts on a side, sometimes more; each of which parts is small like the middle rib, but broad towards, pointed and round, resembling therein a half moon, from whence it took the name; the uppermost parts or divisions being bigger than the lowest. The stalks rise above this leaf two or three inches, bearing many branches of small long tongues, every one like the spiky head of the adders tongues, of a brownish colour, (which whether I shall call them flowers, or the seed, I well know not) which, after they have continued a while, resolve into a mealy dust. The root is small and fibrous. This hath sometimes divers such like leaves as are before described, with so many branches or tops rising from one stalk, each divided from the other.

Place.] It groweth on hills and heaths, yet where there is much grass, for therein it delighteth to grow.

Time.] It is to be found only in April and May, for in June, when any hot weather cometh, for the most part it is withered and gone.

Government and Virtues.] The moon owns the herb. Moonwort is cold, and drying more than adder's tongue, and is therefore held to be more available for all wounds both inward and outward. The leaves boiled in red wine, and drank, stay the immoderate flux of womens courses, and the whites.
It

it also stayeth bleeding, vomiting, and other fluxes. It helpeth all blows and bruises, and to consolidate all fractures and dislocations. It is good for ruptures, but is chiefly used by most with other herbs to make oils or balsams to heal fresh or green wounds (as I said before) either inward or outward, for which it is excellent good.

Moonwort is an herb which (they say) will open locks, and unshoe such horses as tread upon it: This some laugh to scorn, and those no small fools neither; but country people that I know, call it Unshoe the Horse. Besides I have heard commanders say, that on White Down in Devonshire, near Tiverton, there were found thirty horse-shoes, pulled off from the feet of the Earl of Essex's horses, being there drawn up in a body, many of them being but newly shod, and no reason known, which caused much admiration, and the herb described usually grows upon heaths.

Mosses.

I SHALL not trouble the reader with a description of these, since my intent is to speak only of two kinds, as the most principal, viz. Ground Moss and Tree Moss, both which are very well known.

Place] The Ground Moss groweth in our moist woods, and in the bottom of hills, in boggy grounds, and in shadowy ditches, and many other such like places. The Tree Moss groweth only on trees.

Government and Virtues] All sorts of Mosses are under the dominion of Saturn. The Ground Moss is held to be singular good to break the stone, and to expel and drive it forth by urine, being boiled in wine and drank. The herb, being bruised and boiled in water, and applied, easeth all inflammations and pains coming from an hot cause; and is therefore used to ease the pains of the gout.

The Tree Moss is cooling and binding, and partakes of a digesting and mollifying quality withal, as Galen saith. But each moss doth partake of the nature of the tree from whence it is taken; therefore that of the oak is more binding, and is of good effect to stay fluxes in man or woman; as also vomiting or bleeding, the powder thereof being taken in wine. The decoction thereof in wine is very good for women to be bathed, or to sit in, that are troubled with the overflowing
of

of their courses. The same being drank, stayeth the stomach that is troubled with casting, or the hiccough; and, as Avicena saith, it comforteth the heart. The powder thereof taken in drink for some time together, is thought available for the dropsy. The oil that has had fresh Moss steeped therein for a time, and afterwards boiled and applied to the temples and forehead, doth marvellously ease the head ach coming of a hot cause; as also the distillations of hot rheum or humours in the eyes, or other parts. The ancients much used it in their ointments and other medicines against the lassitude, and to strengthen and comfort the sinews: for which, if it was good then, I know no reason but it may be found so still.

Motherwort.

Descript.] THIS hath a hard, square, brownish, rough, strong stalk, rising three or four feet high at least, spreading into many branches, whereon grow leaves on each side, with long foot-stalks, two at every joint, which are somewhat broad and long, as if it were rough or coupled, with many great veins therein of a sad green colour, and deeply dented about the edges, and almost divided. From the middle of the branches up to the tops of them (which are long and small) grow the flowers round them at distances, in sharp pointed, rough, hard husks, of a more red or purple colour than balm or horehound, but in the same manner or form as the horehounds, after which come small, round, blackish seeds in great plenty. The root sendeth forth a number of long strings and small fibres, taking strong hold in the ground, of a dark yellowish or brownish colour, and abideth as the horehound doth; the smell of this not much differeth from it.

Place.] It groweth only in gardens with us in England.

Government and Virtues.] Venus owns the herb, and it is under Leo. There is no better herb to take melancholy vapours from the heart, to strengthen it, and make a merry, chearful, blythe soul than this herb. It may be kept in a syrup or conserve; therefore the Latins called it Cardiaca. Besides, it makes women joyful mothers of children, and settles their wombs as they should be, therefore we call it Motherwort. It is held to be of much use for the trembling of the heart, and faintings and swoonings; from whence it it took the name Cardiaca. The powder thereof, to the quantity of a spoonful, drank in wine, is a wonderful help to women in their sore travail, as also for the suffocating or risings of the mother, and for these effects, it is likely it took the name of Motherwort with us. It also provoketh urine and womens courses, cleanseth the chest of cold phlegm oppressing it, killeth worms in the belly. It is of good use to warm and dry up the humours, to digest and disperse them that are settled in the veins, joints, and sinews of the body, and to help cramps and convulsions.

Mouse-ear.

Descript.] MOUSE-EAR is a low herb, creeping upon the ground by small strings, like the strawberry plant, whereby it shooteth forth small roots, whereat grow upon the ground many small and somewhat short leaves, set in a round form together, and very hairy, which being broken do give a whitish milk: From among these leaves spring up two or three small hoary stalks about a span high, with a few smaller leaves thereon; at the tops whereof standeth usually but one flower, consisting of many pale yellow leaves, broad at the point, and a little dented in, set in three or four rows (the greater uppermost) very like a dandelion flower, and a little reddish underneath about the edges, especially if it grow in a dry ground; which after they have stood long in flower do turn into down, which with the seed is carried away with the wind.

Place.] It groweth on ditch banks, and sometimes in others, if they be dry, and in sandy grounds.

Time.] It flowereth about June or July, and abideth green all the Winter.

Government and Virtues. The Moon owns this herb also; and though authors cry out upon alchymists, for attempting to fix quicksilver by this herb and Moonwort, a Roman would not have judged a thing by the success; if it be to be fixed at all, it is by lunar influence. The juice thereof taken in wine, or the decoction thereof drank, doth help the jaundice, although of long continuance, to drink thereof morning and evening, and abstain from other drink two or three hours after. It is a special remedy against the stone, and the tormenting pains thereof, as also other tortures and griping pains of the bowels. The decoction thereof with succory and

centuary

centuary is held very effectual to help the dropsy, and them that are inclining thereunto, and the diseases of the spleen. It stayeth the fluxes of blood, either at the mouth or nose, and inward bleeding also, for it is a singular wound herb for wounds both inward and outward: It helpeth the bloody-flux, and helpeth the abundance of womens courses. There is a syrup made of the juice thereof, and sugar, by the apothecaries of Italy, and other places, which is of much account with them, to be given to those that are troubled with the cough or phthisic. The same also is singular good for ruptures or burstings. The green herb bruised and presently bound to any cut or wound, doth quickly solder the lips thereof. And the juice, decoction, or powder of the dried herb is most singular to stay malignity of spreading and fretting cankers and ulcers whatsoever, yea, in the mouth and secret parts: The distilled water of the plant is available in all diseases aforesaid, and to wash outward wounds and sores, and apply tents of cloths wet therein.

Mugwort.

Descript] COMMON Mugwort hath divers leaves lying upon the ground, very much divided, or cut deeply in about the brims, somewhat like wormwood, but much larger, of a dark green colour on the upper side, and very hoary white underneath. The stalks rise to be four or five feet high, having on it such like leaves as those below, but somewhat smaller, branching forth very much towards the top, whereon are set very small, pale, yellowish flowers like buttons, which fall away, and after them come small seeds inclosed in round heads. The root is long and hard, with many small fibres growing from it, whereby it taketh strong hold on the ground: but both stalks and leaf do lie down every year, and the root shooteth anew in the spring. The whole plant is of a reasonable scent, and is more easily propagated by the slips than the seed.

Place] It groweth plentifully in many places of this land, by the water sides; as also by small water courses, and in divers other places.

Time] It flowereth and seedeth in the end of Summer

Government and Virtues] This is an herb of Venus, therefore maintaineth the parts of the body she rules, remedies the

the diseases of the parts that are under her signs Taurus and Libra. Mugwort is with good success put among other herbs that are boiled for women to sit over the hot decoction to draw down their courses, to help the delivery of their birth, and expel the after-birth. As also for the obstructions and inflammations of the mother. It breaketh the stone, and causeth one to make water where it is stopped. The juice thereof made up with myrrh, and put under as a pessary, worketh the same effects, and so doth the root also. Being made up with hog's grease into an ointment, it taketh away wens and hard knots and kernels that grow about the neck and throat, and easeth the pains about the neck more effectually, if some field daisies be put with it. The herb itself being fresh, or the juice thereof taken, is a special remedy upon the overmuch taking of opium. Three drams of the powder of the dried leaves taken in wine, is a speedy and the best certain help for the sciatica. A decoction thereof made with camomile and agrimony, and the place bathed therewith while it is warm, taketh away the pains of the sinews, and the cramp.

The Mulberry-tree.

THIS is so well known where it groweth, that it needeth no description.

Time.] It beareth fruit in the month of July and August.

Government and Virtues.] Mercury rules the Tree, therefore are its effects variable as his are. The Mulberry is of different parts, the ripe berries, by reason of their sweetness and slippery moisture, opening the body, and the unripe binding it, especially when they are dried, and then they are good to stay fluxes, lasks, and the abundance of womens courses. The bark of the root killeth the broad worms in the body. The juice or the syrup made of the juice of the berries, helpeth all inflammations or sores in the mouth, or throat, and palate of the mouth when it is fallen down. The juice of the leaves is a remedy against the bitings of serpents, and for those that have taken aconite. The leaves beaten with vinegar, are good to lay on any place that is burnt with fire. A decoction made of the bark and leaves is good to wash the mouth and teeth when they ach. If the root be a little slit or cut, and a small hole made in the ground next thereunto, in the harvest-time, it will give out a certain
juice,

juice, which being hardened the next day, is of good use to help the tooth-ach, to dissolve knots, and purge the belly. The leaves of Mulberries are said to stay bleeding at the mouth or nose, or the bleeding of the piles, or of a wound, being bound unto the places. A branch of the tree taken when the Moon is at the full, and bound to the wrist of a woman's arm, whose courses come down too much, doth stay them in a short space.

Mullein.

Descript.] COMMON White Mullein hath many fair, large, woolly white leaves, lying next the ground, somewhat larger than broad, pointed at the end, and as it were dented about the edges. The stalk riseth up to be four or five feet high, covered over with such like leaves, but lesser, so that no stalk can be seen for the multitude of leaves thereon up to the flowers, which come forth on all sides of the stalk, without any branches for the most part, and are many set together in a long spike, in some of a yellow colour, in others more pale, consisting of five round-pointed leaves, which afterwards have small round heads, wherein small brownish seed is contained. The root is long, white, and woody, perishing after it hath borne seed.

Place.] It groweth by way sides and lanes, in many places of this land.

Time.] It flowereth in July, or thereabouts.

Government and Virtues.] It is under the dominion of Saturn. A small quantity of the root given in wine, is commended by Dioscorides, against lasks and fluxes of the belly. The decoction hereof drank, is profitable for those that are bursten, and for cramps and convulsions, and for those that are troubled with an old cough. The decoction thereof gargled, easeth the pains of the tooth ach. And the oil made by the often infusion of the flowers, is of a very good effect for the piles. The decoction of the root in red wine or in water, (if there be an ague) wherein red hot steel hath been often quenched, doth stay the bloody-flux. The same also openeth obstructions of the bladder and reins when one cannot make water. A decoction of the leaves hereof, and of sage, marjoram, and camomile flowers, and the places bathed therewith, that have sinews stiff with cold or cramps,

doth

doth bring them much ease and comfort. Three ounces of the distilled water of the flowers drank morning and evening for some days together, is said to be the most excellent remedy for the gout. The juice of the leaves and flowers being laid upon rough warts, also the powder of the dried roots rubbed on, doth easily take them away, but doth no good to smooth warts. The powder of the dried flowers is an especial remedy for those that are troubled with the belly-ach, or the pains of the colic. The decoction of the root, and so likewise of the leaves, is of great effect to dissolve the tumours, swellings, or inflammations of the throat. The seed and leaves boiled in wine, and applied, draw forth speedily thorns or splinters gotten into the flesh, ease the pains, and heal them also. The leaves bruised and wrapped in double papers, and covered with hot ashes and embers to bake a while, and then taken forth and laid warm on any blotch or boil happening in the groin or share, doth dissolve and heal them. The seed bruised and boiled in wine, and laid on any member that hath been out of joint, and newly set again, taketh away all swelling and pain thereof.

Mustard.

Descript] OUR common Mustard hath large and broad rough leaves, very much jagged with uneven and unorderly gashes, somewhat like turnip leaves, but lesser and rougher. The stalk riseth to be more than a foot high, and sometimes two feet high, being round, rough and branched at the top, bearing such like leaves thereon as grow below, but lesser, and less divided, and divers yellow flowers one above another at the tops, after which come small rough pods, with small, lank, flat ends, wherein is contained round yellowish seed, sharp, hot, and biting upon the tongue. The root is small, long, and woody when it beareth stalks, and perisheth every year.

Place] This groweth with us in gardens only, and other manured places.

Time.] It is an annual plant, flowering in July, and the seed is ripe in August.

Government and Virtues] It is an excellent sauce for such whose blood wants clarifying, and for weak stomachs, being an herb of Mars, but naught for choleric people, though as good for such as are aged, or troubled with cold diseases.

Aries

Aries claims something to do with it, therefore it strengthens the heart and resisteth poison. Let such whose stomachs are so weak they cannot digest their meat, or appetite it, take of Mustard-seed a dram, cinnamon as much, and having beaten them to powder, and half as much mastick in powder, and with gum arabic dissolved in rose water, make it up into troches, of which they may take one of about half a dram weight, an hour or two before meals; let old men and women make much of this medicine, and they will either give me thanks, or shew manifest ingratitude. Mustard-seed hath the virtue of heat, discussing, rarifying, and drawing out splinters of bones, and other things of the flesh. It is of good effect to bring down womens courses, for the falling sickness or lethargy, drowsy forgetful evil, to use it both inwardly and outwardly, to rub the nostrils, forehead, and temples, to warm and quicken the spirits; for by the fierce sharpness it purgeth the brain by sneezing, and draweth down rheum and other viscous humours, which by their distillations upon the lungs and chest, procure coughing, and therefore, with some honey added thereto, doth much good therein. The decoction of the seed made in wine, and drank, provoketh urine, resisteth the force of poison, the malignity of mushrooms, and venom of scorpions, or other venomous creatures, if it be taken in time; and taken before the cold fits of agues, altereth, lesseneth, and cureth them. The seed taken either by itself, or with other things, either in an electuary or drink, doth mightily stir up bodily lust, and helpeth the spleen and pains in the sides, and gnawings in the bowels; and used as a gargle draweth up the palate of the mouth, being fallen down; and also it dissolveth the swellings about the throat, if it be outwardly applied. Being chewed in the mouth it oftentimes helpeth the tooth ach. The outward application hereof upon the pained place of the sciatica, discusseth the humours, and easeth the pains, as also the gout, and other joint achs; and is much and often used to ease pains in the sides or loins, the shoulders, or other parts of the body, upon the applying thereof to raise blisters, and cureth the disease by drawing it to the outward parts of the body. It is also used to help the falling off of the hair. The seed bruised, mixed with honey, and applied, or made up with wax, taketh away the marks and black and blue

blue spots of bruises, or the like, the roughness or scabbiness of the skin, as also the leprosy, and lousy evil. It helpeth also the crick in the neck. The distilled water of the herb, when it is in the flower, is much used to drink inwardly to help in any of the diseases aforesaid, or to wash the mouth when the palate is down, and for the diseases of the throat to gargle, but outwardly also for scabs, itch, or other the like infirmities, and cleanseth the face from morphew, spots, freckles, and other deformities.

The Hedge-Mustard.

Descript] THIS groweth up usually but with one blackish green stalk, tough easy to bend, but not to break, branched into divers parts, and sometimes with divers stalks, set full of branches, whereon grow long, rough, or hard rugged leaves, very much tore or cut on the edges in many parts, some bigger, and some lesser, of a dirty green colour. The flowers are small and yellow that grow on the tops of the branches in long spikes, flowering by degrees; so that continuing long in flower, the stalk will have small round cods at the bottom, growing upright and close to the stalk, while the top flowers yet shew themselves in which are contained small yellow seed sharp and strong, as the herb is also. The root groweth down slender and woody, yet abiding and springing again every year.

Place] This groweth frequently in this land by the ways and hedge sides, and sometimes in the open fields.

Time] It flowereth most usually about July.

Government and Virtues] Mars owns this herb also. It is singular good in all the diseases of the chest and lungs, hoarseness of voice, and by the use of the decoction thereof for a little space, those have been recovered who had utterly lost their voice, and almost their spirits also. The juice thereof made into a syrup or licking medicine, with honey or sugar, is no less effectual for the same purpose, and for all other coughs, wheezing, and shortness of breath. The same is also profitable for those that have the jaundice, pleurisy, pains in the back and loins, and for torments in the belly, or colic, being also used in clysters. The seed is held to be a special remedy against poison and venom. It is singular good for the sciatica, and in joint achs, ulcers, and cankers in the

K mouth,

mouth, throat, or behind the ears, and no less for the hardness and swelling of the testicles, or of womens breasts.

Nailwort, or Whitlowgrass.

Descript] THIS very small and common herb hath no roots, save only a few strings; neither doth it ever grow to be above a hand's breadth high, the leaves are very small, and somewhat long, not much unlike those of chickweed, among which rise up divers slender stalks, bearing many white flowers one above another, which are exceeding small; after which come small flat pouches containing the seed, which is very small, but of a sharp taste.

Place] It grows commonly upon old stone and brick walls, and sometimes in dry gravelly grounds, especially if there be grass or moss near to shadow it.

Time] They flower very early in the year, sometimes in January, and in February; for before the end of April they are not to be found.

Government and Virtues] It is held to be exceeding good for those imposthumes in the joints, and under the nails, which they call Whitlows, Felons, Andicons, and Nailwheal. Such as would be knowing physicians, let them read those books of mine of the last edition, viz. Reverius, Riolanus, Johnson, Vestingas, Sennertus.

Nep, or Catmint.

Descript.] COMMON Garden Nep shooteth forth hard four square stalks, with a hoariness on them, a yard high or more, full of branches, bearing at every joint two broad leaves like balm, but longer pointed, softer, whiter, and more hoary, nicked about the edges, and of a strong sweet scent. The flowers grow in large tufts at the tops of the branches, and underneath them likewise on the stalks many together, of a whitish purple colour. The roots are composed of many long strings or fibres, fastening themselves stronger in the ground, and abide with green leaves thereon all the Winter.

Place] It is only nursed up in our gardens.

Time] And it flowereth in July, or thereabouts.

Government and Virtues] It is an herb of Venus. Nep is generally used for women to procure their courses, being taken inwardly or outwardly, either alone, or with other convenient herbs in a decoction to bathe them, or sit over the hot fumes thereof; and by the frequent use thereof, it takes away barrenness, and the wind, and pains of the mother. It is also used in pains of the head coming of any cold cause, catarrhs, rheums, and for swimming and giddiness thereof, and is of special use for the windiness of the stomach and belly. It is effectual for any cramp, or cold ache, to dissolve cold and wind that afflicteth the place, and is used for colds, coughs, and shortness of breath. The juice thereof drank in wine, is profitable for those that are bruised by an accident. The green herb bruised and applied to the fundament, and lying there two or three hours, easeth the pains of the piles; the juice also being made up into an ointment, is effectual for the same purpose. The head washed with a decoction thereof, it taketh away scabs, and may be effectual for other parts of the body also.

Nettles.

NETTLES are so well known, that they need no description; they may be found by feeling, in the darkest night.

Government and Virtues] This is also an herb Mars claims dominion over. You know Mars is hot and dry, and you know as well that Winter is cold and moist, then you may know as well the reason why Nettle Tops eaten in the Spring consumeth the phlegmatic superfluities in the body of man, that the coldness and moistness of Winter hath left behind. The roots or leaves boiled, or the juice of either of them, or both made into an electuary with honey and sugar, is a safe and sure medicine to open the pipes and passages of the lungs, which is the cause of wheezing and shortness of breath, and helpeth to expectorate tough phlegm, as also to raise the imposthumed pleurisy; and spend it by spitting; the same helpeth the swelling of the almonds of the throat, the mouth and throat being gargled therewith. The juice is also effectual to settle the palate of the mouth in its place, and to heal and temper the inflammations and soreness of the mouth and throat. The decoction of the leaves in wine, being drank, is singular good to provoke women's courses, and settle the suffocation, strangling of the mother, and all other diseases thereof; as also applied outwardly with a little myrrh. The same also, or the seed, provoketh urine, and expelleth the gravel and stone in the reins or bladder, often proved to be effectual in many that have taken it. The same killeth the worms in children, easeth pains in the sides, and dissolveth the windiness in the spleen, as also in the body, although others think it only powerful to provoke venery. The juice of the leaves taken two or three days together, stayeth bleeding at the mouth. The seed being drank, is a remedy against the stinging of venomous creatures, the biting of mad dogs, the poisonful qualities of hemlock, henbane, nightshade, mandrake, or other such like herbs that stupify or dull the senses; as also the lethargy, especially to use it outwardly, to rub the forehead or temples in the lethargy, and the places stung or bitten with beasts with a little salt. The distilled water of the herb is also effectual (though not so powerful) for the diseases aforesaid, as for outward wounds and sores to wash them, and to cleanse the skin from morphew, leprosy, and other discolourings thereof. The seed or leaves bruised, and put into the nostrils, stayeth the bleeding of them, and taketh away the flesh growing in them called polypus. The juice of the leaves, or the decoction of them, or of the root, is singular good to wash either old, rotten, or stinking sores or fistulas, and gangrenes, and such as fretting, eating, or corroding scabs, manginess, and itch, in any part of the body, as also green wounds by washing them therewith, or applying the green herb bruised thereunto, yea, although the flesh were separated from the bones. the same applied to our wearied members, refresh them, or to place those that have been out of joint, being first set up again, strengtheneth, drieth, and comforteth them. as also those places troubled with achs and gouts, and the defluction of humours upon the joints or sinews; it easeth the pains, and drieth or dissolveth the defluctions. An ointment made of the juice, oil, and a little wax, is singular good to rub cold and benumbed members. An handful of the leaves of green Nettles, and another of Wallwort, or Deanwort, bruised and applied simply themselves to the gout, sciatica, or joint achs in any part, hath been found to be an admirable help thereunto.

Night-

Nightshade.

Descript] COMMON Nightshade hath an upright, round, green, hollow stalk, about a foot or half a yard high, bushing forth in many branches, whereon grow many green leaves, somewhat broad, and pointed at the ends, soft and full of juice, somewhat like unto Bazil, but longer and a little unevenly dented about the edges: At the tops of the stalks and branches come forth three or four more white flowers made of five small pointed leaves a piece, standing on a stalk together one above another, with yellow pointels in the middle, composed of four or five yellow threads set together, which afterwards run into so many pendulous green berries, of the bigness of small peale, full of green juice, and small whitish round flat seed lying within it. The root is white, and a little woody when it hath given flower and fruit, with many small fibres at it. The whole plant is of a waterish insipid taste, but the juice within the berries is somewhat viscous, and of a cooling and binding quality.

Place] It groweth wild with us under our walls, and in rubbish, the common path, and sides of hedges and fields, as also in our gardens here in England, without any planting.

Time] It lieth down every year, and riseth again of its own sowing, but springeth not until the latter end of April at the soonest.

Government and Virtues] It is a cold Saturnine plant. The common Nightshade is wholly used to cool hot inflammations either inwardly or outwardly, being no ways dangerous to any that use it, as most of the rest of the Nightshades are: yet it must be used moderately. The distilled water only of the whole herb is fittest and safest to be taken inwardly: The juice also clarified and taken, being mingled with a little vinegar, is good to wash the mouth and throat that is inflamed. But outwardly the juice of the herbs or berries, with oil of roses, and a little vinegar and ceruse laboured together in a leaden mortar, is very good to anoint all hot inflammations in the eyes. It also doth much good for the shingles, ringworms, and in all running, fretting and corroding ulcers, applied thereunto. A pessary dipped in the juice, and dropped into the matrix, stayeth the immoderate flux of womens courses, a cloth wet therein, and applied to the testicles or cods, upon swelling therein, giveth much ease, also to the gout

gout that cometh of hot and sharp humours. The juice dropped into the ears, easeth pains thereof that arise of heat or inflammations. And Pliny saith, it is good for hot swellings under the throat. Have a care you mistake not the Deadly Nightshade for this; if you know it not, you may let them both alone, and take no harm, having other medicines sufficient in the book.

The Oak.

IT is so well known (the timber thereof being the glory and safety of this nation by sea) that it needeth no description.

Government and Virtues] Jupiter owns the tree. The leaves and bark of the Oak, and the acorn cups, do bind and dry very much. The inner bark of the tree, and the thin skin that covereth the acorn, are most used to stay the spitting of blood, and the bloody flux. The decoction of that bark, and the powder of the cups, do stay vomitings, spitting of blood, bleeding at the mouth, or other flux of blood in men or women, lask also and the involuntary flux of natural seed. The acorn in powder taken in wine provoketh urine, and resisteth the poison of venomous creatures. The decoction of acorns and bark made in milk and taken, resisteth the force of poisonous herbs and medicines, as also the virulency of cantharides, when one by eating them hath his bladder exulcerated, and pisseth blood. Hippocrates saith, he used the fumes of Oak leaves to women that were troubled with the strangling of the mother; and Galen applied them being bruised to cure green wounds. The distilled water of the Oaken bud, before they break out into leaves, is good to be used either inwardly or outwardly, to assuage inflammations and to stop all manner of fluxes in man or woman. The same is singular good in pestilential and hot burning fevers, for it resisteth the force of the infection, and allayeth the heat. It cooleth the heat of the liver, breaketh the stone in the kidneys, and stayeth womens courses. The decoction of the leaves worketh the same effects. The water that is found in the hollow places of old Oaks, is very effectual against any foul or spreading scabs. The distilled water (or concoction, (which is better) of the leaves, is one of the best remedies that I know of for the whites in women.

Oats

Oats.

ARE so well known that they need no description.

Government and Virtues.] Oats fried with bay salt, and applied to the sides, take away the pains of stitches, and wind in the sides of the belly. A poultice made of meal of Oats, and some oil of bays put thereunto, helpeth the itch and the leprosy, as also the fistulas of the fundament, and dissolveth hard imposthumes. The meal of Oats boiled with vinegar, and applied, taketh away freckles and spots in the face, and other parts of the body.

One Bade.

Descript.] THIS small plant never beareth more than one leaf, but only where it riseth up with his stalk which thereon beareth another, and seldom more, which are a bluish green colour, pointed, with many ribs or veins therein, like plantain. At the top of the stalk grow many small white flowers, star fashion, smelling somewhat sweet; after which come small red berries when they are ripe. The root is small, of the bigness of a rush lying and creeping under the upper crust of the earth, shooting forth in divers places.

Place.] It groweth in moist, shadowy, and grassy places of woods, in many places of this land.

Time.] It flowereth about May, and the berries are ripe in June, and then quickly perisheth, until the next year it springeth from the same root again.

Government and Virtues.] It is a precious herb of the Sun. Half a dram, or a dram at most, in powder of the roots hereof taken in wine and vinegar, of each equal parts, and the party laid presently to sweat thereupon, is held to be a sovereign remedy for those that are infected with the plague, and have a sore upon them, by expelling the poison and infection, and defending the heart and spirits from danger. It is a singular good wound herb, and is thereupon used with other the like effects in many compound balms for curing of wounds, be they fresh and green, or old and malignant, and especially if the sinews be hurt.

Orchis.

IT hath gotten almost as many several names attributed to the several sorts of it, as would almost fill a sheet of paper, as dog-stones, goat-stones, fool-stones, fox-stones, satyrion

rion, cullians, together with many others too tedious to rehearse.

Descript.] To describe all the several sorts of it were an endless piece of work; therefore I shall only describe the roots, because they are to be used with some discretion. They have each of them a double root within, some of them are round, in others like a hand; these roots alter every year by course, when the one riseth and waxeth full, the other waxeth lank, and perisheth. Now, it is that which is full which is to be used in medicine, the other being either of no use at all, or else according to the humour of some, it destroys and disannuls the virtue of the other, quite undoing what that doth.

Time.] One or other of them may be found in flower from the beginning of April to the latter end of August.

Temperature and Virtues.] They are hot and moist in operation, under the dominion of Dame Venus, and provoke lust exceedingly, which, they say, the dried and withered root do restrain. They are held to kill worms in children; as also, being bruised and applied to the place, to heal the king's evil.

Onions.

THEY are so well known, that I need not spend time about writing a description of them.

Government and Virtues.] Mars owns them, and they have gotten this quality, to draw any corruption to them, for if you peel one, and lay it upon a dunghill, you will find him rotten in half a day, by drawing putrefaction to it; then being bruised and applied to a plague sore, it is very probable it will do the like. Onions are flatulent, or windy, yet they do somewhat provoke appetite, increase thirst, ease the belly and bowels, provoke womens courses, help the biting of a mad dog, and of other venomous creatures, to be used with honey and rue, increase sperm, especially the seed of them. They also kill worms in children, if they drink the water fasting wherein they have been steeped all night. Being roasted under the embers, and eaten with honey, or sugar and oil, they much conduce to help an inveterate cough, and expectorate the tough phlegm. The juice being snuffed up in the nostrils purgeth the head, and helpeth the lethargy (yet the often eating them is said to procure pains in the head.)

head.) It hath been held by divers country people a great preservative against infection, to eat Onions fasting with bread and salt. As also to make a great Onion hollow, filling the place with good treacle, and after to roast it well under the embers, which, after taking away the outermost skin thereof, being beaten together, is a sovereign salve for either plague or sores, or any other putrified ulcer. The juice of Onions is good for either scalding or burning by fire, water, or gunpowder, and used with vinegar, taketh away all blemishes, spots, and marks in the skin; and dropped in the ears, easeth the pains and noise of them. Applied also with figs beaten together, helpeth to ripen and break imposthumes, and other sores.

Leeks are as like them in quality, as the pome water is like an apple: They are a remedy against a surfeit of mushrooms, being baked under the embers and taken; and being boiled and applied very warm, help the piles. In other things they have the same property as the Onions, although not so effectual.

Orpine.

Descript.] COMMON Orpine riseth up with divers round brittle stalks, thick set with flat and fleshy leaves, without any order, and little or nothing dented about the edges, of a green colour. The flowers are white, or whitish, growing in tufts, after which come small chaffy husks, with seeds like dust in them. The roots are divers, thick round, white tuberous clogs, and the plant groweth not so big in some places as in other where it is found.

Place.] It is frequent in almost every county in this land, and is cherished in gardens with us, where it groweth greater than that which is wild, and groweth in shadowy sides of fields and woods.

Time.] It flowereth about July, and the seed is ripe in August.

Government and Virtues.] The Moon owns the herb, and he that knows her exaltation, knows what I say is true. Orpine is seldom used in inward medicines with us, although Tragus saith from experience in Germany, that the distilled water thereof is profitable for gnawings or excoriations in the stomach or bowels, or for ulcers in the lungs, liver, or other inward parts, as also in the matrix, and helpeth all those diseases, being drank for certain days together. It stayeth the sharpness of humours in the bloody-flux, and other fluxes in the body or in wounds. The root thereof also performeth the like effect. It is used outwardly to cool any heat or inflammation upon any hurt or wound, and easeth the pains of them, as also, to heal scaldings or burnings, the juice thereof being beaten with some green salled oil, and anointed. The leaf bruised, and laid to any green wound in the hands or legs, doth heal them quickly; and being bound to the throat, much helpeth the quinsy; it helpeth also ruptures and burstenness. If you please to make the juice thereof into a syrup with honey or sugar, you may safely take a spoonful or two at a time, (let my author say what he will) for a quinsy, and you shall find the medicine more pleasant, and the cure more speedy, than if you had taken dog's turd, which is the vulgar cure.

Parsley.

THIS is so well known, that it needs no description.
Government and Virtues.] It is under the dominion of Mercury, is very comfortable to the stomach; helpeth to provoke urine and women's courses, to break wind both in the stomach and bowels, and doth a little open the body, but the root much more. It openeth obstructions both of liver and spleen, and is therefore accounted one of the five opening roots. Galen commended it against the fallen sickness, and to provoke urine mightily, especially if the roots be boiled, and eaten like parsnips. The seed is effectual to provoke urine and women's courses, to expel wind, to break the stone, and easeth the pains and torments thereof; it is also effectual against the venom of any poisonous creature, and the danger that cometh to them that have the lethargy, and is as good against the cough. The distilled water of Parsley is a familiar medicine with nurses to give their children when they are troubled with wind in the stomach or belly, which they call the frets; and is also much available to them that are of great years. The leaves of Parsley laid to the eyes that are inflamed with heat, or swollen, doth much help them if it be used with bread and meal; and being fried with butter and

The English *Physician Enlarged.*

applied to womens breasts that are hard through the curdling of their milk, it abateth the hardness quickly, and also it taketh away black and blue marks coming of bruises or falls. The juice thereof dropped into the ears with a little wine, easeth the pains. Tragus setteth down an excellent medicine to help the jaundice and falling-sickness, the dropsy, and stone in the kidneys, in this manner. Take of the seed of Parsley, Fennel, Annise, and Carraways, of each an ounce; of the roots of Parsley, Burnet, Saxifrage, and Carraways, of each an ounce and an half, let the seeds be bruised, and the roots washed and cut small, let them lie all night in steep in a bottle of white wine, and in the morning be boiled in a close earthen vessel until a third part or more be wasted; which being strained and cleared, take four ounces thereof morning and evening first and last, abstaining from drink after it for three hours. This openeth obstructions of the liver and spleen, and expelleth the dropsy or jaundice by urine.

Parsley Piert, or Parsley Breakstone.

Descript] THE root, although it be very small and thready, yet it continues many years, from whence arise many leaves lying along on the ground, each standing upon a long small foot stalk, the leaves as broad as a man's nail, very deeply dented on the edges, somewhat like a parsley leaf, but of a very dusky green colour. The stalks are very weak and slender, about three or four fingers in length, yet so full of leaves that they can hardly be seen, either having no foot stalk at all, or but very short; the flowers are so small they can hardly be seen, and the seed as small as may be.

Place] It is a common herb throughout the nation, and groweth in barren, sandy, moist places. It may be found plentifully about Hampstead Heath, Hyde Park, and in Tothill fields.

Time] It may be found all the Summer-time, even from the beginning of April to the end of October.

Government and Virtues] It is a very good and present to provoke urine, and to break the stone. It is a very good sallad herb. It were good the gentry would pickle it up as they pickle up samphire for their use all the Winter. I cannot teach them how to do it; yet this I can tell them, it is a very wholesome herb. They may also keep the herb dry or in a syrup, if they please. You may take a dram of the powder of it in white wine; it would bring away gravel from the kidneys sensibly, and without pain. It also helps the stranguary.

Parsnip.

THE garden kind thereof is so well known (the root being commonly eaten) that I shall not trouble you with any description of it. But the wild kind being of more physical use, I shall in this place describe it unto you.

Descript.] The wild Parsnip differeth little from the garden, but groweth not so fair and large, nor hath so many leaves, and the root is shorter, more woody, and not so fit to be eaten, and therefore more medicinal.

Place] The name of the first sheweth the place of its growth. The other groweth wild in divers places, as in the marsh by Rochester, and elsewhere, and flowereth in July, the seed being ripe about the beginning of August, the second year after the sowing. For if they do flower the first year, the country people call them Madneps.

Government and Virtues] The garden Parsnips are under Venus. The garden Parsnip nourisheth much, and is good and wholesome nourishment, but a little windy, wherefore it is thought to procure bodily lust; but it fatteneth the body much, if much used. It is conducible to the stomach and reins, and provoketh urine. But the wild Parsnip hath a cutting, attenuating, cleansing, and opening quality therein. It resisteth and helpeth the bitings of serpents, easeth the pains and stitches in the sides, and dissolveth wind both in the stomach and bowels, which is the cholic, and provoketh urine. The root is often used, but the seed much more. The wild being better than the tame, shews Dame Nature to be the best physician.

Cow Parsnip.

Descript.] THIS groweth with three or four large, spread winged, rough leaves, lying often on the ground, or else raised a little from it, with long, round, hairy foot-stalks under them, parted usually into five divisions, the two couple standing each against the other, and one at the end, and each leaf being almost round, yet somewhat deeply
cut

cut in on the edges in some leaves, and not so deep in others, of a whitish green colour, smelling somewhat strongly; among which riseth up a round, crusted, hairy stalk, two or three feet high, with a few joints and leaves thereon, and branched at the top, where stand large umbels of white, and sometimes reddish flowers, and after them flat, whitish, thin, winged seed, two always joined together. The root is long and white, with two or three long strings growing down into the ground, smelling likewise strongly and unpleasant.

Place.] It groweth in moist meadows, and the borders and corners of fields, and near ditches, through this land.

Time.] It flowereth in July, and seedeth in August.

Government and Virtues] Mercury hath the dominion over them. The seed thereof, as Galen saith, is of a sharp and cutting quality, and therefore is a fit medicine for coughs and shortness of breath, the falling sickness and jaundice. The root is available to all the purposes aforesaid, and is also of great use to take away the hard skin that groweth on a fistula, if it be but scraped upon it. The seed hereof being drank, cleanseth the belly from tough phlegmatic water therein, easeth them that are liver grown, womens passions of the mother, as well being drank as the smoke thereof received underneath, and likewise riseth such as are fallen into a deep sleep, or have the lethargy, by burning it under their nose. The seed and root boiled in oil, and the head rubbed therewith, helpeth not only those that are fallen into a frenzy, but also the lethargy or drowsy evil, and those that have been long troubled with the head-ach, if it be likewise used with rue. It helpeth also the running scab and the shingles. The juice of the flowers dropped into the ears that run and are full of matter, cleanseth and healeth them.

The Peach-Tree.

Descript] A Peach Tree groweth not so great as the Apricot-Tree, yet spreadeth branches reasonably well, from whence spring smaller reddish twigs, whereon are set long and narrow green leaves dented about the edges. The blossoms are greater than the plum, and of a light purple colour, the fruit round, and sometimes as big as a reasonable pippin, others smaller, as also differing in colour and taste, as russet, red, or yellow, waterish or firm, with a frize or cotton all over, with a cleft therein like an apricot, and a rugged, furrowed, great stone within it, and a bitter kernel within the stone. It sooner waxeth old, and decayeth, than the apricot, by much.

Place.] They are nursed in gardens and orchards through this land.

Time.] They flower in the Spring, and fructify in Autumn.

Government and Virtues.] Lady Venus owns this Tree, and by it opposeth the ill effects of Mars, and indeed for children and young people nothing is better to purge choler and the jaundice, than the leaves or flowers of this tree, being made into a syrup or conserve: let such as delight to please their lust regard the fruit; but such as have lost their health, and their children let them regard what I say, they may safely give two spoonfuls of the syrup at a time, it is as gentle as Venus herself. The leaves of peaches bruised and laid on the belly, kill worms; and so they do also being boiled in ale and drank, and open the belly likewise; and being dried is a safer medicine to discuss humours. The powder of them strewed upon fresh bleeding wounds stayeth their bleeding and closeth them up. The flowers steeped all night in a little wine standing warm, strained forth in the morning, and drank fasting, doth gently open the belly, and move it downward. A syrup made of them, as the syrup of roses is made, worketh more forcibly than that of roses, for it provoketh vomiting, and spendeth waterish and hydropic humours by the continuance thereof. The flowers made into a conserve, worketh the same effect. The liquor that droppeth from the tree, being wounded, is given in the decoction of Colt-foot, to those that are troubled with the cough or shortness of breath, by adding thereto some sweet wine, and putting some saffron also therein. It is good for those that are hoarse, or have lost their voice; helpeth all defects of the lungs, and those that vomit and spit blood. Two drams hereof given in the juice of lemons, or of radish is good for them that are troubled with the stone. The kernels of the stones do wonderfully ease the pains and wringings of the belly, through wind or sharp humours, and help to make an excellent medicine for the stone upon all occasions, in this manner. I take fifty kernels of peach stones, and one hundred kernels of the cherry stones, a handful of elder flowers fresh or dried, and three pints of muscadel, set them in a close pot into a bed of horse dung for ten days, after which distil in a glass with a gentle fire, and keep it for your use. You may drink upon occasion three or four ounces at a time. The milk or cream of these kernels being drawn forth with some vervain water, and applied to forehead and temples, doth much help to procure rest and sleep to sick persons wanting it. The oil drawn from the kernels, the temples being therewith anointed, doth the like. The said oil put into clysters easeth the pains of the wind colic; and anointed on the lower part of the belly doth the like, and dropped into the ears easeth pains in them; the juice of the leaves doth the like. Being also anointed on the forehead and temples, it helpeth the megrim, and all other parts in the head. If the kernels be bruised and boiled in vinegar, until they become thick, and applied to the head, it marvellously procures the hair to grow again upon bald places, or where it is too thin.

The Pear-Tree.

PEAR-Trees are so well known, that they need no description.

Government and Virtues.] The tree belongs to Venus, and so doth the apple tree. For their physical use they are best discerned by their taste. All the sweet and luscious sorts, whether manured or wild, do help to move the belly downwards, more or less. Those that are hard and sour, do, on the contrary, bind the belly as much, and the leaves do so also. Those that are moist do in some sort cool, but harsh or wild sorts much more, and are very good in repelling medicines; and if the wild sort be boiled with mushrooms, it makes them less dangerous. The said Pears boiled with a little honey helps much the oppressed stomach, as all sorts of them do, some more, some less; but the harsher sorts do more cool and bind, serving well to be bound in green wounds, to cool and stay the blood, and to heal up the wound without farther trouble, or inflammation, as Galen saith he found it by experience. The wild Pears do sooner close up the lips of green wounds than others.

Schola

Schola Salerni adviseth to drink much wine after Pears, or else (say they) they are as bad as poison, nay, and they curse the tree for it too, but if a poor man find his stomach oppressed by eating Pears, it is but working hard, and it will do as well as drinking wine.

Pellitory of Spain.

COMMON Pellitory of Spain, if it be planted in our gardens, will prosper very well, yet there is one sort growing ordinarily here wild, which I esteem to be little inferior to the other, if at all. I shall not deny you the description of them both.

Descript.] Common Pellitory is a very common plant, and will not be kept in our gardens without diligent looking to. The root goes down right into the ground, bearing leaves, being long and finely cut upon the stalk, lying on the ground, much larger than the leaves of the camomile are. At the top it bears one single large flower at a place, having a border of many leaves, white on the upper side, and reddish underneath, with a yellow thrum in the middle, not standing so close as that of camomile doth.

The other common Pellitory which groweth here, hath a root of a sharp biting taste, scarce discernible by the taste from that before described, from whence arise divers brittle stalks, a yard high and more, with narrow long leaves finely dented about the edges, standing one above another up to the tops. The flowers are many and white, standing in tufts like those of yarrow, with a small, yellowish thrum in the middle. The seed is very small.

Place.] The last groweth in fields in the hedges sides and paths almost every where.

Time.] It flowereth at the latter end of June and July.

Government and Virtues.] It is under the government of Mercury, and I am persuaded it is one of the best purgers of the brain that grows. An ounce of the juice taken in a draught of muscadel an hour before the fit of the ague comes, it will assuredly drive away the ague at the second or third time taking at the farthest. Either the herb or root dried and chewed in the mouth, purgeth the brain of phlegmatic humours, thereby not only easing pains in the head and teeth, but also hindereth the distilling of the brain upon the lungs and eyes, thereby preventing coughs, phthisicks and consumptions,

consumptions, the apoplexy and falling sickness. It is an excellent approved remedy in the lethargy. The powder of the herb or root being snuffed up the nostrils, procureth sneezing, and easeth the head ach; being made into an ointment with hog's grease, it takes away black and blue spots occasioned by blows or falls, and helps both the gout and sciatica.

Pellitory of the Wall.

Descript.] IT riseth with brownish, red, tender, weak, clear, and almost transparent stalks, about two feet high, upon which grow at the joints two leaves somewhat broad and long, of a dark green colour, which afterwards turn brownish, smooth on the edges, but rough and hairy, as the stalks are also. At the joints with the leaves from the middle of the stalk upwards, where it spreadeth into branches, stand many small, pale, purplish flowers in hairy rough heads, or husks, after which come small, black, rough seed, which will stick to any cloth or garment that shall touch it. The root is somewhat long, with small fibres thereat, of a dark reddish colour, which abideth the Winter, although the stalks and leaves perish and spring every year.

Place] It groweth wild generally through the land, about the borders of fields, and on the sides of walls, and among rubbish. It will endure well being brought up in gardens, and planted on the shady side, where it will spring of its own sowing.

Time] It flowereth in June and July, and the seed is ripe soon after.

Government and Virtues] It is under the dominion of Mercury. The dried herb Pellitory made up into an electuary with honey, or the juice of the herb, or the decoction thereof made up with sugar or honey, is a singular remedy for an old or dry cough, the shortness of breath, and wheezing in the throat. Three ounces of the juice thereof taken at a time, doth wonderfully help stopping of the urine and to expel the stone or gravel in the kidneys or bladder, and is therefore usually put among other herbs used in clysters, to mitigate pains in the back, sides, or bowels, proceeding of wind, stopping of urine, the gravel or stone as aforesaid. If the bruised herb, sprinkled with some muscadel, be warmed upon a tile, or in a dish upon a few quick coals

coals in a chafing-dish, and applied to the belly, it worketh the same effect. The decoction of the herb, being drank, easeth pains of the mother, and bringeth down women's courses. It also easeth those griefs that arise from obstructions of the liver, spleen and reins. The same decoction, with a little honey added thereto, is good to gargle a sore throat. The juice held a-while in the mouth easeth pains in the teeth. The distilled water of the herb drank with some sugar worketh the same effects, and cleanseth the skin from spots, freckles, purples, wheals, sun burn, morphew, &c. The juice dropped into the ears easeth the noise in them, and taketh away the pricking and shooting pains therein. The same, or the distilled water, assuageth hot and swelling imposthumes, burning, and scaldings by fire or water, as also all other hot tumours and inflammations, or breakings out of heat, being bathed often with wet cloths dipped therein. The said juice made into a liniment with ceruse, and oil of roses, and anointed therewith, cleanseth foul rotten ulcers, and stayeth spreading or creeping ulcers, and running scabs or sores in childrens heads, and helpeth to stay the hair from falling off the head: The said ointment, or the herb applied to the fundament, openeth the piles and easeth their pains; and being mixed with goats tallow, helpeth the gout: The juice is very effectual to cleanse fistulas, and to heal them up safely, or the herb itself bruised and applied with a little salt. It is likewise also effectual to heal any green wound, if it be bruised and bound thereto for three days, you shall need no other medicine to heal it further. A poultice made hereof with mallows, and boiled in wine and wheat bran and bean flower, and some oil put thereto, and applied warm to any bruised sinew, tendon, or muscle, doth in a very short time restore them to their strength, taking away the pains of the bruises, and dissolveth the congealed blood coming of blows, or falls from high places.

The juice of Pellitory of the Wall clarified and boiled in a syrup with honey, and a spoonful of it drank every morning by such as are subject to the dropsy, if continuing that course, though but once a week, if ever they have the dropsy, let them come but to me, and I will cure them gratis.

Penn-

Pennyroyal.

PENNYROYAL is so well known unto all, I mean the common kind, that it needeth no description.

There is a greater kind than the ordinary sort found wild with us, which so abideth being brought into gardens, and differeth not from it, but only in the largeness of the leaves and stalks, in rising higher and not creeping upon the ground so much. The flowers whereof are purple, growing in rundles about the stalks like the other.

Place] The first, which is common in gardens, groweth also in many moist and watery places of this land.

The second is found wild in effect in divers places by the highways from London to Colchester, and thereabouts, more abundantly than in any other countries, and is also planted in the gardens in Essex.

Time] They flower in the latter end of Summer, about August.

Government and Virtues] The herb is under Venus. Dioscorides saith, that Pennyroyal maketh thin tough phlegm, warmeth the coldness of any part whereto it is applied, and digesteth raw or corrupt matter: Being boiled and drank, it provoketh womens courses, and expelleth the dead child and after birth, and stayeth the disposition to vomit being taken in water and vinegar mingled together. And being mingled with honey and salt, it voideth phlegm out of the lungs, and purgeth melancholy by the stool. Drank with wine, it helpeth such as are bitten and stung with venomous beasts, and applied to the nostrils with vinegar, reviveth those that are fainting and swooning. Being dried and burnt, it strengtheneth the gums. It is helpful to those that are troubled with the gout, being applied of itself to the place until it was red, and applied in a plaister, it takes away spots or marks in the face, applied with salt it profiteth those that are splenetic, or liver-grown. The decoction doth help the itch, it washed therewith, being put into baths for women to sit therein, it helpeth the swellings and hardness of the mother. The green herb bruised and put into vinegar cleanseth foul ulcers, and taketh away the marks of bruises and blows about the eyes, and all discolourings of the face by fire, yea, and the leprosy, being drank and outwardly applied. Boiled in wine with honey and salt, it helpeth the toothach. It helpeth the cold griefs of the joints,

taking

taking away the pains, and warmeth the cold part, being fast bound to the place, after a bathing or sweating in an hot house. Pliny addeth, that Pennyroyal and mints together, help faintings, being put into vinegar, and smelled unto, or put into the nostrils or mouth. It easeth head achs, pains of the breast and belly, and gnawing of the stomach; applied with honey, salt, and vinegar, it helpeth cramps, or convulsions of the sinews: Boiled in milk, and drank, it is effectual for the cough, and for ulcers and sores in the mouth; drank in wine it provoketh womens courses, and expelleth the dead child, and after birth. Matthiolus saith, the decoction thereof being drank, helpeth the jaundice and toyle, all pains of the head and sinew that come of a cold cause, and cleareth the eye-sight. It helpeth the lethargy, and applied with barley meal, helpeth burnings; and put into the ears easeth the pains of them.

Male and Female Peony.

Descript.] MALE Peony riseth up with brown stalks, whereon grow green and reddish leaves, upon a stalk without any particular division in the leaf at all. The flowers stand at the top of the stalk, consisting of five or six broad leaves, of a fair purplish red colour, with many yellow threads in the middle standing about the head, which after riseth up to be the seed-vessel, divided into two, three, or four crooked pods like horns, which being full ripe, open and turn themselves down backward, shewing within them divers round, black shining seeds, having also many crimson grains, intermixed with black, whereby it maketh a very pretty shew. The roots are great, thick and long, spreading and running down deep in the ground.

The ordinary Female Peony hath as many stalks, and more leaves on them than the Male; the leaves not so large, but nicked on the edges, some with great and deep, others with smaller cuts and divisions, of a dead green colour. The flowers are of a strong heady scent, usually smaller, and of a more purple colour than the Male, with yellow thrums about the head as the Male hath. The seed vessels are like horns, as in the Male, but smaller, the seed is black, but less shining. The roots consist of many short tuberous clogs, fastened at the end of long things, and all from the heads of the roots, which is thick and short, and of the like scent with the Male.

Place and Time] They grow in gardens, and flower usually about May

Government and Virtues.] It is an herb of the Sun, and under the Lion. Physicians say, Male Peony roots are best; but Dr Reason told me Male Peony was best for men, and Female Peony for women, and he desires to be judged by his brother Dr Experience. The roots are held to be of more virtue than the seed; next the flowers, and last of all, the leaves. The root of the Male Peony, fresh gathered, having been found by experience to cure the falling sickness: but the surest way is, besides hanging it about the neck by which chil ren have been cured, to take the root of the Male Peony washed clean, and stamped somewhat small, and laid to infuse in sack for 24 hours at the least, afterwards strain it, and take it first and last morning and evening, a good draught for sundry days together, before and after a full moon, and this will also cure older persons, if the disease be not grown too old, and past cure, especially if there be a due and orderly preparation of the body with posset drink made of betony &c. The root is also effectual for women that are not sufficiently cleansed after child birth, and such as are troubled with the mother; for which likewise the black seed beaten to powder, and given in wine, is also available. The black seed also taken before bed time and in the morning, is very effectual for such as in their sleep are troubled with the disease called Ephialte, or Incubus, but we do commonly call it the Night mare; a disease which melancholy persons are subject unto. It is also good against melancholy dreams. The distilled water or syrup made of the flowers, worketh the same effects that the root and the seed do, although more weakly. The Female is often used for the purposes aforesaid by reason the Male is so scarce a plant, that it is possessed by few, and those great lovers of rarities in this kind.

Pepperwort, or Dittander.

Descript] OUr common Pepperwort sendeth forth somewhat long and broad leaves of a light bluish greenish colour, finely dented about the edges, and pointed ed at the ends, standing upon round hard stalks, three or four feet high, spreading many branches on all sides, and having many small white flowers at the tops of them, after which follow small seeds in small heads. The root is slender, running much under ground, and shooting up again in many places, and both leaves and roots are very hot and sharp of taste, like pepper, for which cause it took the name.

Place] It groweth naturally in many places of this land, as at Clare in Essex; also near unto Exeter in Devonshire, upon Rochester Common in Kent; in Lancashire, and divers other places; but usually kept in gardens.

Time] It flowereth in the end of June, and in July.

Government and Virtues.] Here is another martial herb for you, make much of it. Pliny and Paulus Ægineta say, that Pepperwort is very successful for the sciatica, or any other gout or pain in the joints, or any other inveterate grief. The leaves hereof to be bruised, and mixed with old hog's grease, and applied to the place, and to continue thereon four hours in men, and two hours in women, the place being afterwards bathed with wine and oil mixed together, and then wrapt up with wool or skins, after they have sweat a little. It also amendeth the deformities or discolourings of the skin, and helpeth to take away marks, scars, and scabs, or the foul marks of burning with fire or iron. The juice hereof is by some used to be given in ale to drink to women with child, to procure them a speedy delivery in travail.

Periwinkle.

Descript] THE common sort hereof hath many branches trailing or running upon the ground shooting out small fibres at the joints as it runneth, taking thereby hold in the ground, and rooteth in divers places. At the joints of these branches stand two small, dark green, shining leaves, somewhat like bay leaves but smaller, and with them come forth also the flowers (one at a joint) standing upon a tender foot stalk, being somewhat long and hollow, parted at the brims sometimes into four, sometimes into five leaves. The most ordinary sorts are of a pale blue colour; some are pure white, and some of a dark reddish purple colour. The root is little bigger than a rush, bushing in the ground, and creeping

creeping with his branches far about, whereby it quickly possesseth a great compass, and is therefore most usually planted under hedges where it may have room to run.

Place.] Those with the pale blue, and those with the white flowers, grow in woods and orchards, by the hedge-sides, in divers places of this land, but those with the purple flowers in gardens only.

Time.] They flower in March and April.

Temperature and Virtues] Venus owns this herb, and saith, That the leaves eaten by man and wife together, cause love between them. The Periwinkle is a great binder, stayeth bleeding both at the mouth and nose, if some of the leaves be chewed. The French use it to stay womens courses. Dioscorides, Galen, and Ægineta, commended it against the lasks and fluxes of the belly to be drank in wine.

St Peter's Wort.

IF Superstition had not been the father of Tradition, as well as Ignorance the mother of Devotion, this herb, (as well as St John's Wort) had found some other name to be known by, but we may say of our forefathers, as St Paul of the Athenians, *I perceive in many things you are too superstitious.* Yet seeing it is come to pass, that custom having got in possession, pleads prescription for the name, I shall let it pass, and come to the description of the herb, which take as followeth.

Descript] It riseth up with square upright stalks for the most part, some greater and higher than St John's Wort (and good reason too, St Peter being the greater apostle, ask the Pope else; for though God would have the saints equal, the Pope is of another opinion) but brown in the same manner, having two leaves at every joint, somewhat like, but larger than St John's Wort, and a little rounder pointed, with few or no holes to be seen thereon, and having sometimes some smaller leaves rising from the bosom of the greater, and sometimes a little hairy also. At the tops of two stalks stand many flat like flowers, with yellow threads in the middle, very like those of St John's Wort, insomuch that this is hardly discerned from it, but only by the largeness and height, the seed being alike also in both. The root abideth long, sending forth new shoots every year.

Place]

Place] It groweth in many groves, and small low woods, in divers places of this land, as in Kent, Huntingdon, Cambridge, and Northamptonshire; as also near water courses in other places.

Time] It flowereth in June and July, and the seed is ripe in August.

Government and Virtues.] There is not a straw to choose between this and St. John's Wort, only St. Peter must have it, lest he should want pot herbs. It is of the same property of St. John's Wort, but somewhat weak, and therefore more seldom used. Two drams of the seed taken at a time in honeyed water, purgeth choleric humours (as saith Dioscorides, Pliny, and Galen) and therefore helpeth those that are troubled with the sciatica. The leaves are used as St John's Wort, to help those places of the body that have been burnt with fire.

Pimpernel.

Descript.] COMMON Pimpernel hath divers weak square stalks lying on the ground, beset all with two small and almost round leaves at every joint, one against another, very like chickweed, but hath no foot-stalks; for the leaves, as it were, compass the stalk. The flower stand singly each by themselves at them and the stalk, consisting of five small round-pointed leaves, of a pale red colour, tending to an orange, with so many threads in the middle, in whose places succeed smooth round heads, wherein is contained small seed. The root is small and fibrous, perishing every year.

Place] It groweth every where almost, as well in the meadows and corn fields, as by the way sides, and in gardens, arising of itself.

Time] It flowereth from May until April, and the seed ripeneth in the mean time, and falleth.

Government and Virtues] It is a gallant solar herb, of a cleansing attractive quality, whereby it draweth forth thorns or splinters, or other such like thing gotten into the flesh; and put up into the nostrils, purgeth the head; and Galen saith also, they have a drying faculty, whereby they are good to solder the lips of wounds, and to cleanse foul ulcers. The distilled water or juice is much esteemed by French dames to cleanse the skin from any roughness,

deformity,

deformity, or discolouring thereof; being boiled in wine and given to drink, it is a good remedy against the plague, and other pestilential fevers, if the party after taking it be warm in his bed, and sweat for two hours after, and use the same for twice at least. It helpeth also all stingings and bitings of venomous beasts, or mad dogs, being used inwardly, and applied outwardly. The same also openeth obstructions of the liver, and is very available against the infirmities of the reins: It provoketh urine, and helpeth to expel the stone and gravel out of the kidneys and bladder, and helpeth much in all inward pains and ulcers. The decoction, or distilled water, is no less effectual to be applied to all wounds that are fresh and green, or old, filthy, fretting, and running ulcers, which it very effectually cureth in a short space. A little mixed with the juce, and dropped into the eyes, cleanseth them from cloudy mists, or thick films which grow over them, and hinder the sight. It helpeth the tooth-ach, being dropped into the ear on the contrary side of the pain. It is also effectual to ease the pains of the hæmorrhoids or piles.

Ground Pine, or Chamepitys.

Descript] OUR common Ground Pine groweth low, seldom rising above an hand's breadth high, shooting forth divers small branches set with slender, small, long, narrow, greyish, or whitish leaves, somewhat hairy, and divided into three parts, many bushing together at a joint, some growing scatteringly upon the stalks, smelling somewhat strong, like unto rosin. The flowers are small, and of a pale yellow colour, growing from the joint of the stalk all along among the leaves, after which come small and round husks. The root is small and woody, perishing every year.

Place] It groweth more plentifully in Kent than any other county of this land, as namely, in many places on this side Dartford, along to Southfleet, Chatham, and Rochester, and upon Chatham Down, hard by the Beacon, and half a mile from Rochester, in a field nigh a house called Selefys.

Time] It flowereth and giveth seed in the summer months.

Government and Virtues] Mars owns the herb. The decoction of Ground Pine drunk, doth wonderfully prevail against the stranguary, or any inward pains arising from the diseases of the reins and urine, and is special good for all obstructions of the liver and spleen, and gently openeth the body; for which purpose they were wont in former times to make pills with the powder thereof, and the pulp of figs. It marvellously helpeth all the diseases of the mother, inwardly or outwardly applied, procuring womens courses, and expelling the dead child and after birth; yea, it is so powerful upon these feminine parts, that it is utterly forbidden for women with child, for it will cause abortion or delivery before the time. The decoction of the herb in wine taken inwardly, or applied outwardly, or both, for some time together, is also effectual in all pains and diseases of the joints, as gouts, cramps, palsies, sciatica, and achs; for which purpose the pills made with powder of Ground Pine, and of hermodactils with Venice turpentine are very effectual. The pills also, continued for some time, are special good for those that have the dropsy, jaundice, and for griping pains of the joints, belly, or inward parts. It helpeth also all diseases of the brain, proceeding of cold and phlegmatic humours and distillations, as also for the falling sickness. It is a special remedy for the poison of the aconites, and other poisonous herbs, as also against the stinging of any venomous creature. It is a good remedy for a cold cough especially in the beginning. For all the purposes aforesaid, the herb being tunned up in new drink and drank, is almost as effectual, but far more acceptable to weak and dainty stomachs. The distilled water of the herb hath the same effects, but more weakly. The conserve of the flowers doth the like, which Matthiolus much commendeth against the palsy. The green herb, or the decoction thereof, being applied, dissolveth the hardness of womens breasts, and all other hard swellings in any other part of the body. The green herb also applied, or the juice thereof with some honey, not only cleanseth putrid, stinking, foul, and malignant ulcers and sores of all sorts, but healeth and soldereth up the lips of green wounds in any part also. Let women forbear, if they be with child, for it works violently upon the feminine part.

Plantain.

THIS groweth usually in meadows and fields, and by path sides, and is so well known, that it needeth no description.

Time)

Time]- It is in its beauty about June, and the seed ripeneth shortly after.

Government and Virtues] It is true, Mizaldus and others, yea, almost all astrology physicians hold this to be an herb of Mars, because it cures the diseases of the head and privities, which are under the houses of Mars, Aries, and Scorpio: The truth is, it is under the command of Venus, and cures the head by antipathy to Mars, and the privities by sympathy to Venus; neither is there hardly a martial disease but it cures.

The juice of Plantain clarified and drank for divers days together, either of itself or in other drink, prevaileth wonderfully against all torments or excoriations in the guts or bowels, helpeth the distillations of rheum from the head, and stayeth all manner of fluxes, even womens courses, when they flow too abundantly. It is good to stay spitting of blood, and other bleedings at the mouth, or the making of foul and bloody water, by reason of any ulcer in the reins or bladder, and also stayeth the too free bleeding of wounds. It is held an especial remedy for those that are troubled with the phthisic, or consumption of the lungs, or ulcers of the lungs, or coughs that come of heat. The decoction or powder of the roots or seeds is much more binding for all the purposes aforesaid than the leaves. Dioscorides saith, that the roots boiled in wine and taken, helpeth the tertian ague and for the quartan ague (but letting the number pass as fabulous) I conceive the decoction of divers roots may be effectual. The herb (but especially the seed) is held to be profitable against the dropsy, the falling sickness, the yellow jaundice, and stoppings of the liver and reins. The roots of Plantain, and Pellitory of Spain, beaten into powder, and put into the hollow teeth, taketh away the pains of them. The clarified juice or distilled water dropped into the eyes, cooleth the inflammations in them, and taketh away the pin and web; and dropped into the ears, easeth the pains in them, and helpeth and removeth the heat. The same also with the juice of houseleek is profitable against all inflammations and breakings out of the skin, and against burnings and scaldings by fire and water. The juice or decoction made either of itself, or other things of the like nature, is of much use and good effect for old and hollow ulcers that are hard to be cured, and for cankers and sores in the mouth or privy parts of man or woman, and helpeth also the pains of the piles in the fundament. The juice mixed with oil of roses, and the temples and forehead anointed therewith, easeth the pains of the head proceeding from heat, and helpeth lunatic and frantic persons very much; as also the biting of serpents, or a mad dog. The same also is profitably applied to all hot gouts in the feet or hands, especially in the beginning. It is also good to be applied where any bone is out of joint, to hinder inflammations, swellings, and pain that presently rise thereupon. The powder of the dried leaves taken in drink killeth the worms of the belly, and boiled in wine, killeth worms that breed in old and foul ulcers. One part of Plantain water, and two parts of the brine of powdered beef, boiled together and clarified, is a most sure remedy to heal all spreading scabs or itch in the head and body, all manner of tetters, ringworms, the shingles, and all other running and fretting sores. Briefly, the Plantains are singular good wound herbs to heal fresh or old wounds or sores, either inward or outward.

Plums.

ARE so well known, that they need no description.
Government and Virtues] All Plums are under Venus, and are like women, some better, some worse. As there is great diversity of kinds, so there is in the operation of Plums, for some that are sweet moisten the stomach, and make the belly soluble, those that are sour quench thirst more, and bind the belly; the moist and waterish do sooner corrupt in the stomach, but the firm do nourish more, and offend less. The dried fruit sold by the grocers under the name of Damask Prunes, do somewhat loosen the belly, and being stewed, are often used, both in health and sickness, to relish the mouth and stomach, to procure appetite, and a little to open the body, allay choler, and cool the stomach. Plum tree leaves boiled in wine, are good to wash and gargle the mouth and throat, to dry the flux of rheum coming to the palate, gums, or almonds of the ears. The gum of the tree is good to break the stone. The gum of leaves boiled in vinegar, and applied, kills tetters and ringworms. Matthiolus saith, the oil pressed out of the kernels of the stone, as oil of almonds is made, is good against the inflamed piles,

and

and tumours or swellings of ulcers, hoarseness of the voice, roughness of the tongue and throat, and likewise the pains in the ears. And that five ounces of the said oil taken with one ounce of muscadel, driveth forth the stone, and helpeth the colic.

Polypody of the Oak.

Descript] THIS is a small herb consisting of nothing but roots and leaves, bearing neither stalk, flower, nor seed, as it is thought. It hath three or four leaves rising from the root, every one single by itself, of about a hand length, are winged, consisting of many small narrow leaves, cut into the middle rib, standing on each side of the stalk, large below and smaller up to the top, not dented nor notched at the edges at all, as the male fern hath, of a sad green colour, and smooth on the upper side, but on the other side somewhat rough by reason of some yellowish spots set thereon. The root is smaller than one's little finger, lying aslope, or creeping along under the upper crust of the earth, brownish on the outside and greenish within, of a sweetish harshness in taste, set with certain rough knags on each side thereof, having also much mossiness or yellow hairiness upon it, and some fibres underneath it, whereby it is nourished.

Place] It groweth as well upon old rotten stumps, or trunks of trees, as oak, beech, hazel, willow, or any other, as in the woods under them, and upon old mud walls, as also in mossy, stoney, and gravelly places near unto wood. That which groweth upon oak is accounted the best; but the quantity thereof is scarce sufficient for the common use.

Time] It being always green, may be gathered for use at any time.

Government and Virtues] And why, I pray, must Polypodium of the Oak only be used, gentle college of physicians? Can you give me but a glimpse of reason for it? It is only because it is dearest. Will you never leave your covetousness till your lives leave you? The truth is, that which grows upon the earth is best ('tis an herb of Saturn, and he seldom climbs trees) to purge melancholy; if the humour be otherwise, chuse you Polypodium accordingly. Meuse (who is called the physician's evangelist, for the certainty of his medicines, and the truth of his opinion) saith, That it drieth up thin humours, digesteth thick and tough, and purgeth burnt choler, especially tough and thick phlegm, and thin phlegm also, even from the joints, and therefore good for those that are troubled with melancholy, or quartan agues, especially if it be taken in whey or honeyed water, or in barley water, or the broth of a chicken with epithymum, or with beets and mallows. It is good for the hardness of the spleen, and for prickings or stitches in the sides, as also for the colic. Some use to put to it some fennel seeds, or annise seeds, or ginger, to correct that loathing it bringeth to the stomach which is more than it needeth, being a safe and gentle medicine, fit for all persons which daily experience confirmeth, and an ounce of it may be given at a time in a decoction, if there be not senna, or some other strong purger put with it. A dram or two of the powder of the dried roots taken fasting in a cup of honeyed water worketh gently, and for the purposes aforesaid. The distilled water, both of roots and leaves, is much more commended for the quartan ague, to be taken for many days together, as also against melancholy, or fearful and troublesome sleeps or dreams; and with some sugar candy dissolved therein, is good against the cough, shortness of breath, and wheezings, and those distillations of thin rheum upon the lungs, which cause phthisics, and oftentimes consumptions. The fresh roots beaten small, or the powder of the dried roots mixed with honey, and applied to the member that is out of joint, doth much help it; and applied also to the nose, cureth the disease called Polypus, which is a piece of flesh growing therein, and in time stoppeth the passage of breath through that nostril; and it helpeth those clefts or chops that come between the fingers or toes.

The Poplar Tree.

THERE are two sorts of Poplars, which are most familiar with us, viz. the Black and White, both which I shall here describe unto you.

Descript.] The white Poplar groweth great and reasonably high, covered with thick, smooth, white bark, especially the branches, having long leaves cut into several divisions almost like a vine leaf, but not of so deep a green on the upper side, and hoary white underneath, of a reasonable good

good scent, the whole form representing the form of Colts-foot. The catkins which it bringeth forth before the leaves, are long, and of a faint reddish colour, which fall away, bearing seldom good seed with them. The wood hereof is smooth, soft, and white, very finely waved, whereby it is much esteemed.

The Black Poplar groweth higher and straiter than the White, with a greyish bark bearing broad green leaves, somewhat like ivy leaves, not cut in on the edges like the White, but whole and dented, ending in a point, and not white underneath, hanging by slender long foot stalks, which with the air are continually shaken like as the aspen leaves are. The catkins hereof are greater than those of the white, composed of many round green berries, as if they were set together in a long cluster, containing much downy matter, which being ripe is blown away with the wind. The clammy buds hereof, before they spread into leaves, are gathered to make Unguentum Populneum, and are of a yellowish green colour, and small, somewhat sweet, but strong. The wood is smooth, tough and white, and easy to be cloven. On both these trees groweth a sweet kind of musk, which in former times was used to put into sweet ointments.

Place] They grow in moist woods, and by water sides in sundry places of this land, yet the White is not so frequent as the other.

Time] Their time is likewise expressed before. The catkins coming forth before the leaves in the end of Summer.

Government and Virtues] Saturn hath dominion over both. White Poplar, saith Galen, is of a cleansing property. The weight of one ounce in powder of the bark thereof being drank, saith Dioscorides, is a remedy for those that are troubled with the sciatica, or the stranguary. The juice of the leaves dropped warm into the ears, easeth the pains in them. The young clammy buds or eyes before they break out into leaves, bruised, and a little honey put to them, is a good medicine for a dull sight. The Black Poplar is held to be more cooling than the white, and therefore the leaves bruised with vinegar and applied, help the gout. The seed drank in vinegar, is held good against the falling sickness. The water that droppeth from the hollow places of this tree taketh away warts, pushes, wheals, and other the like breakings out of the body. The young Black Poplar buds, saith

Matthiolus,

Matthiolus, are much used by women to beautify their hair, bruising them with fresh butter, straining them after they have been kept for some time in the Sun. The ointment called Populneum, which is made of this Poplar, is singular good for all heat and inflammations in any part of the body, and tempereth the heat of wounds. It is much used to dry up the milk of womens breasts, when they have weaned their children.

Poppy.

OF this I shall describe three kinds, viz. the white and black of the garden, and the Erratick Wild Poppy, or Corn Rose.

Descript] The White Poppy hath at first four or five whitish green leaves lying upon the ground, which rise with the stalk, compassing it at the bottom of them, and are very large, much cut or torn on the edges, and dented also besides. The stalk, which is usually four or five feet high, hath sometimes no branches at the top, and usually but two or three at most, bearing every one but one head wrapped up in a thin skin, which boweth down before it is ready to blow, and then rising, and being broken, the flower within it spreading itself open, and consisting of four very large, white round leaves, with many whitish round threads in the middle, set about a small, round, green head, having a crown, or star like cover at the head thereof, which growing ripe, becomes as large as a great apple, wherein are contained a great number of small round seeds in several partitions or divisions next unto the shell, the middle thereof remaining hollow and empty. The whole plant, both leaves, stalks and heads, while they are fresh, young and green, yield a milk when they are broken, of an unpleasant bitter taste, almost ready to provoke casting, and of a strong heady smell, which being condensate, is called Opium. The root is white and woody, perishing as soon as it hath given ripe seed.

The Black Poppy little differeth from the former, until it beareth its flower, which is somewhat less, and of a black purplish colour, but without any purple spots in the bottom of the leaf. The head of the seed is much less than the former, and openeth itself a little round about the top under the crown, so that the seed, which is very black, will fall out, if one turn the head thereof downward.

The Wild Poppy, or Corn Rose, hath long and narrow leaves, very much cut in on the edges into many divisions, of a light green colour, sometimes hairy withal. The stalk is blackish and hairy also, but not so tall as the garden kind, having some such like leaves thereon to grow below, parted into three or four branches sometimes, whereon grow small hairy heads bowing down before the skin break, wherein the flower is inclosed, which when it is full blown open, is of a fair yellowish red or crimson colour, and in some much paler, without any spot in the bottom of the leaves, having many black soft threads in the middle, compassing a small green head, which when it is ripe, is not bigger than one's little finger's end, wherein is contained much black seed, smaller by half than that of the garden. The root perisheth every year, and springeth again of its own sowing. Of this kind there is one lesser in all the parts thereof, and differeth in nothing else.

Place.] The garden kinds do not naturally grow wild in any place, but are all sown in gardens where they grow.

The Wild Poppy, or Corn Rose is plentiful enough, and many times too much in the corn fields of all counties through this land, and also upon ditch banks, and by hedge sides. The smaller wild kind is also found in corn fields, and also in some other places, but not so plentifully as the former.

Time.] The garden kinds are usually sown in the Spring, which then flower about the end of May, and somewhat earlier, if they spring of their own sowing.

The Wild kind flower usually from May until July, and the seed of them is ripe soon after the flowering.

Government and Virtues.] The herb is Lunar, and of the juice of it is made opium, only for lucre of money they cheat you, and tell you it is a kind of tear, or some such like thing, that drops from poppies when they weep, and that is somewhere beyond the sea. I know not where beyond the Moon. The garden poppy heads with seeds made into a syrup is frequently, and to good effect, used to procure rest and sleep in the sick and weak, and to stay catarrhs and defluction of thin rheums from the head into the stomach and lungs, causing a continual cough the fore-runner of a consumption; it helpeth also hoarseness of the throat, and when one hath lost their voice, which the oil of the seed doth likewise. The black seed boiled in wine, and drank, is said also to stay the flux of the belly, and womens courses. The empty shells, or poppy heads, are usually boiled in water, and given to procure rest and sleep: So do the leaves in the same manner; as also if the head and temples be bathed with the decoction warm, or with the oil of poppies, the green leaves or heads bruised, and applied with a little vinegar, or made into a poultice with barley-meal or hog's grease, cooleth and tempereth all inflammations, as also the disease called St Anthony's fire. It is generally used in treacle and mithridate, and in all other medicines that are made to procure rest and sleep, and to ease pains in the head as well as in other parts. It is also used to cool inflammations, agues, or frenzies, or to stay defluctions which cause a cough or consumption, and also other fluxes of the belly, or womens courses, it is also put into hollow teeth, to ease the pain, and hath been found by experience to ease pains of the gout.

The Wild Poppy, or Corn Rose, (as Mathiolus saith) is good to prevent the falling sickness. The syrup made with the flower, is with good effect given to those that have the pleurisy; and the dried flowers also, either boiled in water, or made into powder and drank, either in the distilled water of them, or some other drink, worketh the like effect. The distilled water of the flowers is held to be of much good use against surfeits, being drank evening and morning: It is also more cooling than any of the other poppies, and therefore cannot but be as effectual in hot agues, frenzies, and other inflammations either inward or outward. Galen saith, the seed is dangerous to be used inwardly.

Purslane.

GARDEN Purslane (being used as a sallad herb) is so well known that it needeth no description; I shall therefore only speak of its virtues as followeth.

Government and Virtues] 'Tis an herb of the Moon. It is good to cool any heat in the liver, blood, reins, and stomach, and in hot agues nothing better: It stayeth hot and choleric fluxes of the belly, womens courses, the whites, and gonorrhea, or running of the reins, the distillation from the head, and pains therein proceeding from heat, want of sleep, or the frenzy. The seed is more effectual than the herb, and is of singular good use to cool the heat and sharpness of urine, and the outrageous lust of the body, venereous dreams, and the like: insomuch that the over frequent use hereof extinguisheth the heat and virtue of natural procreation. The seed bruised and boiled in wine, and given to children, expelleth the worms. The juice of the herb is held effectual to all the purposes aforesaid; as also to stay vomitings, and taken with some sugar or honey, helpeth an old and dry cough, shortness of breath, and the phthisic, and stayeth immoderate thirst. The distilled water of the herb is used by many (as the more pleasing) with a little sugar to work the same effects. The juice also is singular good in the inflammations and ulcers in the secret parts of man or woman, as also the bowels and hæmorrhoids, when they are ulcerous, or excoriations in them. The herb bruised and applied to the forehead and temples, allays excessive heat therein, that hinders rest and sleep, and applied to the eyes taketh away the redness and inflammation in them, and those other parts where pushes, wheals, pimples, St Anthony's fire, and the like, break forth: if a little vinegar be put to it, and laid to the neck, with as much of galls and linseed together, it taketh away the pains therein, and the crick in the neck. The juice is used with oil of roses for the same causes, or for blasting by lightning, and burnings by gunpowder, or for womens sore breasts, and to allay the heat in all other sores or hurts; applied also to the navels of children that stick forth, it helpeth them; it is also good for sore mouths and gums that are swollen, and to fasten loose teeth. Camerarius saith, that the distilled water used by some, took away the pain of their teeth, when all other remedies failed, and the thickened juice made into pills with the powder of gum tragacanth and arabick, being taken, prevaileth much to help those that make bloody water. Applied to the gout it easeth pains thereof, and helpeth the hardness of the sinews, if it come not of the cramp, or a cold cause.

Primroses.

THEY are so well known, that they need no description. Of the leaves of Primroses are made as fine a salve to heal wounds as any that I know. You shall be taught to make salves of any herb at the latter end of the book; make this as you are taught there, and do not (you that have any ingenuity in you) see your poor neighbours go with wounded limbs when an halfpenny cost will heal them.

Privet.

Descript.] OUR common Privet is carried up with many slender branches to a reasonable height and breadth, to cover arbours, bowers, and banquetting houses, and brought, wrought, and cut into so many forms of men, horses, birds, &c. which though at first supported, groweth afterwards strong of itself. It beareth long and narrow green leaves by the couples, and sweet smelling white flowers in tufts at the end of the branches, which turn into small black berries that have a purplish juice with them, and some seeds that are flat on the one side, with a hole or dent therein.

Place.] It groweth in this land, in divers woods.

Time.] Our Privet flowereth in June and July, the berries are ripe in August and September.

Government and Virtues.] The Moon is lady of this. It is little used in physic with us in these times, more than in lotions to wash sores, and sore mouths, and to cool inflammations, and dry up fluxes. Yet Matthiolus saith it serveth to all the uses for the which cypress, or the East Privet is appointed by Dioscorides and Galen. He farther saith, That the oil that is made of the flowers of Privet infused therein, and set in the sun, is singular good for the inflammations of wounds, and for the head ach coming of an hot cause. There is a sweet water also distilled from the flowers, that is good for all those diseases that need cooling and drying, and therefore helpeth all fluxes of the belly and stomach, bloody fluxes, and womens courses, being either drank or applied, as all those that void blood at the mouth, or any other place, and for distillations of rheum in the eyes, especially if it be used with tutia.

Queen of the Meadows, Meadow Sweet, or Mead Sweet.

Descript.] THE stalks of this are reddish, rising to be three feet high, sometimes four or five feet, having at the joints thereof large winged leaves, standing one

one above another at distances, consisting of many and somewhat broad leaves, set on each side of a middle rib, being hard, rough, or rugged, crumpled much like unto elm leaves, having also some smaller leaves with them, (as agrimony hath) somewhat deeply dented about the edges of a sad green colour on the upper side and greyish underneath, of a pretty sharp scent and taste, somewhat like unto the burnet, and a leaf hereof put into a cup of claret wine, giveth also a fine relish to it. At the tops of the stalks and branches stand many tufts of small white flowers thrust thick together, which smell much sweeter than the leaves, and in their places, being fallen, some crooked and cornered seed. The root is somewhat woody, and blackish on the outside, and brownish within, with divers great strings, and lesser fibres set thereat, of a strong scent, but nothing so pleasant as the flowers and leaves, and perisheth not, but abideth many years, shooting forth anew every Spring.

Place] It groweth in moist meadows that lie much wet, or near the courses of water.

Time] It flowereth in some places or other all the three Summer months, that is, June, July, and August, and the seed is ripe soon after.

Government and Virtues.] Venus claims dominion over the herb. It is used to stay all manner of bleedings, fluxes, vomitings, and womens courses, as also their whites. It is said to alter and take away the fits of the quartan agues, and to make a merry heart, for which purpose some use the flowers, and some the leaves. It helpeth speedily those that are troubled with the colic, being boiled in wine, and with a little honey taken warm, it openeth the belly, but boiled in red wine, and drank, it stayeth the flux of the belly. Outwardly applied, it helpeth old ulcers that are cankerous, or hollow and fistulous, for which it is by many much commended, as also for sores in the mouth, or secret parts. The leaves, when they are full grown, being laid on the skin, will, in a short time, raise blisters thereon, as Tragus saith. The water thereof helpeth the heat and inflammation in the eyes.

The Quince-Tree.

Descript] THE ordinary Quince-Tree groweth often to the height and bigness of a reasonable apple-tree,

tree, but more usually lower, and crooked, with a rough bark, spreading arms and branches far abroad. The leaves are somewhat like those of the apple tree, but thicker, broader, and fuller of veins, and whiter on the other side, not dented at all about the edges. The flowers are large and white, some times dashed over with a blush. The fruit that followeth is yellow, being near ripe, and covered with a white freeze, or cotton, thick set on the young and growing less as they grow to be thorough ripe, bunched out oftentimes in some places, some being like an apple, and some like a pear, of a strong heady scent, and not durable to keep, and is sour, harsh, and of an unpleasant taste to eat fresh, but being scalded, roasted, baked, or preserved, becometh more pleasant.

Place and Time] It best likes to grow near ponds and water-sides, and is frequent through this land, and floureth not until the leaves be come forth. The fruit is ripe in September or October.

Government and Virtues] Old Saturn owns the tree. Quinces, when they are green, help all sorts of fluxes in men or women, and choleric lasks, casting, and whatever needeth astriction, more than any way prepared by fire, yet the syrup of the juice, or the conserve, are much conducible, much of the binding quality being consumed by the fire; if a little vinegar be added, it stirreth up the languishing appetite, and the stomach given to casting; some spices being added, comforteth and strengtheneth the decaying and fainting spirits, and helpeth the liver oppressed, that it cannot perfect the digestion, or correcteth choler and phlegm. If you would have them purging, put honey to them instead of sugar, and if more laxative, for choler, rhubarb, for phlegm, turbith, for watery humours, scammony: but if more forcibly to bind, use the unripe Quinces, with roses and acacia, hypocistis, and some torrefied rhubarb. To take the crude juice of Quinces, is held a preservative against the force of deadly poison, for it hath been found most certainly true, that the very smell of a Quince hath taken away all the strength of the poison of white hellebore. If there be need of any outwardly binding and cooling of hot fluxes, the oil of Quinces, or other medicines that may be made thereof are very available to anoint the belly or other parts therewith; it likewise strengtheneth the stomach and belly, and the sinews that

loose and

loosened by sharp humours falling on them, and restraineth immoderate sweatings. The mucilage taken from the seeds of Quinces, and boiled in a little water, is very good to cool the heat, and heal the sore breasts of women. The same with a little sugar, is good to lenify the harshness and hoarseness of the throat, and roughness of the tongue. The cotton or down of Quinces boiled and applied to plague-sores healeth them up, and laid as a plaister, made up with wax, it bringeth hair to them that are bald, and keepeth it from falling, if it be ready to shed.

Raddish, or Horse-Raddish.

THE garden Raddish is so well known, that it needeth no description.

Descript] The Horse-Raddish hath its first leaves that rise before Winter, about a foot and a half long, very much cut in or torn on the edges into many parts, of a dark green colour, with a greater rib in the middle; after these have been up a while, others follow, which are greater, rougher, broader and longer, whole and not divided at first, but only somewhat rougher dented about the edges; the stalks when it beareth flowers (which is seldom) are great, rising up with some few lesser leaves thereon, to three or four feet high, spreading at the top many small branches of whitish flowers, made of four leaves a piece, after which come small pods, like those of shepherd's purse, but seldom with any seed in them. The root is great, long, white and rugged, shooting up divers heads of leaves, which may be parted for increase, but it doth not creep in the ground, nor run above ground, and is of a strong, sharp and bitter taste, almost like mustard.

Place.] It is found wild in some places, but is chiefly planted in gardens, and joyeth in moist and shadowy places.

Time] It seldom flowereth, but when it doth, it is in July.

Government and Virtues] They are both under Mars. The juice of Horse-raddish given to drink, is held to be very effectual for the scurvy. It killeth the worms in children, being drank, and also laid upon the belly. The root bruised and laid to the place grieved with the sciatica, joint-ach, or the hard swellings of the liver and spleen, doth wonderfully help them all. The distilled water of the herb and root is more familiar to be taken with a little sugar for all the purposes aforesaid.

Garden Radishes are in wantonness by the gentry eaten as a sallad, but they breed but scurvy humours in the stomach, and corrupt the blood, and then send for a physician as fast as you can: this is one cause makes the owners of such nice palates so unhealthful, yet for such as are troubled with the gravel, stone, or stoppage of urine, they are good physic, if the body be strong that takes them, you may make the juice of the roots into a syrup if you please, for that use. They purge by urine exceedingly.

Ragwort.

IT is called also St. James's-wort, and Stagger-wort, and Summer-wort, and Segrum.

Descript.] The greater common Ragwort hath many large and long dark green leaves lying on the ground, very much rent and torn on the sides in many places, from among which rise up sometimes but one, and sometimes two or three square or crested blackish or brownish stalks, three or four feet high, sometimes branched, bearing divers such like leaves upon them, at several distances unto the top, where it branches forth into many stalks bearing yellow flowers, consisting of divers leaves, set as a pale or border, with a dark yellow thrum in the middle, which do abide a great while, but at last are turned into down, and with the small blackish grey seed, are carried away with the wind. The root is made of many fibres, whereby it is firmly fastened into the ground, and abideth many years.

There is another sort thereof different from the former only in this, that it riseth not so high, the leaves are not so finely jagged, nor of so dark a green colour, but rather somewhat whitish, soft and woolly, and the flowers usually paler.

Place.] They grow both of them wild in pastures, and untilled grounds in many places, and oftentimes both in one field.

Time.] They flower in June and July, and the seed is ripe in August.

Government and Virtues.] Ragwort is under the command of Dame Venus, and cleanseth, digesteth, and discusseth. The decoction of the herb is good to wash the mouth or throat that hath ulcers or sores therein, and in

swelling,

swellings, hardness, or imposthumations for it thoroughly cleanseth and healeth them, as also the quinsey, and the king's-evil. It helpeth to stay catarrhs, thin rheums, and defluctions from the head into the eyes, nose, or lungs. The juice is found by experience to be singular good to heal green wounds, and to cleanse and heal all old and filthy ulcers in the privities and in other parts of the body, as also inward wounds and ulcers; stayeth the malignity of fretting and running cankers, and hollow fistulas, not suffering them to spread farther. It is also much commended to help achs and pains either in the fleshy part, or in the nerves and sinews; as also the sciatica, or pain of the hips or huckle bone, to bathe the places with the decoction of the herb, or to anoint them with an ointment made of the herb, bruised and boiled in old hog's suet, with some mastick and olibanum in powder added unto it after it is strained forth. In Sussex we call it Ragwee.

Rattle Grass.

OF this there are two kinds which I shall speak of, *viz.* the red and yellow.

Descript.] The common Red Rattle hath sundry reddish, hollow stalks, and sometimes green, rising from the root, lying for the most part on the ground, some growing more upright, with many small reddish or green leaves set on both sides of a middle rib, finely dented about the edges: The flowers stand at the tops of the stalks and branches, of a fine purplish red colour, like small gaping hooks; after which come blackish seed in small husks, which lying loose therein, will rattle with shaking. The root consists of two or three small whitish strings with some fibres thereat.

The common Yellow Rattle hath seldom above one round great stalk, rising from the root, about half a yard, or two feet high, and but few branches thereon, having two long and somewhat broad leaves set at a joint, deeply cut in on the edges, resembling the comb of a cock, broadest next to the stalk, and smaller to the end. The flowers grow at the tops of the stalks with some shorter leaves with them, hooded after the same manner that the others are, but of a fair yellow colour, or in some paler, and in some more white. The seed is contained in large husks, and being ripe, will rattle or make a noise with lying loose in them. The root is small and slender, perishing every year.

Place]

Place] They grow in meadows and woods generally thro' this land.

Time] They are in flower from Midsummer until August be..., sometimes.

Government and Virtues] They are both of them under the dominion of the Moon. The Red Rattle is accounted profitable to heal up fistulas and hollow ulcers, and to ... the flux of humours in them, as also the abundance of womens courses, or any other flux of blood, being boiled in red wine, and drank.

The Yellow Rattle, or Cock's Comb, is held to be good for those that are troubled with a cough, or dimness of sight, if the herb, being boiled with beans, and some honey put thereto, be drank or dropped into the eyes. The whole seed being put into the eyes, draweth forth any skin, dimness or film, from the sight, without trouble or pain.

Rest Harrow, or Cammock.

Descript] COMMON Rest Harrow riseth up with divers rough woody twigs half a yard, or a yard high, set at the joints without order, with little round-ish leaves, sometime more than two or three at a place, of a dark green colour, without thorns while they are young, but afterwards armed in sundry places with short and sharp thorns. The flowers come forth at the tops of the twigs and branches, whereof it is full fashioned like pease or bean blossoms, but lesser, flatter, and somewhat closer, of a faint purplish colour; after which come small pods containing small, flat round seed. The root is blackish on the outside, and whitish within, very tough, and hard to break when it is fresh and green, and as hard as an horn when it is dried, thrusting down deep into the ground, and spreading likewise, every piece being apt to grow again if it be left in the ground.

Place] It groweth in many places of this land, as well in the arable as waste ground.

Time] It flowereth about the beginning or middle of July, and the seed is ripe in August.

Government and Virtues] It is under the dominion of Mars. It is singular good to provoke urine when it is stopped, and to break and drive forth the Stone, which the powder of the bark of the root taken in wine performeth effectually. Matthiolus saith, The same helpeth the disease called Her-

Carnosa, the fleshy rupture, by taking the said powder for some months together constantly, and that it hath cured some which seemed incurable by any other means than by cutting or burning. The decoction thereof made with some vinegar, gargled in the mouth, easeth the tooth ach, especially when it comes of rheum; and the said decoction is very powerful to open obstruction of the liver and spleen, and other parts. A distilled water in *Balneo Mariæ*, with four pounds of the root hereof first sliced small, and afterwards steeped in a gallon of Canary wine, is singular good for all the purposes aforesaid, and to cleanse the passages of the urine. The powder of the said root made into an electuary, or lozenges, with sugar, as also the bark of the fresh roots boiled tender and afterwards beaten to a conserve with sugar, work the like effect. The powder of the roots strewed upon the brims of ulcers, or mixed with any other convenient thing, and applied, consumeth the hardness, and causeth them to heal the better.

Rocket.

IN regard the Garden Rocket is rather used as a sallad herb than to any physical purposes, I shall omit it, and only speak of the common wild Rocket. The description whereof take as followeth:

Descript.] The common wild Rocket hath longer and narrower leaves, much more divided into slender cuts and jags on both sides the middle rib than the garden kinds have, of a sad green colour, from among which rise up divers stalks, two or three feet high, sometimes set with the like leaves, but smaller and smaller upwards, branched from the middle into divers stiff stalks, bearing sundry yellow flowers on them, made of four leaves a piece, as the others are, which afterwards yield them small reddish seed, in small long pods, of a more bitter and hot biting taste than the garden kinds, as the leaves are also.

Place] It is found wild in divers places of this land.

Time] It flowereth about June or July, and the seed is ripe in August.

Government and Virtues] The wild Rockets are forbidden to be used alone, in regard their sharpness fumeth into the head causing achs and pains therein, and are less hurtful to hot and cholerick persons, for fear of inflaming their blood, and

and therefore, for such we may say a little doth but a little harm, for angry Mars rules them, and he sometimes will be rusty when he meets with fools. The wild Rocket is more strong and effectual to increase sperm and venerous qualities, whereunto all the seed is more effectual than the garden kind, it serveth also to help digestion, and provoketh urine exceedingly. The seed is used to cure the bitings of serpents, the scorpion, and the shrew mouse, and other poisons, and expelleth worms, and other noisome creatures that breed in the belly. The herb boiled or stewed, and some sugar put thereto, helpeth the cough in children, being taken often. The seed also taken in drink, taketh away the ill scent of the arm pits, increaseth milk in nurses, and wasteth the spleen. The seed mixed with honey, and used on the face, cleanseth the skin from morphew, and used with vinegar, taketh away freckles and redness in the face, or other parts; and with the gall of an ox, it mendeth foul scars, black and blue spots, and the marks of the small-pox.

Winter-Rocket, or Cresses.

Descript.] WINTER Rocket, or Winter Cresses, hath divers somewhat large sad green leaves lying upon the ground, torn or cut in divers parts, somewhat like unto Rocket or turnip leaves, with smaller pieces next the bottom, and broad at the ends, which so abide all the Winter, (if it spring up in Autumn, when it is used to be eaten) from among which rise up divers small round stalks, full of branches, bearing many small yellow flowers of four leaves a piece, after which come small pods, with reddish seed in them. The root is somewhat stringy, and perisheth every year after the seed is ripe.

Place.] It groweth of its own accord in gardens and fields, by the way sides, in divers places, and particularly in the next pasture to the Conduit head behind Gray's Inn, that brings water to Mr Lamb's Conduit in Holburn.

Time.] It flowereth in May, seedeth in June, and then perisheth.

Government and Virtues.] This is profitable to provoke urine, to help stranguary, and expel gravel and the stone. It is good for the scurvy, and found by experience to be a singular good wound herb to cleanse inward wounds, the juice or decoction being drank, or outwardly applied to wash foul ulcers and sores, cleansing them by sharpness, and hindering or abating the dead flesh from growing therein, and healing them by the drying quality.

Roses.

I HOLD it altogether needless to trouble the reader with a description of any of these, since both the garden Roses, and the Roses of the briars, are well enough known; take therefore the virtue of them as followeth. And first I shall begin with the garden kinds.

Government and Virtues.] What a pother have authors made with Roses! What a racket have they kept? I shall add, red Roses are under Jupiter, Damask under Venus, White under the Moon, and Provence under the King of France. The white and red Roses are cooling and drying, and yet the white is taken to exceed the red in both the properties, but is seldom used inwardly in any medicine: The bitterness in the Roses when they are fresh, especially the juice, purgeth choler, and watery humours; but being dried, and that heat which caused the bitterness being consumed, they have then a binding and astringent quality: Those also that are not full blown do both cool and bind more than those that are full blown, and the white Rose more than the Red. The decoction of red Roses made with wine and used, is very good for the head-ach, and pains in the eyes, ears, throat and gums, as also for the fundament, the lower parts of the belly and the matrix being bathed or put into them. The same decoction with the roots remaining in it, is profitably applied to the region of the heart to ease the inflammation therein, as also St. Anthony's fire, and other diseases of the stomach. Being dried and beaten to powder, and taken in steeled wine or water, it helpeth to stay womens courses. The yellow threads in the middle of the Roses (which are erroneously called the Rose Seed) being powdered and drank in the distilled water of quince, stayeth the overflowing of womens courses, and doth wonderfully stay the defluctions of rheum upon the gums and teeth, preserving them from corruption, and fastening them if they be loose, being washed and gargled therewith, and some vinegar of squills added thereto. The heads with the seed being used in powder, or in a decoction, stayeth the lask and spitting of blood. Red Roses doth strengthen the heart, the stomach and the liver, and the retentive faculty: They mitigate the pains that arise from heat, assuage inflammations, procure rest and sleep, stay both whites and reds in women, the gonorrhea, or running of the reins, and fluxes of the belly; the juice of them doth purge and cleanse the body from choler and phlegm. The husk of the roses, with the beards and nails of the Roses, are binding and cooling, and the distilled water of either of them is good for the heat and redness in the eyes, and to stay and dry up the rheums and watering of them. Of the red Roses are usually made many compositions, all serving to sundry good uses, viz. Electuary of Roses, conserve, both moist and dry, which is more usually called Sugar of Roses. Syrup of dry Roses, and Honey of Roses. The cordial powder called *Diaribodon Abbatis*, and *Aromatica Rosarum*. The distilled water of Roses, vinegar of Roses, ointment, and oil of Roses, and the Rose leaves dried, are of very great use and effect. To write at large of every one of these would make my book swell too big, it being sufficient for a volume of itself, to speak fully of them. But briefly the electuary is purging, whereof two or three drams taken by itself in some convenient liquor, is a purge sufficient for a weak constitution, but may be increased to six drams, according to the strength of the patient. It purgeth choler without trouble, and it is good in hot fevers, and pains of the head arising from hot choleric humours, and heat in the eyes, the jaundice also, and joint aches proceeding of hot humours. The moist conserve is of much use, both binding and cordial; for until it be about two years old, it is more binding than cordial, and after that, more cordial than binding. Some of the younger conserve taken with mithridate mixed together, is good for those that are troubled with distillations of rheum from the brain to the nose, and defluctions of rheum into the eyes; as also for fluxes and lasks of the belly; and being mixed with the powder of mastick is very good for the running of the reins, and for the looseness of humours in the body. The old conserve against faintings, swooning, weakness and trembling of the heart, strengthens both it and a weak stomach, helpeth digestion, stayeth casting, and is a very good preservative in the time of infection.

fection. The dry conserve, which is called the Sugar of Roses, is a very good cordial to strengthen the heart and spirits; as also to stay defluctions. The syrup of dried red Roses strengthens a stomach given to casting, cooleth an overheated liver, and the blood in agues, comforteth the heart, and resisteth putrefaction and infection, and helpeth to stay lasks and fluxes. Honey of Roses is much used in gargles and lotions to wash sores, either in the mouth, throat, or other parts, both to cleanse and heal them, and to stay the fluxes of humours falling upon them. It is also used in clysters both to cool and cleanse. The cordial powders, called Diarrhodon Abbatis and Aromatica Rosarum, do comfort and strengthen the heart and stomach, procure an appetite, help digestion, stay vomiting, and are very good for those that have slippery bowels, to strengthen them, and to dry up their moisture: Red Rose water is well known, and of a familiar use on all occasions, and better than damask Rosewater, being cooling and cordial, refreshing, quickening the weak and faint spirits, used either in meats or broths, to wash the temples, to smell at the nose, or to smell the sweet vapours thereof out of a perfuming pot, or cast into a hot fire shovel. It is also of much good use against the redness and inflammations of the eyes to bathe them therewith, and the temples of the head, as also against pain and ach, for which purpose also vinegar of Roses is of much good use, and to procure rest and sleep, if some thereof, and Rose-water together, be used to smell unto, or the nose and temples moistened therewith, but more usually to moisten a piece of a red Rose cake, cut for the purpose, and heated between a double-folded cloth, with a little beaten nutmeg, and poppy-seed strewed on the side that must lie next to the forehead and temples, and bound so thereto all night. The ointment of Roses is much used against heat and inflammations in the head, to anoint the forehead and temples, and being mixt with *Unguentum Populneum*, to procure rest, it is also used for the heat of the liver, the back and reins, and to cool and heal pushes, wheals, and other red pimples rising in the face or other parts. Oil of Roses is not only used by itself to cool any hot swellings or inflammations, and to bind and stay fluxes of humours unto sores, but is also put into ointments and plaisters that are cooling and binding, and restraining the flux of humours. The dried leaves of the red

Roses

Roses are used both inwardly and outwardly, both cooling, binding, and cordial, for with them are made both *Aromaticum Rosarum*, *Diarrhodon Abbatis*, and *Saccharum Rosarum*, each of whose properties are before declared. Rose leaves and mint, heated and applied outwardly to the stomach, stay castings, and very much strengthen a weak stomach, and applied as a fomentation to the region of the liver and heart, do much cool and temper them, and also serve instead of a Rose cake (as is said before) to quiet the over-hot spirits, and cause rest and sleep. The syrup of damask Roses is both simple and compound, and made with agarick. The simple solutive syrup is a familiar, safe, gentle and easy medicine, purging choler, taken from one ounce to three or four, yet this is remarkable herein, that the distilled water of this syrup should notably bind the belly. The syrup with agarick is more strong and effectual, for one ounce thereof by itself will open the body more than the other, and worketh as much on phlegm as choler. The compound syrup is more forcible in working on melancholic humours, and available against the leprosy, itch, tetters, &c. and the French disease. Also honey of Roses solutive is made of the same infusions that the syrup is made of, and therefore worketh the same effect, both opening and purging, but is oftener given to phlegmatic than choleric persons, and is more used in clysters than in potions, as the syrup made with sugar is. The conserve and preserved leaves of those Roses are also operative in gently opening the belly.

The simple water of the damask Roses is chiefly used for fumes to sweeten things, as the dried leaves thereof to make sweet powders, and fill sweet bags; and little use they are put to in physic, although they have some purging quality, the wild Roses also are few or none of them used in physic, but are generally held to come near the nature of the manured Roses. The fruit of the wild briar which are called Hips, being thoroughly ripe, and made into a conserve with sugar, besides the pleasantness of the taste, doth gently bind the belly, and stay defluctions from the head upon the stomach drying up the moisture thereof, and helpeth digestion. The pulp of the hips dried into a hard consistence, like to the juice of liquorice, or so dried that it may be made into powder and taken in drink, stayeth speedily the whites in women. The briar ball is often used, being made into

powder

powder and drank, to break the stone, to provoke urine when it is stopped, and to ease and help the cholic; some appoint it to be burnt, and then taken for the same purpose. In the middle of the balls are often found certain white worms, which being dried and made into powder and some of it drank, is found by the experience of many to kill and drive forth the worms of the belly.

Rosa Solis, or Sun Dew.

Descript] It hath divers small, round, hollow leaves somewhat greenish, but full of certain red hairs, which make them seem red, every one standing upon his own foot stalk, reddish, hairy likewise. The leaves are continually moist in the hottest day, yea, the hotter the sun shines on them, the moister they are, with a clamminess that will rope (as we say), the small hairs always holding this moisture. Among these leaves rise up slender stalks, reddish also, three or four fingers high, bearing divers small white knobs one above another, which are flowers; after which in the heads are contained small seeds. The root is a few small hairs.

Place] It groweth usually in bogs and wet places, and sometimes in moist woods.

Time] It flowereth in June, and then the leaves are fittest to be gathered.

Government and Virtues] The Sun rules it, and it is under the sign Cancer. Rosa Solis is accounted good to help those that have a salt rheum distilling on the lungs, which breedeth a consumption, and therefore the distilled water thereof in wine is held fit and profitable for such to drink, which water will be of a good yellow colour. The same water is held to be good for all other diseases of the lungs, as phthisics, wheezings, shortness of breath, or the cough; as also to heal the ulcers that happen in the lungs, and it comforteth the heart and fainting spirits. The leaves outwardly applied to the skin will raise blisters, which has caused some to think it dangerous to be taken inwardly; but there are other things which will also draw blisters, yet nothing dangerous to be taken inwardly. There is an usual drink made thereof with aqua vitæ and spices frequently, and without any offence or danger, but to good purpose used in qualms and passions of the heart.

Rosemary.

OUR garden Rosemary is so well known, that I need not describe it.

Time.] It flowereth in April and May with us, sometimes again in August.

Government and Virtues.] The Sun claims privilege in it, and it is under the celestial Ram. It is an herb of as great use with us in these days as any whatsoever, not only for physical but civil purposes. The physical use of it being my present task, is very much both for inward and outward diseases, for by the warming and comforting heat thereof it helpeth all cold diseases, both of the head, stomach, liver, and belly. The decoction thereof in wine helpeth the cold distillations of rheums into the eyes, and all other cold diseases of the head and brain, as the giddiness or swimming therein, drowsiness or dullness of the mind and senses like a stupidness, the dumb palsy, or loss of speech, the lethargy, and falling sickness, to be both drank, and the temples bathed therewith. It helpeth the pains in the gums and teeth, by rheum falling into them, not by putrefaction, causing an evil smell from them, or a stinking breath. It helpeth a weak memory, and quickeneth the senses. It is very comfortable to the stomach in all the cold griefs thereof, helpeth both retention of meat and digestion, the decoction of powder being taken in wine. It is a remedy for the windiness in the stomach, bowels, and spleen, and expels it powerfully. It helpeth those that are liver grown, by opening the obstructions thereof. It helpeth dim eyes, and procureth a clear sight, the flowers thereof being taken all the while it is flowering, every morning fasting, with bread and salt. Both Dioscorides and Galen say, That if a decoction be made thereof with water, and they that have the yellow jaundice exercise their bodies presently after the taking thereof, it will certainly cure them. The flowers, and conserve made of them, are singular good to comfort the heart, and to expel the contagion of the pestilence; to burn the herb in houses and chambers, correcteth the air in them. Both the flowers and leaves are very profitable for women that are troubled with the whites, if they be daily taken. The dried leaves shred small, and taken in a pipe, as tobacco is taken helpeth those that have any cough, phthisic, or consumption, by warming and drying the thin distillations which cause those diseases. The leaves are very much used in bathings; and made into ointments or oil, are singular good to help cold benumbed joints, sinews, or members. The chymical oil drawn from the leaves and flowers, is a sovereign help for all the diseases aforesaid, to touch the temples and nostrils with two or three drops for all the diseases of the head and brain spoken of before; as also to take one drop, two or three, as the case requireth, for the inward griefs: Yet must it be done with discretion, for it is very quick and piercing, and therefore but a very little must be taken at a time. There is also another oil made by insolation in this manner. Take what quantity you will of the flowers, and put them into a strong glass close stopped, tie a fine linen cloth over the mouth, and turn the mouth down into another strong glass, which being set in the sun, an oil will distil down into the lower glass, to be preserved as precious for divers uses, both inward and outward, as a sovereign balm to heal the diseases beforementioned, to clear dim sights, and take away spots, marks, and scars in the skin.

Rhubarb, or Raphontick.

DO not start, and say, This grows you know not how far off, and then ask me, How it comes to pass that I bring it among our English simples? For though the name may speak it foreign, yet it grows with us in England, and that frequent enough in our gardens; and when you have thoroughly perused its virtues, you will conclude it nothing inferior to that which is brought out of China, and by that time this hath been as much used as that hath been, the name which the other hath gotten will be eclipsed by the fame of this; take therefore a description at large of it as followeth:

Descript.] At the first appearing out of the ground, when the Winter is past, it hath a great round brownish head, rising from the middle or sides of the root, which openeth itself into sundry leaves one after another, very much crumpled or folded together at the first, and brownish; but afterwards it spreadeth itself, and becometh smooth, very large and almost round, every one standing on a brownish stalk of the thickness of a man's thumb, when they are grown to their fulness, and most of them two feet and more in length, especially when they grow in any moist or good ground; and the stalk of the leaf, from the bottom thereof to the leaf itself, being also two feet, the breadth thereof from edge to edge, in the broadest place, being also two feet, of a sad or dark green colour, of a fine tart or smooth taste, much more pleasant than the garden or wood sorrel. From among these riseth up some, but not every year, strong thick stalks, not growing so high as the Patience, or Garden Dock with such round leaves as grow below, but smaller at every joint up to the top, and among the flowers, which are white, spreading forth into many branches, consisting of five or six small leaves a piece, hardly to be discerned from the threads of the middle, and seeming to be all threads, after which come brownish three-square seeds, like unto other docks, but larger, whereby it may be plainly known to be a dock. The root grows in time to be very great, with divers and sundry great spreading branches from it, of a dark brownish or reddish colour on the outside, with a pale yellow skin under it, which covereth the inner substance or root, which rind and skin being pared away, the root appears of so fresh and lively a colour, with fresh coloured veins running thro' it, that the choicest of that Rhubarb that is brought us from beyond the seas cannot excel it, which root, if it be dried carefully, and as it ought (which must be in our country by the gentle heat of a fire, in regard the sun is not enough here to do it, and every piece kept from touching one another) will hold its colour almost as well as when it is fresh, and is has been approved of, and commended by those who have often times used them.

Place] It groweth in gardens, and flowereth about the beginning or middle of June, and the seed is ripe in July.

Time] The roots that are to be dried and kept all the year following, are not to be taken up before the stalk and leaves be quite withered and gone, and that is not until the middle or end of October, and if they be taken a little before the leaves do spring, or when they are sprung up, the roots will not have half so good a colour in them.

I have given the precedence unto this, because in virtues
also

also it hath the pre-eminence. I come now to describe unto you that which is called Patience, or Monk's Rhubarb; and next unto that, the great round leaved Dock, or Bastard Rhubarb, for the one of these may happily supply in the absence of the other, being not much unlike in their virtues, only one more powerful and efficacious than the other. And lastly, shall shew you the virtues of all the three sorts.

Garden-Patience, or Monk's Rhubarb.

Descrip] THIS is a Dock bearing the name of Rhubarb for some purging quality therein, and groweth up with large tall stalks, set with somewhat broad and long fair green leaves, not dented at all. The tops of the stalks being divided into many small branches, bear reddish or purplish flowers, and three-square seed, like unto other docks. The root is long, great and yellow, like unto the wild docks, but a little redder; and if it be a little dried, sheweth less store of discoloured veins than the next doth when it is dry.

Great round-leaved Dock, or Bastard Rhubarb.

Descript.] THIS hath divers large, round, thin, yellowish green leaves rising from the root, a little waved about the edges, every one standing upon a reasonable thick and long brown ish foot stalk, from among which riseth up a pretty big stalk, about two feet high with some such like leaves growing thereon, but smaller, at the top whereof stand in a long spike many small brownish flowers, which turn into a hard three square shining brown seed, like the garden Patience before described. The root groweth greater than that, with many branches of great fibres thereat yellow on the outside, and somewhat pale, yellow within with some discoloured veins like to the Rhubarb which I first described, but much less than it, especially when it is dry.

Place and Time] These also grow in gardens, and flower and seed at or near the same time that our true Rhubarb doth, viz. they flower in June, and the seed is ripe in July.

Temperature and Virtues.] Mars claims predominacy over all these wholesome herbs. You cry out upon him for an unfortunate, when God created him for your good (only he is angry with fools.) What dishonour is this, not to Man, but to God himself? A dram of the dried root of Monk's Rhubarb, with a scruple of ginger made into powder, and taken fasting in a draught or mess of warm broth, purgeth choler and phlegm downwards very gently and safely, without danger. The seed thereof contrary doth bind the belly, and helpeth to stay any sort of lasks or bloody flux. The distilled water thereof is very profitably used to heal scabs; also foul ulcerous sores, and to lay the inflammation of them: the juice of the leaves or roots, or the decoction of them in vinegar, is used as a most effectual remedy to heal scabs and running sores.

The Bastard Rhubarb hath all the properties of the Monk's Rhubarb, but more effectual for both inward and outward diseases. The decoction thereof without vinegar dropped into the ears, taketh away the pains; gargled in the mouth, taketh away the tooth-ach; and being drank, healeth the jaundice. The seed thereof taken, easeth the gnawing and griping pains of the stomach, and taketh away the loathing thereof unto meat. The root thereof helpeth the ruggedness of the nails, and being boiled in wine, helpeth the swelling of the throat, commonly called the King's evil, as also the swellings of the kernels of the ears. It helpeth them that are troubled with the stone, provoketh urine, and helpeth the dimness of the sight. The roots of this Bastard Rhubarb are used in opening and purging diet drinks, with other things, to open the liver, and to cleanse and cool the blood.

The properties of that which is called the English Rhubarb, are the same with the former, but much more effectual, and hath all the properties of the true Italian Rhubarbs, except the force in purging, wherein it is but half the strength thereof, and therefore a double quantity must be used. It likewise hath not that bitterness and astriction; in other things it worketh almost in an equal quantity, which are these. It purgeth the body of choler and phlegm, being either taken of itself, made into powder, and drank in a draught of white wine, or steeped therein all night, and taken fasting, or put among other purges, as shall be thought convenient, cleansing the stomach, liver, and blood, opening obstructions, and helpeth those griefs that come thereof, as the jaundice, dropsy, swelling of the spleen, tertian, and daily agues, and pricking pains of the sides; and also it

stayeth

stayeth spitting of blood. The powder taken with cassia dissolved, and washed Venice turpentine, cleanseth the reins, and strengtheneth them afterwards, and is very effectual to stay the running of the reins, or gonorrhea. It is also given for the pains and swellings in the head, for those that are troubled with melancholy, and helpeth the sciatica, gout, and the cramp. The powder of the Rhubarb taken with a little mummia and madder roots in some red wine, dissolveth clotted blood in the body, happening by any fall or bruise, and helpeth burstings and broken parts, as well inward as outward. The oil likewise wherein it hath been boiled, worketh the like effects, being anointed. It is used to heal those ulcers that happen in the eyes or eyelids, being steeped and strained; as also to assuage the swellings and inflammations; and applied with honey, boiled in wine, it taketh away all blue spots or marks that happen therein. Whey or white wine are the best liquors to steep it in, and thereby it worketh more effectually in opening obstructions, and purging the stomach and liver. Many do use a little Indian spikenard as the best corrector thereof.

Meadow Rue.

Descript.] MEADOW Rue riseth up with a yellow stringy root, much spreading in the ground, shooting forth new sprouts and round about, with many green stalks, two feet high, crested all the length of them, set with joints here and there, and many large leaves on them, above as well as below, being divided into smaller leaves, nicked or dented in the fore part of them, of a red green colour on the upper side, and pale green underneath. Toward the top of the stalk there shooteth forth divers short branches, on every one whereof stand two, or three, or four small heads, or buttons, which breaking the skin that incloseth them, shooteth forth a tuft of pale greenish yellow threads, which falling away, there come in their places small three cornered cods, wherein is contained small, long and round seed. The whole plant hath a strong unpleasant scent.

Place.] It groweth in many places of this land, in the borders of moist meadows, and ditch sides.

Time.] It flowereth about July, or the beginning of August.

Government and Virtues.] Dioscorides saith, That this herb bruised and applied, perfectly healeth old sores, and the distilled water of the herb and flowers doth the like. It is used by some among other pot-herbs to open the body, and make it soluble; but the roots washed clean, and boiled in ale and drank, provoke to stool more than the leaves, but yet very gently. The root boiled in water, and the places of the body most troubled with vermin and lice washed therewith while it is warm, destroyeth them utterly. In Italy it is used against the plague, and in Saxony against the jaundice, as *Camerarius* saith.

Garden Rue.

GARDEN Rue is so well known by this name, and the name Herb of Grace, that I shall not need to write any further description of it, but shall only shew you the virtue of it, as followeth.

Government and Virtues.] It is an herb of the Sun, and under Leo. It provoketh urine and womens courses, being taken either in meat or drink. The seed thereof taken in wine, is an antidote against all dangerous medicines or deadly poisons. The leaves taken either by themselves, or with figs and walnuts, is called Mithridate's counter poison against the plague, and causeth all venomous things to become harmless; being often taken in meat and drink, it abateth venery, and destroyeth the ability to get children. A decoction made thereof with some dried dill-leaves and flowers, easeth all pains and torments inwardly to be drank, and outwardly to be applied warm to the place grieved. The same being drank, helpeth the pain both of the chest and sides, as also coughs and hardness of breathing, the inflammations of the lungs, and the tormenting pains of the sciatica and the joints, being anointed, or laid to the places; as also the shaking fits of agues, to take a draught before the fit comes; being boiled or infused in oil, it is good to help the wind cholic, the hardness and windiness of the mother, and freeth women from the strangling or suffocation thereof, if the share and the parts thereabouts be anointed therewith: It killeth and driveth forth the worms of the belly, if it be drank after it is boiled in wine to the half, with a little honey; it helpeth the gout or pains in the joints, hands, feet or knees, applied there-

thereunto; and with figs it helpeth the dropsy, being bathed therewith: Being bruised and put into the nostrils, it stayeth the bleeding thereof; it helpeth the swelling of the cods, if they be bathed with a decoction of Rue and Bay leaves. It taketh away wheals and pimples, if being bruised with a few myrtle leaves, it be made up with wax, and applied. It cureth the morphew, and taketh away all sorts of warts, if boiled in wine with some pepper and nitre, and the place rubbed therewith, and with almond and honey, helpeth the dry scabs, or any tetter or ring worm. The juice thereof warmed in a pomegranate shell or rind, and dropped into the ears, helpeth the pains of them. The juice of it and fennel, with a little honey, and the gall of a cock put thereunto, helpeth the dimness of the eye sight. An ointment made of the juice thereof with oil of roses, ceruse, and a little vinegar, and anointed, cureth St Anthony's fire, and all running sores in the head: and the stinking ulcers of the nose, or other parts. The antidote used by Mithridates, every morning fasting, to secure himself from any poison or infection, was this. Take twenty leaves of rue, a little salt, a couple of walnuts, and a couple of figs, beaten together into a mess, with twenty juniper berries, which is the quantity appointed for every day. Another electuary is made thus. Take of nitre, pepper, and cummin seed, of each equal parts; of the leaves of Rue clean picked, as much in weight as all the other three weighed; beat them well together, and put as much honey as will make it up into an electuary (but you must first steep your cummin seed in vinegar twenty-four hours, and then dry it, or rather roast it in a hot fire shovel, or in an oven) and is a remedy for the pains or griefs in the chest or stomach, of the spleen, belly, or sides, by wind or stitches: of the liver by obstructions; of the reins and bladder by the stopping of urine; and helpeth also to extenuate fat corpulent bodies. What an infamy is cast upon the ashes of Mithridates, or Methridates (as the Augustines read his name) by unworthy people. They that deserve no good report themselves, love to give none to others, viz. That renowned King of Pontus fortified his body by poison against poison. (*He cast out devils by Beelzebub, prince of the devils.*) What a sot is he that knows not he had accustomed his body to cold poisons, hot poisons would have dispatched him? On the contrary, if not, corrosions would

would have done it. The whole world is at this present time beholden to him for his studies in physic, and he that useth the quantity but of an hazel nut of that receipt every morning, to which his name is adjoined, shall to admiration preserve his body in health, if he do but consider that Rue is an herb of the Sun, and under Leo, and gather it and the rest accordingly.

Rupture-Wort.

Descript.] THIS spreads very many thready branches round about upon the ground, about a span long, divided into many other smaller parts full of small joints set very thick together, whereat come forth two very small leaves of a French yellow, green coloured branches and all, where groweth forth also a number of exceeding small yellowish flowers, scarce to be discerned from the stalk and leaves, which turn into seeds as small as the very dust. The root is very long and small, thrusting down deep in the ground. This hath neither smell nor taste at first, but afterwards hath a little astringent taste, without any manifest heat: yet a little bitter and sharp withal.

Place.] It groweth in dry, sandy, and rocky places.

Time.] It is fresh and green all the Summer.

Government and Virtues.] They say Saturn causeth ruptures: if he doth, he does no more than he can cure; if you want wit, he will teach you, though to your cost. This herb is Saturn's own, and is a noble antivenerean. Rupture-wort hath not its name in vain; for it is found by experience to cure the rupture, not only in children, but also in elder persons, if the disease be not too inveterate, by taking a dram of the powder of the dried herb every day in wine, or a decoction made and drank for certain days together. The juice of distilled water of the green herb, taken in the same manner, helpeth all other fluxes either of man or woman; vomiting also, and the gonorrhea or running of the reins, being taken any of the ways aforesaid. It doth also most assuredly help those that have the stranguary, or are troubled with the stone or gravel in the reins or bladder. The same helpeth stitches in the sides, griping pains of the stomach or belly, the obstructions of the liver, and cureth the yellow jaundice; likewise it kills also the worms in children. Being outwardly applied,

applied, it conglutinateth wounds notably, and helpeth much to stay defluctions of rheum from the head to the eyes, nose and teeth, being bruised green, and bound thereto; or the forehead, temples, or the nape of the neck behind, bathed with the decoction of the dried herb. It also drieth up the moisture of fistulous ulcers, or any other that are foul and spreading.

Rushes.

ALTHOUGH there are many kinds of Rushes, yet I shall only here insist upon those which are best known, and most medicinal; as the bulrushes, and other of the soft and smooth kinds, which grow so commonly in almost every part of this land, and are so generally noted, that I suppose it needless to trouble you with any description of them; briefly then to take the virtues of them as followeth:

Government and Virtues.] The seed of the soft Rushes, (saith Dioscorides and Galen, toasted, saith Pliny) being drank in wine and water, stayeth the lask and womens courses, when they come down too abundantly; but it causeth head-ach: It provoketh sleep likewise, but must be given with caution. The root boiled in water, to the consumption of one third, helpeth the cough.

Thus you see that conveniencies have their inconveniencies, and virtue is seldom unaccompanied with some vices. What I have written concerning Rushes, is to satisfy my countrymens question. *Are our Rushes good for nothing?* Yes, and as good let them alone as taken. There are remedies enough without them for any disease, and therefore as the proverb is, I care not a Rush for them; or rather, they will do you as much good as if one had given you a Rush.

Rye.

THIS is so well known in all the counties of this land, and especially to the country people, who feed much thereon, that if I did describe it, they would presently say, I might as well have spared that labour. Its virtues follow:

Government and Virtues.] Rye is more digesting than wheat; the bread and leaven thereof ripeneth and breaketh imposthumes, boils, and other swellings: The meal of Rye put between a double cloth, and moistened with a little vinegar, and heated in a pewter dish, set over a chaffing dish of coals, and bound fast to the head while it is hot, doth much ease the continual pains of the head. Matthiolus saith, That the ashes of Rye straw put into water, and steeped therein a day and a night, and the chops of the hands or feet washed therewith, doth heal them.

Saffron.

THE herb needs no description, it being known generally where it grows.

Place] It grows frequently at Walden in Essex, and in Cambridgeshire

Government and Virtues] It is an herb of the Sun, and under the Lion, and therefore you need not demand a reason why it strengthens the heart so exceedingly. Let not above ten grains be given at one time, for the Sun, which is the fountain of light, may dazzle the eyes, and make them blind, a cordial being taken in an immoderate quantity, hurts the heart instead of helping it. It quickeneth the brain, for the Sun is exalted in Aries, as well as he hath his house in Leo: It helpeth consumptions of the lungs, and difficulty of breathing: It is excellent in epidemical diseases, as pestilence, small pox, and measles. It is a notable expulsive medicine, and a notable remedy for the yellow jaundice. My opinion is, (but I have no author for it) that hermodactyls are nothing else but the roots of Saffron dried; and my reason is, that the roots of all crocus, both white and yellow, purge phlegm as hermodactyls do; and if you please to dry the roots of any crocus, neither your eyes nor your taste shall distinguish them from hermodactyls.

Sage.

OUR ordinary garden Sage needeth no description.

Time.] It flowereth in or about July.

Government and Virtues.] Jupiter claims this, and bids me tell you, it is good for the liver, and to breed blood. A decoction of the leaves and branches of Sage made and drank, saith Dioscorides, provokes urine, bringeth down womens courses, helps to expel the dead child, and causeth the hair to become black. It stayeth the bleeding of wounds, and cleanseth foul ulcers and sores. The decoction made in wine

taketh

taketh away the itching of the cods, if they be bathed therewith. Agrippa faith, that if women that cannot conceive by reason of the moist slipperiness of their wombs, shall take a quantity of the juice of Sage, with a little salt, for four days before they company with their husbands, it will help them not only to conceive, but also to retain the birth without miscarrying. Orpheus faith, three spoonfuls of the juice of Sage taken fasting, with a little honey, doth presently stay the spitting or casting of blood in them that are in a consumption. These pills are much commended: Take of spikenard, ginger, of each two drams; of the seed of Sage toasted at the fire, eight drams, of the long pepper 2 drams; all these being brought into powder, put thereto so much juice of Sage as may make them into a mass of pills, taking a dram of them every morning fasting, and so likewise at night, drinking a little pure water after them. Matthiolus faith, it is very profitable for all manner of pains in the head coming of cold and rheumatic humours; as also for all pains of the joints, whether inwardly or outwardly, and therefore helpeth the falling sickness, the lethargy, such as are dull and heavy of spirit, the palsy, and is of much use in all defluctions of rheum from the head, and for the diseases of the chest or breast. The leaves of Sage and nettles bruised together, and laid upon the imposthume that riseth behind the ears, doth assuage it much. The juice of Sage taken in warm water, helpeth a hoarseness and a cough. The leaves sodden in wine, and laid upon the place affected with the palsy, helpeth much, if the decoction be drank: Also, Sage taken with wormwood is good for the bloody flux. Pliny faith, it procures womens courses, and stayeth them coming down too fast; helpeth the stinging and biting of serpents, and killeth the worms that breed in the ear, and in sores Sage is of excellent use to help the memory, warming and quickening the senses; and the conserve made of the flowers is used to the same purpose, and also for all the former recited diseases. The juice of Sage drank with vinegar, hath been of good use in time of the plague at all times. Gargles likewise are made with Sage, rosemary, honeysuckles, and plantain, boiled in wine or water, with some honey or allum put thereto, to wash sore mouths and throats, cankers, or the secret parts of man or woman, as need requireth. And with other hot and comfortable herbs, Sage is

boiled

boiled to bathe the body and the legs in the Summer time, especially to warm cold joints or sinews, troubled with the palsy and cramp, and to comfort and strengthen the parts. It is much commended against the stitch, or pains in the side coming of wind, if the place be fomented warm with the decoction thereof in wine, and the herb also after boiling be laid warm thereunto.

Wood-Sage.

Descript.] WOOD Sage riseth up with square hoary stalks, two feet high at the least, with two leaves set at every joint, somewhat like other Sage leaves, but smaller, softer, whiter, and rounder, and a little dented about the edges, and smelling somewhat stronger. At the tops of the stalks and branches stand the flowers, on a slender like spike, turning themselves all one way when they blow, and are of a pale and whitish colour, smaller than Sage, but hooded and gaping like unto them. The seed is blackish and round; four usually seem in a husk together; the root is long and stringy, with divers fibres thereat, and abideth many years.

Place.] It groweth in woods, and by wood-sides; as also in divers fields and bye lanes in the land.

Time] It flowereth in June, July, and August.

Government and Virtues] The herb is under Venus. The decoction of the Wood Sage provoketh urine and womens courses: It also provoketh sweat, digesteth humours, and discusseth swellings and nodes in the flesh, and is therefore thought to be good against the French pox. The decoction of the green herb, made with wine, is a safe and sure remedy for those who by falls, bruises or blows, suspect some vein to be inwardly broken, to disperse and void the congealed blood, and to consolidate the veins. The drink used inwardly, and the herb used outwardly, is good for such as are inwardly bursten, and is found to be a sure remedy for the palsy. The juice of the herb, or the powder thereof dried, is good for moist ulcers and sores in the legs, and other parts, to dry them, and cause them to heal more speedily. It is no less effectual also in green wounds, to be used upon any occasion.

Solomon's

Solomon's Seal.

Descript.] THE common Solomon's Seal riseth up with a round stalk half a yard high, bowing or bending down to the ground, set with single leaves one above another, somewhat large, and like the leaves of the lily-convally, or May lily, with an eye of bluish upon the green, with some ribs therein, and more yellowish underneath. At the foot of every leaf, almost from the bottom up to the top of the stalk, come forth small, long, white and hollow pendulous flowers, somewhat like the flowers of May-lily, but ending in five long points, for the most part two together, at the end of a long foot-stalk, and sometimes but one, and sometimes also two stalks, with flowers at the foot of a leaf, which are without any scent at all, and stand on one side of the stalk. After they are past, come in their places small round berries, great at the first, and blackish green, tending to blueness when they are ripe, wherein lie small, white, hard, and stony seeds. The root is of the thickness of one's finger or thumb, white and knotted in some places, a flat round circle representing a Seal, whereof it took the name, lying along under the upper crust of the earth, and not growing downward, but with many fibres underneath.

Place] It is frequent in divers places of this land; as, namely, in a wood two miles from Canterbury, by Fish Pool Hill, as also in Bushy Close belonging to the parsonage of Alderbury, near Clarendon, two miles from Salisbury; in Cheffon-wood, or Cheffon Hill, between Newington and Sittingbourn in Kent, and divers other places in Essex, and other counties.

Time.] It flowereth about May: The root abideth and shooteth anew every year.

Government and Virtues] Saturn owns the plant, for he loves his bones well. The root of Solomon's Seal is found by experience to be available in wounds, hurts, and outward sores, to heal and close up the lips of those that are green, and to dry up and restrain the flux of humours to those that are old. It is singularly good to stay vomitings and bleeding wheresoever, as also all fluxes in man or woman, whether whites or reds in women, or the running of the reins in men; also to knit any joint, which by weakness useth to be often out of place, or will not stay in long when it is set; also, to knit and join broken bones in any part of the body, the roots being bruised and applied to the places, yea, it hath been found by late experience, that the decoction of the root in wine, or the bruised root put into wine or other drink, and after a night's infusion, strained forth hard and drank, hath helped both man and beast, whose bones hath been broken by any occasion, which is the most assured refuge of help to people of divers counties of the land that they can have: It is no less effectual to help ruptures and burstings, the decoction in wine, or the powder in broth or drink, being inwardly taken, and outwardly applied to the place. The same is also available for inward or outward bruises, falls or blows, both to dispel the congealed blood, and to take away both the pains and the black and blue marks that abide after the hurt. The same also, or the distilled water of the whole plant, used to the face, or other parts of the skin, cleanseth it from morphew, freckles, spots, or marks whatsoever, leaving the place fresh fair, and lovely, for which purpose it is much used by the Italian Dames.

Samphire.

Descript.] ROCK Samphire groweth up with a tender green stalk about half a yard, or two feet high at the most, branching forth almost from the very bottom, and stored with sundry thick and almost round (somewhat long) leaves, of a deep green colour, sometimes two together, and sometimes more on a stalk, and sappy, and of a pleasant, hot, and spicy taste. At the top of the stalks and branches stand umbels of white flowers, and after them come large seed bigger than fennel seed, yet somewhat like it. The root is great, white, and long, continuing many years, and is of an hot and spicy taste also.

Place.] It groweth on the rocks that are often moistened at the least, if not overflowed with the sea water.

Time.] And it flowereth and seedeth in the end of July and August.

Government and Virtues] It is an herb of Jupiter, and was in former times wont to be used more than it is now, the more is the pity. It is well known almost to every body, that ill digestions and obstructions are the cause of most of the diseases which the frail nature of man is subject to, both which might be remedied by a more frequent use of this herb.

herb. If people would have sauce to their meat, they may take some for profit as well as for pleasure. It is a safe herb, very pleasant both to taste and stomach, helping digestion, and in some sort opening obstructions of the liver and spleen; provoketh urine, and helpeth thereby to wash away the gravel and stone engendered in the kidneys or bladder.

Sanicle.

Descript.] ORDINARY Sanicle sendeth forth many great round leaves, standing upon long brownish stalks, every one somewhat deeply cut or divided into five or six parts, and some of these also cut in somewhat like the leaf of crow's foot, or dove's-foot, and finely dented about the edges, smooth, and of a dark shining colour, and sometimes reddish about the brim; from among which arise up small, round green stalks, without any joint or leaf thereof, saving at the top, where it branches forth into flowers, having a leaf divided into three or four parts at that joint with the flowers, which are small and white, starting out of small round greenish yellow heads, many standing together in a tuft, in which afterwards are the seeds contained, which are small round burs, somewhat like the leaves of clevers, and stick in the same manner upon any thing that they touch. The root is composed of many blackish strings or fibres, set together at a little long head which abideth with green leaves all the Winter, and perisheth not.

Place] It is found in many shadowy woods, and other places of this land.

Time] It flowereth in June, and the seed is ripe shortly after.

Government and Virtues] This is one of Venus's herbs, to cure the wounds or mischiefs Mars inflicteth upon the body of man. It heals green wounds speedily, or any ulcers, imposthumes, or bleedings inward, also tumours in any part of the body; for the decoction or powder in drink taken, and the juice used outwardly, dissipateth the humours; and there is not found any herb that can give such present help either to man or beast, when the disease falleth upon the lungs or throat, and to heal up putrid malignant ulcers in the mouth, throat and privities, by gargling or washing with the decoction of the leaves and roots made in water, and a little honey put thereto. It helpeth to stay womens courses,

and

and all other fluxes of blood, either by the mouth, urine, or stool, and lasks of the belly; the ulcerations of the kidneys also, and the pains in the bowels, and gonorrhea, or running of the reins, being boiled in wine or water, and drank. The same also is no less powerful to help any rupture or burstings, used both inwardly and outwardly: And briefly, it is as effectual in binding, restraining, consolidating, heating, drying and healing, as comfrey, bugle, self-heal, or any other of the vulnerary herbs whatsoever.

Saracens Confound, or Saracens Woundwort.

Descript.] THIS groweth high sometimes, with brownish stalks, and other whiles with green, to a man's height, having narrow green leaves snipped about the edges, somewhat like those of the peach tree, or willow leaves, but not of such a white green colour. The tops of the stalks are furnished with many yellow star-like flowers, standing in green heads, which when they are fallen, and the seed ripe, which is somewhat long, small and of a brown colour, wrapped in down, is therewith carried away with the wind. The root is composed of fibres set together at a head, which perishing not in Winter, although the stalks dry away, and no leaf appeareth in the Winter. The taste hereof is strong and unpleasant; and so is the smell also.

Place.] It groweth in moist and wet grounds by wood sides, and sometimes in the moist places of shadowy groves, as also by the water side.

Time.] It flowereth in July, and the seed is soon ripe, and carried away with the wind.

Government and Virtues.] Saturn owns the herb, and it is of a sober condition like him. Among the Germans this wound herb is preferred before all others of the same quality. Being boiled in wine, and drank, it helpeth the indisposition of the liver, and freeth the gall from obstructions; whereby it is good for the yellow jaundice, and for the dropsy in the beginning of it; for all inward ulcers of the reins, mouth or throat, and inward wounds and bruises, likewise for such sores as happen in the privy parts of men or women; being steeped in wine, and then distilled, the water thereof drank, is singular good to ease all gnawings in the stomach, or other pains of the body, as also the pains of the

mother

mother: And being boiled in water, it helpeth continual agues; and the said water, or the simple water of the herb distilled, or the juice or decoction, are very effectual to heal any green wound, or old sore or ulcer whatsoever, cleansing them from corruption, and quickly healing them up: Briefly, whatsoever hath been said of bugle or sanicle, may be found herein.

Sauce-alone, or Jack by the Hedge-side.

Descript.] THE lower leaves of this are rounder than those that grow towards the tops of the stalks, and are set singly on the joint, being somewhat round and broad, pointed at the ends, dented also about the edges, somewhat resembling nettle leaves for the form, but of a fresher green colour, not rough or pricking: The flowers are white, growing at the top of the stalks one above another, which being past, follow small round pods, wherein are contained round seed somewhat blackish. The root stringy and thready, perisheth every year after it hath given seed, and raiseth itself again of its own sowing. The plant, or any part thereof, being bruised, smelleth of garlic, but more pleasantly, and tasteth somewhat hot and sharp, almost like unto rocket.

Place.] It groweth under walls, and by hedge sides, and path ways in fields in many places.

Time] It flowereth in June, July, and August.

Government and Virtues] It is an herb of Mercury. This is eaten by many country people as sauce to their salt fish, and helpeth well to digest the crudities and other corrupt humours engendered thereby: It warmeth also the stomach, and causeth digestion. The juice thereof boiled with honey is accounted to be as good as hedge mustard for the cough, to cut and expectorate the tough phlegm. The seed bruised and boiled in wine, is a singular good remedy for the wind colic, or the stone, being drank warm. It is also given to women troubled with the mother, both to drink, and the seed put into a cloth, and applied while it is warm, is of singular good use. The leaves also, or the seed boiled, is good to be used in clysters to ease the pains of the stone. The green leaves are held to be good to heal the ulcers in the legs.

Winter

Winter and Summer Savory.

BOTH these are so well known, (being entertained as constant inhabitants in our gardens) that they need no description.

Government and Virtues.] Mercury claims the dominion over this herb, neither is there a better remedy against the colic and iliac passion, than this herb, keep it dry by you all the year, if you love yourself and your ease, and it is a hundred pounds to a penny if you do not; keep it dry, make conserves and syrups of it for your use, and withal, take notice that the Summer kind is the best. They are both of them hot and dry, especially the Summer kind, which is both sharp and quick in taste, expelling wind in the stomach and bowels, and is a present help for the rising of the mother procured by wind; provoketh urine and womens courses, and is much commended for women with child to take inwardly, and to smell often unto. It cureth tough phlegm in the chest and lungs, and helpeth to expectorate it the more easily; quickens the dull spirits in the lethargy, the juice thereof being snuffed up into the nostrils. The juice dropped into the eyes, cleareth a dull sight, if it proceed of thin cold humours distilled from the brain. The juice heated with oil of Roses, and dropped into the ears, easeth them of the noise and singing in them, and of deafness also. Outwardly applied with wheat flour, in manner of a poultice, it giveth ease to them, and taketh away their pains. It also taketh away the pain that comes by stinging of bees, wasps, &c.

Savine.

TO describe a plant so well known is needless, it being nursed up almost in every garden, and abiding green all the Winter.

Government and Virtues] It is under the dominion of Mars, being hot and dry in the third degree, and being of exceeding clean parts, is of a very digesting quality. If you dry the herb into powder, and mix it with honey, it is an excellent remedy to cleanse old filthy ulcers and fistulas, but it hinders them from healing. The same is excellent good to break carbuncles and plague sores; also helpeth the king's evil, being applied to the place. Being spread over

a piece

a piece of leather, and applied to the navel, kills the worms in the belly, helps scabs and itch, running sores, cankers, tetters, and ringworms; and being applied to the place, may haply cure venereal sores. This I thought good to speak of, as it may be safely used outwardly, for inwardly it cannot be taken without manifest danger.

The common White Saxifrage.

Descript.] THIS hath a few small reddish kernels of roots covered with some skins, lying among divers small blackish fibres, which send forth divers round, faint or yellow green leaves, and greyish underneath, lying above the ground, unevenly dented about the edges, and somewhat hairy, every one upon a little foot-stalk, from whence riseth up round, brownish hairy, green stalks, two or three feet high, with a few such like round leaves as grow below, but smaller, and somewhat branched at the top, whereon stand pretty large white flowers of five leaves a-piece, with some yellow threads in the middle, standing in a long crested, brownish, green husk. After the flowers are past, there ariseth sometimes a round hard head, forked at the top, wherein is contained small black seed, but usually they fall away without any seed, and it is the kernels or grains of the root which are usually called the White Saxifrage-seed, and so used.

Place] It groweth in many places of this land, as well in the lowermost as in the upper dry corners of meadows, and grassy sandy places. It used to grow near Lamb's conduit, on the backside of Gray's Inn.

Time] It flowereth in May, and then gathered, as well for that which is called the seed, as to distil, for it quickly perisheth down to the ground when any hot weather comes.

Government and Virtues] It is very effectual to cleanse the reins and bladder, and to dissolve the stone engendered in them, and to expel it and the gravel by urine, to help the stranguary; for which purpose the decoction of the herb or roots in white wine is most usual, or the powder of the small kernelly root, which is called the seed, taken in white wine, or in the same decoction made with white wine, is most usual. The distilled water of the whole herb, root and flowers, is most familiar to be taken. It provoketh also womens courses, and freeth and cleanseth the stomach and lungs

lungs from thick and tough phlegm that trouble them. There are not many better medicines to break the stone than this.

Burnet Saxifrage.

Descript.] THE greater sort of our English Burnet Saxifrage groweth up with divers long stalks of winged leaves, set directly opposite one to another on both sides, each being somewhat broad, and a little pointed and dented about the edges, of a sad green colour. At the top of the stalks stand umbels of white flowers, after which come small and blackish seed. The root is long and whitish, abiding long. Our lesser Burnet Saxifrage hath much finer leaves than the former, and very small, and set one against another, deeply jagged about the edges, and of the same colour as the former. The umbels of the flowers are white, and the seed very small, and so is the root, being also somewhat hot and quick in taste.

Place] These grow in moist meadows of this land, and are easy to be found, being well sought for among the grass, wherein many times they lay hid scarcely to be discerned

Time.] They flower about July, and their seed is ripe in August.

Government and Virtues.] They are both of them herbs of the moon. The Saxifrages are hot as pepper; and Tragus saith, by his experience, that they are wholesome. They have the same properties the parsleys have, but in provoking urine, and easing the pains thereof, and of the wind and colic, are much more effectual, the roots or seed being used either in powder, or in decoctions, or any other way; and likewise helpeth the windy pains of the mother, and to procure their courses, and to break and void the stone in the kidneys, to digest cold, viscous, and tough phlegm in the stomach, and is an especial remedy against all kind of venom. Castoreum being boiled in the distilled water thereof, is singular good to be given to those that are troubled with cramps and convulsions. Some do use to make the seeds into comfits (as they do carraway seeds) which is effectual to all the purposes aforesaid. The juice of the herb dropped into the most grievous wounds of the head drieth up their moisture, and healeth them quickly. Some women use the distilled water to take away freckles or spots in the skin or face;

face; and to drink the same sweetened with sugar for all the purposes aforesaid.

Scabious, three Sorts.

Descript] COMMON Field Scabious groweth up with many hairy, soft, whitish green leaves, some whereof are very little, if at all jagged on the edges, others very much rent and torn on the sides, and have threads in them, which upon breaking may be plainly seen; from among which rise up divers hairy green stalks, three or four feet high, with such like hairy green leaves on them, but more deeply and finely divided, branched forth a little: At the tops thereof, which are naked and bare of leaves for a good space, stand round heads of flowers, of a pale bluish colour, set together in a head, the outermost whereof are larger than the inward, with many threads also in the middle, somewhat flat at the top, as the head with the seed is likewise, the root is great, white and thick, growing down deep into the ground, and abideth many years.

There is another sort of Field Scabious different in nothing from the former, but only it is smaller in all respects.

The Corn Scabious differeth little from the first, but that it is greater in all respects, and the flowers more inclining to purple, and the root creepeth under the upper crust of the earth and runneth not deep into the ground as the first doth.

Place] The first groweth more usually in meadows, especially about London every where.

The second in some of the dry fields about this city, but not so plentifully as the former.

The third in standing corn, or fallow fields, and the borders of such like fields.

Time] They flower in June and July, and some abide flowering until it be late in August, and the seed is ripe in the mean time.

There are many other sorts of Scabious, but I take these which I have here described to be most familiar with us. The virtues of both these and the rest, being much alike, take them as followeth.

Government and Virtues] Mercury owns the plant Scabious is very effectual for all sorts of coughs, shortness of breath, and all other diseases of the breasts and lungs, ripening

ing and digesting cold phlegm, and other tough humour, voideth them forth by coughing and spitting: It ripeneth also all sorts of inward ulcers and imposthumes, pleurisy also, if the decoction of the herb dry or green be made in wine, and drank for some time together. Four ounces of the clarified juice of Scabious taken in the morning fasting, with a dram of mithridate, or Venice treacle, freeth the heart from any infection of pestilence, if after the taking of it the party sweat two hours in bed, and this medicine be again, and again repeated, if need require. The green herb bruised and applied to any carbuncle or plague sore, is found by certain experience to dissolve and break it in three hours space. The same decoction also drank, helpeth the pains and stitches in the side. The decoction of the roots taken for forty days together, or a dram of the powder of them taken at a time in whey, doth (as Matthiolus saith) wonderfully help those that are troubled with running or spreading scabs, tetters, ringworms, yea, although they proceed from the French pox, which he saith, he hath tried by experience. The juice or decoction drank helpeth also scabs and breakings out of the itch, and the like. The juice also made up into an ointment and used, is effectual for the same purpose. The same also healeth all inward wounds by the drying, cleansing, and healing quality therein: And a syrup made of the juice and sugar, is very effectual to all the purposes aforesaid, and so is the distilled water of the herb and flowers made in due season, especially to be used when the green herb is not in force to be taken. The decoction of the herb and roots outwardly applied, doth wonderfully help all sorts of hard or cold swellings in any part of the body, is effectual for shrunk sinews or veins, and healeth green wounds, old sores and ulcers. The juice of Scabious, made up with the powder of Borax and Samphire, cleanseth the skin of the face or other parts of the body, not only from freckles and pimples, but also from morphew and leprosy; the head washed with the decoction, cleanseth from dandruff, scurf, sores, itch, and the like, used warm. The herb bruised and applied, doth in a short time loosen and draw forth any splinter, broken bone, arrow head, or other such like thing lying in the flesh.

Scurvy

Scurvygrass.

Descript.] OUR ordinary English Scurvygrass hath many thick flat leaves, more long than broad, and sometimes longer and narrower; sometimes also smooth on the edges, and sometimes a little waved, sometimes plain, smooth and pointed, of a sad green, and sometimes a bluish colour, every one standing by itself upon a long foot-stalk, which is brownish or greenish also, from among which arise many slender stalks, bearing few leaves thereon like the other, but longer and lesser for the most part. At the tops whereof grow many whitish flowers, with yellow threads in the middle, standing about a green head, which becometh the seed vessel, which will be somewhat flat when it is ripe, wherein is contained reddish seed, tasting somewhat hot. The root is made of many white strings, which stick deeply into the mud, wherein it chiefly delights, yet it will well abide in the more upland and drier ground, and tasteth a little brackish and salt even there, but not so much as where it hath the salt water to feed upon.

Place.] It groweth all along the Thames side, both on the Essex and Kentish shores, from Woolwich round about the sea coasts to Dover, Portsmouth, and even to Bristol, where it is had in plenty; the other with round leaves groweth in the marshes in Holland, in Lincolnshire, and other places of Lincolnshire by the sea side.

Descript.] There is also another sort called Dutch Scurvygrass, which is most known, and frequent in gardens, and hath fresh, green, and almost round leaves rising from the root, not so thick as the former, yet in some rich ground, very large, even twice as big as in others, not dented about the edges, or hollow in the middle, standing on a long foot stalk, from among these rise long slender stalks, higher than the former, with more white flowers at the tops of them, which turn into small pods, and smaller brownish seed than the former. The root is white, small, and thready. The taste is nothing salt at all; it hath a hot, aromatical, spicy taste.

Time.] It flowereth in April and May, and giveth seed ripe quickly after.

Government and Virtues.] It is an herb of Jupiter. The English Scurvygrass, is more used for the salt taste it beareth, which doth somewhat open and cleanse; but the Dutch vygrafs is of better effect, and chiefly used (if it may be had by those that have the scurvy,) and is of singular good effect to cleanse the blood, liver, and spleen, taking the juice in the Spring every morning fasting in a cup of drink. The decoction is good for the same purpose, and openeth obstructions, evacuating cold, clammy, and phlegmatic humours both from the liver and the spleen, and bringing the body to a more lively colour. The juice also helpeth all foul ulcers and sores in the mouth, gargled therewith; and used outwardly, cleanseth the skin from spots, marks, or scars that happen therein.

Self-Heal. Called also Prunel, Carpenter's Herb, Hook-Heal, and Sickle-wort.

Descript.] THE common Self Heal is a small, low, creeping herb, having many small, round-pointed leaves, like leaves of wild mint, of a dark green colour, without dents on the edges, from among which rise square hairy stalks, scarce a foot high, which spread sometimes into branches with small leaves set thereon, up to the tops, where stand brown spiked heads of small brownish leaves like scales and flowers together, almost like the head of cassidony, which flowers are gaping, and of a bluish purple or more pale blue in some places sweet, but not so in others. The root consists of many fibres downward, and spreading strings also whereby it increaseth. The small stalks with the leaves creeping on the ground, shoot forth fibres taking hold on the ground, whereby it is made a great tuft in a short time.

Place] It is found in woods and fields everywhere.

Time.] It flowereth in May, and sometimes in April.

Government and Virtues] Here is another herb of Venus, Self Heal, whereby when you are hurt you may heal yourself. It is a special herb for inward and outward wounds. Take it inwardly in syrup for inward wounds; outwardly in unguents and plaisters for outward. As Self-Heal is like Bugle in form, so also in the qualities and virtues, serving for all the purposes whereto Bugle is applied with good success, either inwardly or outwardly, for inward wounds or ulcers whatsoever within the body, for bruises, falls, and such like hurts. If it be accompanied with Bugle,

Sanicle, and other the like wound-herbs, it will be more effectual to wash or inject into ulcers in the parts outwardly. Where there is cause to repress the heat and sharpness of humours flowing to any sores, ulcers, inflammations, swellings, or the like, or to stay the flux of blood in any wound or part, this is used with some good success, as also to cleanse the foulness of sores, and cause them more speedily to be healed. It is an especial remedy for all green wounds, to solder the lips of them, and to keep the place from any further inconveniencies. The juice hereof used with oil of roses to anoint the temples and forehead, is very effectual to remove the head ach, and the same mixed with honey of roses, cleanseth and healeth all ulcers in the mouth and throat, and those also in the secret parts. And the proverb of the Germans, French, and others, is verified in this, *That he needeth neither physician nor surgeon that hath* Self-Heal *and* Sanicle *to help himself.*

The Service-Tree.

IT is so well known in the place where it grows, that it needeth no description.

Time] It flowereth before the end of May, and the fruit is ripe in October.

Government and Virtues.] Services, when they are mellow, are fit to be taken to stay fluxes, scouring, and casting, yet less than medlars. If they be dried before they be mellow, and kept all the year, they may be used in decoctions for the said purpose, either to drink or to bathe the parts requiring it; and are profitably used in that manner to stay the bleeding of wounds, and of the mouth or nose, to be applied to the forehead, and nape of the neck; and are under the dominion of Saturn.

Shepherd's Purse.

IT is called Whoreman's Permacety, Shepherd's Scrip, Shepherd's Pounce, Toywort, Pickpurse, and Ca'swort.

Descript] The root is small, white, and perisheth every year. The leaves are small and long, of a pale green colour, and deeply cut in on both sides, among which spring up a stalk which is small and round, containing small leaves upon it even to the top. The flowers are white and very small, after which come the little cases which hold the seed, which are flat, almost in the form of a heart.

Place.] They are frequent in this nation, almost by every path-side.

Time.] They flower all the Summer long: nay, some of them are so fruitful that they flower twice a year.

Government and Virtues.] It is under the dominion of Saturn, and of a cold, dry, and binding nature, like to him. It helps all fluxes of blood, either caused by inward or outward wounds; as also flux of the belly, and bloody-flux, spitting and pissing of blood, stops the terms in women, being bound to the wrists of the hands, and the soles of the feet, it helps the yellow-jaundice. The herb being made into a poultice, helps inflammations and St Anthony's fire. The juice being dropped into the ears heals the pains, noise, and mutterings thereof. A good ointment may be made of it for all wounds, especially wounds in the head.

Smallage.

THIS is also very well known, and therefore I shall not trouble the reader with any description thereof.

Place] It groweth naturally in dry and marshy ground; but if it be sown in gardens, it there prospereth very well.

Time.] It abideth green all the Winter, and seedeth in August.

Government and Virtues] It is an herb of Mercury. Smallage is hotter, drier, and much more medicinal than parsley, for it much more openeth obstructions of the liver and spleen, rarifieth thick phlegm, and cleanseth it and the blood withal. It provoketh urine and women's courses, and is singular good against the yellow jaundice, tertian and quartan agues, if the juice thereof be taken, but especially made up into a syrup. The juice also put to honey of roses, and barley water is very good to gargle the mouth and throat of those that have sores and ulcers in them, and will quickly heal them. The same lotion also cleanseth and healeth all other foul ulcers and cankers elsewhere, if they be washed therewith. The seed is especially used to break and expel wind, to kill worms, and to help a stinking breath. The root is effectual to all the purposes aforesaid, and is held to be stronger in operation than the herb, but especially to open obstructions, and to rid away any ague, if the juice thereof be taken in wine, or the decoction thereof in wine be used.

Sopewort,

Sopewort, or Bruisewort.

Descript.] The root creepeth under ground far and near, with many joints therein, of a brown colour on the outside, and yellow within, shooting forth in divers places weak round stalks, full of joints, set with two leaves a piece at every one of them on the contrary side, which are ribbed somewhat like the plantain, and fashioned like the common field white campion leaves, seldom having any branches from the sides of the stalks, but set with flowers at the top, standing in long husk, like the wild campions, made of five leaves a piece, round at the ends, and dented in the middle, of a rose colour, almost white, sometimes deeper, sometimes paler, of a reasonable scent.

Place.] It groweth wild in many low and wet grounds of this land, by brooks and the sides of running waters.

Time.] It flowereth usually in July, and so continueth all August and part of September, before they be quite spent.

Temperature and Virtues.] Venus owns it. The country people in divers places do use to bruise the leaves of Sopewort, and lay it to their fingers, hands or legs, when they are cut, to heal them up again. Some make great boast thereof, that it is diuretical to provoke urine, and thereby to expel gravel and the stone in the reins or kidneys, and do also account it singular good to void hydropical waters; and they no less extol it to perform an absolute cure in the French pox, more than either sarsaparilla, guiacum, or China can do; which, how true it is, I leave others to judge.

Sorrel.

OUR ordinary Sorrel, which grows in gardens, and also wild in the fields, is so well known, that it needeth no description.

Government and Virtues.] It is under the dominion of Venus. Sorrel is prevalent in all hot diseases, to cool any inflammation and heat of blood in agues, pestilential or choleric, or sickness and fainting, arising from heat, and to refresh the overspent spirits with the violence of furious or fiery fits of ague, to quench thirst, and procure an appetite in fainting or decaying stomachs. For it resisteth the putrefaction of the blood, killeth worms, and is a cordial to the heart, which the seed doth more effectually, being more drying and binding, and thereby stayeth the hot fluxes of womens courses, or of humours in the bloody-flux, or that of the stomach. The root also in a decoction, or in powder, is effectual for all the said purposes. Both roots and seed, as well as the herb, are held powerful to resist the poison of the scorpion. The decoction of the roots is taken to help the jaundice, and to expel the gravel and the stone in the reins or kidneys. The decoction of the flowers made with wine and drank, helpeth the black jaundice, as also the inward ulcers of the body and bowels. A syrup made with the juice of Sorrel and fumitory is a sovereign help to kill those sharp humours that cause the itch. The juice thereof, with a little vinegar, serveth well to be used outwardly for the same cause, and is also profitable for tetters, ringworms, &c. It helpeth also to discuss the kernels in the throat; and the juice gargled in the mouth, helpeth the sores therein. The leaves wrapt in a colewort leaf and roasted in the embers, and applied to a hard imposthume, blotch, boil, or plague sore, doth both ripen and break it. The distilled water of the herb is of much good use for all the purposes aforesaid.

Wood Sorrel.

Descript.] THIS groweth upon the ground, having a number of leaves coming from the root made of three leaves, like a trefoil, but broad at the ends, and cut in the middle, of a yellowish green colour, every one standing on a long foot stalk, which at their first coming up are close folded together to the stalk, but opening themselves afterwards, and are of a fine sour relish, and yielding a juice which will turn red when it is clarified, and maketh a most dainty clear syrup. Among these leaves rise up divers tender, weak foot stalks, with every one of them a flower at the top, consisting of five small-pointed leaves, star-fashion, of a white colour in most places, and in some dashed over with a small show of bluish on the back side only. After the flowers are past, follow small round heads, with small yellow seed in them. The roots are nothing but small strings fastened to the end of a small long piece; all of them being of a yellowish colour.

Place.] It groweth in many places of our land, in woods and wood-sides where they be moist and shadowed, and in other places not too much open to the sun.

Time]

Time.] It flowereth in April and May.

Government and Virtues.] Venus owns it. Wood Sorrel serveth for all the purposes that the other Sorrels do, and is more effectual in hindering putrefaction of blood, and ulcers in the mouth and body, and to quench thirst, to strengthen a weak stomach, to procure an appetite, to stay vomiting, and very excellent in any contagious sickness or pestilential fevers. The syrup made of the juice is effectual in all the cases aforesaid, and so is the distilled water of the herb. Spunges or linen cloths wet in the juice, and applied outwardly to any hot swelling or inflammations, doth much cool and help them. The same juice taken and gargled in the mouth, and after it is spit forth, taken afresh, doth wonderfully help a foul stinking canker or ulcers therein. It is singular good to heal wounds, or to stay the bleeding of thrusts or stabs in the body.

Sow Thistle.

SOW Thistles are generally so well known, that they need no description

Place] They grow in gardens and manured grounds, sometimes by old walls, path sides of fields and highways.

Government and Virtues.] This and the former are under the influence of Venus. Sow Thistles are cooling, and somewhat binding, and are very fit to cool a hot stomach, and ease the pains thereof. The herb boiled in wine, is very helpful to stay the dissolution of the stomach, and the milk that is taken from the stalks when they are broken, given in drink, is beneficial to those that are short-winded, and have a wheezing. Pliny saith, That it hath caused the gravel and stone to be voided by urine, and that the eating thereof helpeth a stinking breath. The decoction of the leaves and stalks causeth abundance of milk in nurses, and their children to be well coloured. The juice or distilled water is good for all hot inflammations, wheals, and eruptions or heat in the skin, itching of the hæmorrhoids. The juice boiled or thoroughly heated in a little oil of bitter almond or the peel of a pomegranate, and dropped into the ears, is a sure remedy for deafness, singings, &c. Three spoonfuls of the juice taken warmed in white wine, and some wine put thereto, causeth women in travail to have so easy and speedy delivery, that they may be able to walk presently after. It is wonderfully good for women to wash their faces with, to clear the skin, and give it a lustre.

Southern Wood.

SOUTHERN Wood is so well known to be an ordinary inhabitant in our gardens, that I shall not need to trouble you with any description thereof.

Time] It flowereth for the most part in July and August.

Government and Virtues] It is a gallant mercurial plant, worthy of more esteem than it hath. Dioscorides saith, That the seed bruised, heated in warm water, and drank, helpeth those that are bursten, or troubled with cramps or convulsions of the sinews, the sciatica, or difficulty in making water, and bringeth down womens courses. The same taken in wine is an antidote, or counter poison, against all deadly poison, and driveth away serpents and other venomous creatures; as also the smell of the herb, being burnt, doth the same. The oil thereof anointed on the back bone before the fits of the agues come, taketh them away: It taketh away inflammations in the eyes, if it be put with some part of roasted quince, and boiled with a few crumbs of bread, and applied. Boiled with barley meal, it taketh away pimples, pushes, or wheal, that arise in the face, or other parts of the body. The seed as well as the dried herb, is often given to kill worms in children: The herb bruised and laid to, helpeth to draw forth splinters and thorns out of the flesh. The ashes thereof drieth up and healeth old ulcers, that are without inflammation, although by the sharpness thereof it biteth sore, and putteth them to sore pains; as also the sores in the privy parts of man or woman. The ashes mingled with old sallad oil, helpeth those that have hair fallen, and are bald, causing the hair to grow again either on the head or beard. Daranters saith, That the oil made of Southern Wood, and put among the ointments that are used against the French disease, is very effectual, and likewise killeth lice in the head. The distilled water of the herb is said to help them much that are troubled with the stone, as also for the diseases of the spleen and mother. The Germans commend it for a singular wound herb, and therefore call it Stabwort. It is held by all writers, ancient and modern, to be more offensive to the stomach than worm wood.

Spignel.

Spignel.

Descript] THE roots of common Spignel do spread much and deep in the ground, many strings of branches growing from one head, which is hairy at the top, of a blackish brown colour on the outside, and white within, smelling well, and of an aromatical taste, from whence rise sundry long stalks of most fine cut leaves like hair, smaller than dill, set thick on both sides of the stalks, and of a good scent. Among these leaves rise up round stiff stalks, with a few joints and leaves on them, and at the tops an umbel of fine pale white flowers; at the edges whereof sometimes will be seen a shew of the reddish bluish colour, especially before they be full blown, and are succeeded by small, somewhat round seeds, bigger than the ordinary fennel, and of a brown colour, divided into two parts, and crusted on the back, as most of the umbelliferous seeds are.

Place] It groweth wild in Lancashire, Yorkshire, and other northern counties, and is also planted in gardens.

Government and Virtues.] It is an herb of Venus. Galen saith, The roots of Spignel are available to provoke urine, and women's courses, but if too much thereof be taken, it causeth head-ach. The roots boiled in wine or water, and drank, helpeth the stranguary and stoppings of the urine, the wind, swellings and pains in the stomach, pains of the mother, and all joint aches. If the powder of the root be mixed with honey, and the same taken as a licking medicine, it breaketh tough phlegm, and drieth up the rheum that falleth on the lungs. The roots are accounted very effectual against the stinging or biting of any venomous creature, and is one of the ingredients in Mithridate, and other antidotes of the same.

Spleenwort, or Ceterach.

Descript] THIS smooth Spleenwort, from a black, thready and bushy root, sendeth forth many long, single leaves, cut in on both sides into round dents almost to the middle, which is not so hard as that of Polypody, each division being not always set opposite unto the other, cut between each, smooth, and of a light green on the upper side, and a dark yellowish roughness on the back, folding or rolling itself inward at the first springing up.

Place] It groweth as well upon stone walls, as moist and

shadowy places, about Bristol, and other the west parts plentifully; as also on Framlingham-Castle, on Beaconsfield church in Berkshire, at Stroude in Kent, and elsewhere, and abideth green all the Winter.

Government and Virtues] Saturn owns it. It is generally used against infirmities of the spleen: It helpeth the stranguary, and wasteth the stone in the bladder, and is good against the yellow-jaundice, and the hiccough; but the juice of it in women hindereth conception. Matthiolus saith, That if a dram of the dust that is on the back side of the leaves be mixed with half a dram of amber in powder, and taken with the juice of purslain or plantain, it helps the running of the reins speedily, and that the herb and root being boiled and taken, helpeth all melancholy diseases, and those especially that arise from the French disease. Camerarius saith, That the distilled water thereof being drank, is very effectual against the stone in the reins and bladder; and that the lee that is made of the ashes thereof being drank for some time together, helpeth splenetic persons. It is used in outward remedies for the same purpose.

Star Thistle.

Descript] A COMMON Star Thistle hath divers narrow leaves lying next the ground, cut on the edges somewhat deeply into many parts, soft or a little woolly, all over green, among which rise up divers weak stalks parted into many branches, all lying down to the ground, that it seemeth a pretty bush, set with divers the like divided leaves up to the tops, where severally do stand small whitish green heads, set with sharp white pricks, (no part of the plant else being prickly) which are somewhat yellowish; out of the middle whereof riseth the flowers, composed of many small reddish purple threads; and in the heads, after the flowers are past, come small whitish round seed, lying down as others do. The root is small, long and woody, perishing every year, and rising again of their own sowing.

Place] It groweth wild in the fields about London in many places, as at Mile End Green, in Finsbury Fields beyond the Windmills, and many other places.

Time] It flowereth early, and seedeth in July, and sometimes in August.

Government and Virtues.] This, as almost all Thistles are, is under Mars. The seed of this Star Thistle made into powder, and drank in wine, provoketh urine, and helpeth to break the stone, and driveth it forth. The root in powder, and given in wine and drank, is good against the plague and pestilence, and drank in the morning fasting for some time together, it is very profitable for a fistula in any part of the body. Baptista Sardas doth much commend the distilled water hereof, being drank to help the French disease, to open the obstructions of the liver, and cleanse the blood from corrupted humours, and is profitable against the quotidian or tertian ague.

Strawberries.

THESE are so well known through this land, that they need no description.

Time] They flower in May ordinarily, and the fruit is ripe shortly after.

Government and Virtues.] Venus owns the herb. Strawberries, when they are green, are cool and dry; but when they are ripe they are cool and moist: The berries are excellent good to cool the liver, the blood, and the spleen, or an hot choleric stomach; to refresh and comfort the fainting spirits, and quench thirst: They are good also for other inflammations; yet it is not amiss to refrain from them in a fever, lest by their putrifying in the stomach they increase the fits. The leaves and roots boiled in wine and water, and drank, do likewise cool the liver and blood, and assuage all inflammations in the reins and bladder, provoke urine, and allay the heat and sharpness thereof. The same also being drank stayeth the bloody flux and womens courses, and helps the swelling of the spleen. The water of the berries carefully distilled, is a sovereign remedy and cordial in the panting and beating of the heart, and is good for the yellow jaundice. The juice dropped into foul ulcers, or they washed therewith, or the decoction of the herb and root, doth wonderfully cleanse and help to cure them. Lotions and gargles for sore mouths, or ulcers therein or in the privy parts or elsewhere, are made with the leaves and roots thereof; which is also good to fasten loose teeth, and to heal spungy foul gums. It helpeth also to stay catarrhs, or defluxions of rheum in the mouth, throat, teeth, or eyes. The juice or water is singular good for hot and red inflamed eyes,

eyes, if dropped into them, or they bathed therewith. It is also of excellent property for all pushes, wheals, and other breakings forth of hot and sharp humours in the face and hands, and other parts of the body, to bathe them therewith, and to take away any redness in the face, or spots, or other deformities in the skin, and to make it clear and smooth. Some use this medicine: Take so many Strawberries as you shall think fitting, and put them into a distillatory, or body of glass fit for them, which being well closed, let it in a bed of horse dung for your use. It is an excellent water for hot inflamed eyes, and to take away a film, or skin that beginneth to grow over them, and for such other defects in them as may be helped by any outward medicine.

Succory.

Descript.] THE garden Succory hath longer and narrower leaves than the Endive, and more cut in, torn on the edges, and the root abideth many years. It beareth also blue flowers like Endive, and the seed is hardly distinguished from the seed of the smooth or ordinary Endive.

The wild Succory hath divers long leaves lying on the ground, very much cut in or torn on the edges, on both sides, even to the middle rib, ending in a point; sometimes it hath a rib down to the middle of the leaves, from among which riseth up a hard, round, woody stalk, spreading into many branches, set with smaller and lesser divided leaves on them up to the tops, where stand the flowers, which are like the garden kind, and the seed is also (only take notice that the flowers of the garden kind are gone in on a sunny day, they being so cold, that they are not able to endure the beams of the sun, and therefore more delight in the shade) the root is white, but more hard and woody than the garden kind. The whole plant is exceeding bitter

Place] This groweth in many places of our land in waste untilled and barren fields. The other in gardens.

Government and Virtues] It is an herb of Jupiter. Garden Succory, as it is more dry and less cold than Endive, so it openeth more. An handful of the leaves, or roots boiled in wine or water, and a draught thereof drank fasting driveth forth choleric and phlegmatic humours, openeth obstructions of the liver, gall and spleen, helpeth the yellow jaundice, the heat of the reins, and of the urine; the dropsy also; and those that have an evil disposition in their bodies, by reason of long sickness, evil diet, &c. which the Greeks call Cachexia. A decoction thereof made with wine, and drank, is very effectual against long lingering agues; and a dram of the seed in powder, drank in wine, before the fit of the ague, helpeth to drive it away. The distilled water of the herb and flowers (if you can take them in time) hath the like properties, and is especially good for hot stomachs, and in agues, either pestilential or of long continuance; for swoonings and passions of the heart, for the heat and head-ach in children, and for the blood and liver. The said water, or the juice, or the bruised leaves applied outwardly, allays swellings, inflammations, St Anthony's fire, pushes, wheals and pimples, especially used with a little vinegar; as also to wash pestiferous sores. The said water is very effectual for sore eyes that are inflamed with redness, for nurses breasts that are pained by the abundance of milk.

The wild Succory, as it is more bitter, so it is more strengthening to the stomach and liver.

Stone-Crop, Prick-Madam, or Small-Housleek.

Descript] It groweth with divers trailing branches upon the ground, set with many thick, flat, roundish, whitish green leaves, pointed at the ends. The flowers stand many of them together, somewhat loosely. The roots are small, and run creeping under ground.

Place.] It groweth upon the stone walls and mud walls, upon the tiles of houses, and pent-houses, and amongst rubbish, and in other gravelly places.

Time] It flowereth in June and July, and the leaves are green all the Winter.

Government and Virtues.] It is under the dominion of the Moon, cold in quality, and something binding. And therefore very good to stay defluctions, especially such as fall upon the eyes. It stops bleeding, both inward and outward, helps cankers, and all fretting sores and ulcers. It abates the heat of choler, thereby preventing diseases arising from choleric humours. It expels poison much, resisteth pestilential fevers, being exceeding good also for tertian agues:

You may drink the decoction of it, if you please, for all the foregoing infirmities. It is so harmless an herb, you can scarce use it amiss: Being bruised and applied to the place, it helps the king's evil, and any other knots or kernels in the flesh; as also the piles.

English Tobacco.

Descript] THIS riseth up with a round thick stalk, about two feet high, whereon do grow thick, flat green leaves, nothing so large as the other Indian kind, somewhat round-pointed also, and nothing dented about the edges. The stalk branches forth, and beareth at the tops divers flowers set on great husks like the other, but nothing so large: scarce standing above the brims of the husks, round pointed also, and of a greenish yellow colour. The seed that followeth is not so bright, but larger, contained in the like great heads. The roots are neither so great nor woody; it perisheth every year with the hard frosts in Winter, but riseth generally of its own sowing.

Place] This came from some parts of Brasil, as it is thought, and is more familiar in our country than any of the other sorts; early giving ripe seed, which the other seldom do.

Time] It flowereth from June, sometimes to the end of August, or later, and the seed ripeneth in the meantime.

Government and Virtues.] It is a martial plant. It is found by good experience to be available to expectorate tough phlegm from the stomach, chest and lungs. The juice thereof made into a syrup, or the distilled water of the herb drank with some sugar, or without, if you will, or the smoke taken by a pipe, as is usual, but fasting, helpeth to expel worms in the stomach and belly, and to ease the pains in the head, or megrim, and the griping pains in the bowels. It is profitable for those that are troubled with the stone in the kidneys, both to ease the pains by provoking urine, and also to expel gravel and the stone engendered therein, and hath been found very effectual to expel windiness, and other humours, which cause the strangling of the mother. The seed hereof is very effectual to expel the tooth ach, and the ashes of the burnt herb to cleanse the gums, and make the teeth white. The herb bruised and applied to the place grieved

with

with the king's-evil, helpeth it in nine or ten days effectually. Monardus faith, It is a counter poison against the biting of any venomous creature, the herb also being outwardly applied to the hurt place. The distilled water is often given with some sugar before the fit of an ague, to lessen it, and take it away in three or four times using. If the distilled fæces of the herb, having been bruised before the distillation, and not distilled dry, be set in warm dung for fourteen days, and afterwards be hung up in a bag in a wine cellar, the liquor that distilleth therefrom is singularly good to use for cramps, achs, the gout and sciatica, and to heal itches, scabs, and running ulcers, cankers, and all foul sores whatsoever. The juice is also good for all the said griefs, and likewise to kill lice in children's heads. The green herb bruised and applied to any green wounds, cureth any fresh wound or cut whatsoever; and the juice put into old sores, both cleanseth and healeth them. There is also made hereof a singular good salve to help imposthumes, hard tumours, and other swellings by blows and falls.

The Tamarisk-Tree.

IT is so well known in the places where it grows, that it needeth no description.

Time] It flowereth about the end of May, or in June, and the seed is ripe and blown away in the beginning of September.

Government and Virtues] A gallant Saturnine herb it is. The root, leaves, young branches, or bark boiled in wine, and drank, stays the bleeding of the hæmorrhoidal veins, the spitting of blood, the too abounding of womens courses, the jaundice, the colic, and the biting of all venomous serpents, except the asp; and outwardly applied, is very powerful against the hardness of the spleen, and the tooth-ach, pains in the ears, red and watering eyes. The decoction, with some honey put thereto, is good to stay gangrenes and fretting ulcers, and to wash those that are subject to nits and lice. Alpinus and Vestingius affirm, That the Egyptians do with good-success use the wood of it to cure the French disease, as others do with lignum vitæ or guiacum; and give it also to those who have the leprosy, scabs, ulcers, or the like. Its ashes doth quickly heal blisters raised by burnings or scaldings. It helps the dropsy, arising from hardness of the spleen, and therefore to drink out of cups made of the wood is good for splenetic persons. It is also helpful for melancholy, and the black jaundice that ariseth thereof.

Garden Tansy.

GARDEN Tansy is so well known, that it needeth no description.

Time.] It flowereth in June or July.

Government and Virtues.] Dame Venus was minded to pleasure women with child by this herb, for there grows not an herb fitter for their use than this, it is just as though it were cut out for the purpose. This herb bruised and applied to the navel, stays miscarriages; I know no herb like it for that use. Boiled in ordinary beer, and the decoction drank, doth the like: and if her womb be not as she would have it, this decoction will make it so. Let those women that desire children love this herb, it is their best companion, (their husbands excepted.) Also it consumes the phlegmatic humours, the cold and moist constitution of Winter most usually affects the body of man with, and that was the first reason of eating tansies in the Spring. At last the world being over run with Popery, a monster called Superstition, peeks up his head, and, as a judgment of God, obscures the bright beams of knowledge by his dismal looks; (physicians seeing the Pope and his imps selfish, they began to do so too) and now forsooth Tansies must be eaten only on Palm and Easter Sundays, and their neighbour days. At last superstition being too hot to hold, and the selfishness of physicians walking in the clouds, after the Friars and Monks had made the people ignorant, the superstition of the time was found out, by the virtue of the herb hidden, and now it is almost, if not altogether, left off. Surely our physicians are beholden to none so much as they are to Monks and Friars. For want of eating this herb in Spring, maketh people sickly in Summer; and that makes work for the physician. If it be against any man or woman's conscience to eat Tansy in the Spring, I am as unwilling to burthen their conscience, as I am that they should burthen mine; they may boil it in wine and drink the decoction, it will work the same effect. The decoction of the common Tansy, or the juice drank in wine

wine, is a singular remedy for all the griefs that come by stopping of the urine, helpeth the stranguary, and those that have weak reins and kidneys. It is also very profitable to dissolve and expel wind in the stomach, belly or bowels, to procure womens courses, and expel windiness in the matrix, if it be bruised and often smelled unto, as also applied to the lower part of the belly. It is also very profitable for such women as are given to miscarry in child bearing, to cause them to go out their full time: It is used also against the stone in the reins, especially to men. The herb fryed with eggs (as it is accustomed in the Spring time) which is called a Tansy, helpeth to digest and carry downward those bad humours that trouble the stomach. The seed is very profitably given to children for the worms, and the juice in drink is as effectual. Being boiled in oil, it is good for the sinews shrunk by cramps, or pained with colds, if thereto applied.

Wild Tansy, or Silver Weed.

THIS is also so well known, that it needeth no description.

Place] It groweth almost in every place.

Time] It flowereth in June and July.

Government and Virtues.] Now Dame Venus hath fitted women with two herbs of one name, one to help conception, the other to maintain beauty, and what more can be expected of her? What now remains for you, but to love your husbands, and not to be wanting to your poor neighbours? Wild Tansy stayeth the lask, and all the fluxes of blood in men and women, which some say it will do, if the green herb be worn in the shoes, so it be next the skin; and it is true enough, that it will stop the terms if worn so, and the whites too, for aught I know. It stayeth also spitting or vomiting of blood. The powder of the herb taken in some of the distilled water helpeth the whites in women, but more especially if a little coral and ivory in powder be put to it. It is also commended to help children that are bursten, and have a rupture, being boiled in water and salt. Being boiled in water and drank, it easeth the griping pains of the bowels, and is good for the sciatica and joint achs. The same boiled in vinegar, with honey and allum, and gargled in the mouth,

mouth, easeth the pains of the tooth ach, fasteneth loose teeth, helpeth the gums that are sore, and settleth the palate of the mouth in its place, when it is fallen down. It cleanseth and healeth ulcers in the mouth or secret parts, and is very good for inward wounds, and to close the lips of green wounds, and to heal old, moist, and corrupt running sores in the legs or elsewhere. Being bruised and applied to the soles of the feet and hand wrists, it wonderfully cooleth the hot fits of the agues, be they never so violent. The distilled water cleanseth the skin of all discolourings therein, as morphew, sun burnings, &c. as also pimples, freckles, and the like; and dropped into the eyes, or cloths wet therein and applied, taketh away the heat and inflammations in them.

Thistles.

OF these are many kinds growing here in England, which are so well known, that they need no description: Their difference are easily known by the places where they grow, viz.

Place] Some grow in fields, some in meadows, and some among the corn; others on heaths, greens, and waste grounds in many places.

Time] They flower in June and August, and their seed is ripe quickly after.

Government and Virtues.] Surely Mars rules it, it is such a prickly business All these Thistles are good to provoke urine, and to mend the stinking smell thereof, as also the rank smell of the arm pits, or the whole body, being boiled in wine and drank, and are said also to help a stinking breath, and to strengthen the stomach Pliny saith, That the juice bathed on the place that wanteth hair, it being fallen off, will cause it to grow again speedily.

The Melancholy Thistle.

Descript] IT riseth up with tender single hoary green stalks, bearing thereon four or five green leaves, dented above the edges; the points thereof are little or nothing prickly, and at the top usually but one head, yet sometimes from the bosom of the uppermost leaves there shooteth forth another small head, scaly and
prickly,

prickly, with many reddish thrumbs or threads in the middle, which being gathered fresh, will keep the colour a long time, and fadeth not from the stalk for a long time, while it perfects the seed, which is of a mean bigness lying in the down. The root hath many strings fastened to the head, or upper part, which is blackish, and perisheth not.

There is another sort, little differing from the former, but that the leaves are more green above, and more hoary underneath, and the stalk being about two feet high, beareth but one scaly head, with threads and seeds as the former.

Place] They grow in many moist meadows of this land, as well in the southern, as in the northern parts.

Time.] They flower about July or August, and their seed ripeneth quickly after.

Government and Virtues.] It is under Capricorn, and therefore under both Saturn and Mars; one rids melancholy by sympathy, the other by antipathy. Their virtues are but few, but those not to be despised; for the decoction of the thistle in wine being drank, expels superfluous melancholy out of the body, and makes a man as merry as a cricket; superfluous melancholy causeth care, fear, sadness, despair, envy, and many evils more besides; but religion teacheth to wait upon God's providence, and cast our care upon him who careth for us. What a fine thing were it if men and women could live so? And yet seven years care and fear makes a man never the wiser, nor a farthing richer. Dioscorides saith, the root borne about one doth the like, and removes all diseases of melancholy. Modern writers laugh at him: *Let them laugh that win*, my opinion is, that it is the best remedy against all melancholy diseases that grows; they that please to use it.

Our Lady's Thistle.

Descript.] OUR Lady's Thistle hath divers very large and broad leaves lying on the ground cut in, and as it were crumpled, but somewhat hairy on the edges, of a white green shining colour, wherein are many lines and streaks of a milk-white colour running all over, and set with many sharp and stiff prickles all about, among which riseth up one or more strong, round and prickly stalks, set full of the like leaves up to the top, where, at the end of every branch, comes forth a great prickly Thistle-like

like head, strongly armed with prickles, and with bright purple thrumbs rising out of the middle. After they are past, the seed groweth in the said heads, lying in soft white down, which is somewhat flatish in the ground, and many string and fibres fastened thereunto. All the whole plant is bitter in taste.

Place] It is frequent on the banks of almost every ditch.

Time] It flowereth and seedeth in June, July, and August.

Government and Virtues] Our Lady's Thistle is under Jupiter, and thought to be as effectual as Carduus Benedictus for agues, and to prevent and cure the infection of the plague; as also to open the obstructions of the liver and spleen, and thereby is good against the jaundice. It provoketh urine, breaketh and expelleth the stone, and is good for the dropsy. It is effectual also for the pains in the sides, and many other inward pains and gripings. The seed and distilled water are held powerful to all the purposes aforesaid, and besides, it is often applied both outwardly with cloths or spunges, to the region of the liver, to cool the distemper thereof, and to the region of the heart, against swoonings and passions of it. It cleanseth the blood exceedingly; and in Spring, if you please to boil the tender plant (but cut off the prickles, unless you have a mind to choak yourself) it will change your blood as the season changeth, and that is the way to be safe.

The Woolen, or Cotton Thistle.

Descript.] THIS hath many large leaves lying upon the ground, somewhat cut in, and as it were crumpled on the edges, of a green colour on the upper side, but covered over with a long hairy wool or cotton down, set with most sharp and cruel pricks, from the middle of whose heads of flowers come forth many purplish crimson threads, and sometimes white, although but seldom. The seed that followeth in those white downy heads, is somewhat large and round, resembling the seed of Lady's Thistle, but paler. The root is great and thick, spreading much, yet usually dieth after seed time.

Place] It groweth on divers ditch-banks, and in the corn-fields and highways, generally throughout the land, and is often growing in gardens.

Government and Virtues.] It is a plant of Mars. Dioscorides and

and Pliny write, That the leaves and roots hereof taken in drink, helpeth those that have a crick in their neck, that they cannot turn it, unless they turn their whole body. Galen saith, That the roots and leaves hereof are good for such persons that have their bodies drawn together by some spasm or convulsion, or other infirmities; as the rickets (or as the college of physicians would have it, Rachites, about which name they have quarrelled sufficiently) in children, being a disease that hindereth their growth, by binding their nerves, ligaments, and whole structure of their body.

The Fuller's Thistle, or Teasle.

IT is so well known, that it needs no description, being used with the cloth-workers.

The wild Teasle is in all things like the former, but that the prickles are small, soft, and upright, not hooked or stiff, and the flowers of this are of a fine bluish, or pale carnation colour, but of the manured kind, whitish.

Place] The first groweth, being sown in gardens or fields, for the use of cloth workers: The other near ditches and rills of water in many places of this land.

Time.] They flower in July, and are ripe in the end of August.

Government and Virtues.] It is an herb of Venus. Dioscorides saith, That the root bruised and boiled in wine, till it be thick, and kept in a brazen vessel, and after spread as a salve, and applied to the fundament, doth heal the cleft thereof, cankers and fistulas therein, also taketh away warts and wens. The juice of the leaves dropped into the ears, killeth worms in them. The distilled water of the leaves dropped into the eyes, taketh away redness and mists in them that hinder the sight, and is often used by women to preserve their beauty, and to take away redness and inflammations, and all other heat or discolourings.

Treacle Mustard.

Descript.] IT riseth with a hard round stalk, about a foot high, parted into some branches, having divers soft green leaves, long and narrow, set thereon, waved, but not cut into the edges, broadest towards the ends, somewhat round pointed; the flowers are white that grow at the

the tops of the branches, spike fashion, one above another; after which come round pouches, parted in the middle with a furrow, having one blackish brown seed on either side, somewhat sharp in taste, and smelling of garlic, especially in the fields where it is natural, but not so much in gardens. The roots are small and thready, perishing every year.

Give me leave here to add Mithridate Mustard, although it may seem more properly by the name to belong to M, in the alphabet.

Mithridate Mustard.

Descript.] THIS groweth higher than the former, spreading more and higher branches, whose leaves are smaller and narrower, sometimes unevenly dented about the edges. The flowers are small and white, growing on long branches, with much smaller and rounder vessels after them, and parted in the same manner, having smaller brown seeds than the former, and much sharper in taste. The root perisheth after seed time, but abideth the first Winter after springing.

Place] They grow in sundry places in this land, as half a mile from Hatfield, by the river side, under a hedge as you go to Hatfield, and in the street of Peckham on Surry side.

Time] They flower and seed from May to August.

Government and Virtues.] Both of them are herbs of Mars. The Mustards are said to purge the body both upwards and downwards, and procureth womens courses so abundantly, that it suffocateth the birth. It breaketh inward imposthumes, being taken inwardly; and used in clysters, helpeth the sciatica. The seed applied doth the same. It is an especial ingredient unto mithridate and treacle, being of itself an antidote resisting poison, venom, and putrefaction. It also is available in many cases for which the common Mustard is used, but somewhat weaker.

The Black Thorn, or Sloe-Bush.

IT is so well known, that it needeth no description.

Place] It groweth in every country in the hedges and borders of fields.

Time] It flowereth in April, and sometimes in March, but

but the fruit ripeneth after all other plums whatsoever, and is not fit to be eaten until the Autumn frost mellow them.

Government and Virtues.] All the parts of the Sloe Bush are binding, cooling and dry, and all effectual to stay bleeding at the nose and mouth, or any other place; the lask of the belly or stomach, or bloody flux, the too much abounding of womens courses, and helpeth to ease the pains of the sides, bowels, and guts, that come by overmuch scouring, to drink the decoction of the bark of the roots, or more usually the decoction of the berries, either fresh or dried. The conserve also is of very much use, and more familiarly taken for the purpose aforesaid. But the distilled water of the flowers first steeped in sack for a night, and drawn therefrom by the heat of the Balneum Anglice, a bath, is a most certain remedy, tried and approved, to ease all manner of gnawings in the stomach, the sides and bowels, or any griping pains in any of them, to drink a small quantity when the extremity of the pain is upon them. The leaves also are good to make lotions to gargle and wash the mouth and throat wherein are swellings, sores, or kernels; and to stay the defluctions of rheum to the eyes, or other parts, as also to cool the heat and inflammations of them, and ease hot pains of the head, to bathe the forehead and temples therewith. The simple distilled water of the flowers is very effectual for the said purposes, and the condensate juice of the Sloes. The distilled water of the green berries is used also for the said effects.

Thorough Wax, or Thorough Leaf.

Descript.] COMMON Thorough Wax sendeth forth a strait round stalk, two feet high, or better, whose lower leaves being of a bluish colour, are smaller and narrower than those up higher, and stand close thereto, not compassing it; but as they grow higher, they do more encompass the stalk, until it wholly pass through them, branching toward the top into many parts, where the leaves grow smaller again, every one standing single, and never two at a joint. The flowers are small and yellow, standing in tufts at the heads of the branches, where afterwards grow the seed, being blackish, many thick thrust together. The root is small, long and woody, perishing every year, after seed time, and rising again plentifully of its own sowing.

Place.] It is found growing in many cornfields, and pasture-grounds in this land.

Time.

Time.] It flowereth in July, and the seed is ripe in August.

Temperature and Virtues.] Both this and the former are under the influence of Saturn. Thorough Wax is of singular good use for all sorts of bruises and wounds either inward or outward, and old ulcers and sores likewise, if the decoction of the herb with water and wine be drank, and the place washed therewith, or the juice of the green herb bruised or boiled either by itself, or with other herbs, in oil or hog's grease, to be made into an ointment to serve all the year. The decoction of the herb, or powder of the dried herb, taken inwardly, and the same or the leaves bruised, and applied outwardly, is singular good for all ruptures and burstings, especially in children before they be too old. Being applied with a little flour and wax to childrens navels that stick forth, it helpeth them.

Thyme.

IT is in vain to describe an herb so commonly known.

Government and Virtues.] It is a noble strengthener of the lungs, as notable a one as grows; neither is there scarce a better remedy growing for that disease in children which they commonly call the Chincough, than it is. It purgeth the body of phlegm, and is an excellent remedy for shortness of breath. It kills worms in the belly, and being a notable herb of Venus, provokes the terms, gives safe and speedy delivery to women in travail, and brings away the after birth. It is so harmless you need not fear the use of it. An ointment made of it takes away hot swellings and warts, helps the sciatica and dulness of sight, and takes away pains and hardness of the spleen: 'Tis excellent for those that are troubled with the gout; as also, to anoint the cods that are swelled. It easeth pains in the loins and hips. The herb taken any way inwardly, comforts the stomach much, and expels wind.

Wild Thyme, or Mother of Thyme.

WILD Thyme also is so well known, that it needeth no description.

Place.] It may be found commonly in commons and other barren places throughout the nation.

Government and Virtues.] It is under the dominion of Venus, and under the sign Aries, and therefore chiefly appropriated

priated to the head. It provoketh urine and the terms, and easeth the griping pain of the belly, cramps, ruptures, and inflammations of the liver. If you make a vinegar of the herb, as vinegar of roses is made (you may find out the way in my translation of the London Dispensatory) and anoint the head with it, it presently stops the pains thereof. It is excellent good to be given either in phrenzy or lethargy, although they are two contrary diseases: It helps spitting and pissing of blood, coughing, and vomiting; it comforts and strengthens the head, stomach, reins, and womb, expels wind, and breaks the stone.

Tormentil, or Septfoil.

Descript] THIS hath reddish, slender, weak branches rising from the root, lying on the ground, rather leaning than standing upright, with many short leaves that stand closer to the stalks than Cinquefoil (to which this is very like) with the foot-stalk compassing the branches in several places; but those that grow to the ground are set upon long foot-stalks, each whereof are like the leaves of Cinquefoil, but somewhat long and lesser, dented about the edges, many of them divided but into five leaves, but most of them into seven, whence it is also called Septfoil; yet some may have six, and some eight, according to the fertility of the soil. At the tops of the branches stand divers small yellow flowers, consisting of five leaves, like those of Cinquefoil, but smaller. The root is smaller than bistort, somewhat thick, but blacker without and not so red within, yet sometimes a little crooked, having blackish fibres thereat.

Place] It groweth as well in woods and shady places, as in the open champian country, about the borders of fields in many places of this land, and almost in every *oom ast* in Sussex.

Time] It flowereth all the Summer long.

Government and Virtues] This is a gallant herb of the Sun. Tormentil is most excellent to stay all kinds of fluxes of blood or humours in man or woman, whether at nose, mouth, or belly. The juice of the herb and root, or the decoction thereof, taken with some Venice treacle, and the person laid to sweat, expel any venom or poison, or the plague, fever, or other contagious diseases as the pox, measles, &c. for it is an ingredient in all antidotes or counter poisons.

Valesius is of opinion, that the decoction of this root is no less effectual to cure the French pox than Guiacum or China; and it is not unlikely, because it so mightily resisteth putrefaction. The root taken inwardly is most effectual to help any flux of the belly, stomach, spleen, or blood; and the juice wonderfully opens obstructions of the liver and lungs, and thereby helpeth the yellow jaundice. The powder or decoction drank, or to sit thereon as a bath, is an assured remedy against abortion in women, if it proceed from the over flexibility or weakness of the inward retentive faculty, as also a plaister made therewith, and vinegar applied to the reins of the back, doth much help not only this, but also those that cannot hold their water, the powder being taken in the juice of plantain, and is commended against the worms in children. It is very powerful to ruptures and burstings, as also for bruises and falls, to be used as well outwardly as inwardly. The root hereof made up with pellitory of Spain and allum, and put into a hollow tooth, not only assuageth the pain, but stayeth the flux of humours which causeth it. Tormentil is no less effectual and powerful a remedy against outward wounds, sores and hurts, than for inward, and is therefore a special ingredient to be used in wound drinks, lotions and injections, for foul corrupt rotten sores and ulcers of the mouth, secrets, or other parts of the body. The juice or powder of the root put in ointments, plaisters, and such things that are applied to wounds or sores, is very effectual, as the juice of the leaves, and the root bruised and applied to the throat, or jaws, healeth the king's evil, and easeth the pain of the sciatica, the same used with a little vinegar, is a special remedy against the running sores of the head or other parts; scabs also, and the itch, or any such eruptions in the skin, proceeding of salt and sharp humour. The same is also effectual for the piles or hæmorrhoids, if they be washed or bathed therewith, or with the distilled water of the herb and roots. It is found also helpful to dry up any sharp rheum that distilleth from the head into the eyes, causing redness, pain, watchings, itching, or the like, if a little prepared tutia, or white amber, be used with the distilled water thereof. Many women use this water as a secret to help themselves and others, when they are troubled with too much flowing of the whites or reds, both to drink it, or inject it with a syringe. And here is enough, only remember the Sun challengeth this herb. Turn-

Turnsole, or Heliotropium.

Descript.] THE greater Turnsole riseth with one upright stalk, about a foot high, or more, dividing itself almost from the bottom, into divers small branches, of a hoary colour, at each joint of the stalk and branches grow small broad leaves, somewhat white and hoary. At the tops of the stalks and branches stand small white flowers, consisting of four, and sometimes five small leaves, set in order one above another, upon a small crooked spike which turneth inwards like a bowed finger, opening by degrees as the flowers blow open; after which in their place come forth cornered seed, four for the most part standing together; the root is small and thready, perishing every year, and the seed shedding every year, raiseth it again the next Spring.

Place] It groweth in gardens, and flowereth and seedeth with us, notwithstanding it is not natural to this land, but to Spain and France, where it grows plentifully.

Government and Virtues] It is an herb of the Sun, and a good one too. Dioscorides saith, That a good handful of this, which is called the Great Turnsole, boiled in water, and drank, purgeth both choler and phlegm; and boiled with cummin, helpeth the stone in the reins, kidneys, or bladder, provoketh urine and womens courses, and causeth an easy and speedy delivery in childbirth. The leaves bruised and applied to places pained with the gout, or that have been out of joint, and newly set, and full of pain, do give much ease; the seed and juice of the leaves also being rubbed with a little salt upon warts or wens, and other kernels in the face, eye lids, or any other part of the body, will, by often using, take them away.

Meadow Trefoil, or Honeysuckles.

IT is so well known, especially by the name of Honeysuckles, white and red, that I need not describe them.

Place] They grow almost every where in this land.

Government and Virtues] Mercury hath dominion over the common sorts. Dodoneus saith, The leaves and flowers are good to ease the griping pains of the gout, the herb being boiled and used in a clyster. If the herb be made into a poultice, and applied to inflammations, it will ease them.

The juice dropped in the eyes, is a familiar medicine with many country people, to take away the pin and web (as they call it) in the eyes; it also allayeth the heat and blood shooting of them. Country people do also in many places drink the juice thereof against the biting of an adder; and having boiled the herb in water, they first wash the place with the decoction, and then lay some of the herb also to the hurt place. The herb also boiled in swine's grease, and so made into an ointment, is good to apply to the biting of any venomous creatures. The herb also bruised and heated between tiles, and applied hot to the share, causeth them to make water who had it stopt before. It is held likewise to be good for wounds, and to take away seed. The decoction of the herb and flowers, with the seed and root, taken for some time, helpeth women that are troubled with the whites. The seed and flowers boiled in water, and after made into a poultice with some oil, and applied, helpeth hard swellings and imposthumes.

Heart Trefoil.

BESIDES the ordinary sort of Trefoil, here are two more remarkable, and one of which may be probably called Heart Trefoil, not only because the leaf is triangular, like the heart of a man, but also because each leaf contains the perfect icon of a heart, and that in its proper colours, viz. a flesh colour.

Place] It groweth between Longford and Bow, and beyond Southwark, by the highway and parts adjacent.

Government and Virtues] It is under the dominion of the Sun, and if it were used, it would be found as great a strengthener of the heart and cherisher of the vital spirits as grows, relieving the body against fainting and swoonings, for using it against poison and pestilence, defending the heart against the noisome vapours of the spleen.

Pearl Trefoil.

IT differs not from the common sort, save only in this one particular, it hath a white spot in the leaf like a pearl. It is particularly under the dominion of the Moon, and its icon sheweth that it is of a singular virtue against the pearl, or pin and web in the eyes.

Tutsan, or Park Leaves.

Descript.] It hath brownish shining round stalks, crested the length thereof, rising two by two, and sometimes three feet high, branching forth even from the bottom, having divers joints, and at each of them two fair large leaves standing, of a dark bluish green colour on the upper side, and of a yellowish green underneath, turning reddish toward Autumn. At the top of the stalks stand large yellow flowers, and heads with seed, which being greenish at the first, and afterwards reddish, turn to be of a blackish purple colour when they are ripe, with small brownish seed within them, and they yield a reddish juice or liquor, somewhat resinous and of a harsh and styptic taste, as the leaves also and the flowers be, although much less, but do not yield such a clear claret wine colour as some say it doth; the root is brownish, somewhat great, hard, and woody, spreading well in the ground.

Place.] It groweth in many woods, groves, and woody grounds, as parks and forests, and by hedge sides in many places in this land, as in Hampstead wood, by Ratley in Essex, in the wilds of Kent, and in many other places needless to recite.

Time.] It floweth later than St. John's or St. Peter's wort.

Government and Virtues.] It is an herb of Saturn, and a most noble antivenerean. Tutsan purgeth cholerick humours, as St. Peter's wort is said to do, for therein it worketh the same effects, both to help the sciatica and gout, and to heal burnings by fire; it staieth all the bleedings of wounds, if either the green herb be bruised, or the powder of the dry be applied thereto. It hath been accounted, and certainly it is a sovereign herb to heal either wound or sore, either outwardly or inwardly, and therefore always used in drinks, lotions, balms, oils, ointments, or any other sorts of green wounds, old ulcers or sores, in all which the continual experience of former ages hath confirmed the use thereof to be admirable good, though it be not so much in use now, as when physicians and surgeons were so wise to use herbs more than now they do.

Garden Valerian.

Descript.] This hath a thick short greyish root, lying for the most part above ground, shooting forth on all other sides such like small pieces of roots, which have all of them many long green strings and fibres under them in the ground, whereby it draweth nourishment. From the head of these roots spring up many green leaves, which at first are somewhat broad and long, without any divisions at all in them, or denting on the edges; but those that rise up after are more and more divided on each side, some to the middle rib, being winged, as made of many leaves together on a stalk, and those upon a stalk in like manner more divided, but smaller towards the top than below. The stalk riseth to be a yard high or more, sometimes branched at the top, with many small whitish flowers, sometimes dashed over at the edges with a pale purplish colour of a little scent which passing away, there followeth small brownish white seed, that is easily carried away with the wind. The root smelleth more strong than either leaf or flower, and is of more use in medicines.

Place] It is generally kept with us in gardens.

Time] It flowereth in June and July, and continueth flowering until the frost pull it down.

Government and Virtues] This is under the influence of Mercury. Dioscorides saith, That the Garden Valerian hath a warming faculty, and that being dried and given to drink, it provoketh urine, and helpeth the stranguary. The decoction thereof taken, doth the like also, and taketh away pains of the sides, provoketh womens courses, and is used in antidotes. Pliny saith, That the powder of the root given in drink, or the decoction thereof taken, helpeth all stoppings and stranglings in any part of the body, whether they proceed of pains in the chest or sides, and taketh them away. The root of Valerian boiled with liquorice, raisins, and anniseed, is singular good for those that are short winded, and for those that are troubled with the cough, and helpeth to open the passages, and to expectorate phlegm easily. It is given to those that are bitten or stung by any venomous creature, being boiled in wine. It is of a special virtue against the plague, the decoction thereof being drunk, and the root being used to smell to. It helpeth to expel the wind in the belly. The green herb with the root taken fresh, being bruised and applied to the head, taketh away the pains and pricking there, stayeth rheum and thin distillations, and being boiled in white wine, and a drop thereof put into the eyes, taketh

away

away the dimness of the sight, or any pin or web therein: It is of excellent property to heal any inward sores or wounds, and also for outward hurts or wounds, and drawing away splinters or thorns out of the flesh.

Vervain.

Descript] THE common Vervain hath somewhat long broad leaves next the ground deeply gashed about the edges, and some only deeply dented, or cut all alike, of a blackish green colour on the upper side, somewhat grey underneath. The stalk is square, branched into several parts, rising about two feet high, especially if you reckon the long spike of flowers at the tops of them, which are set on all sides one above another, and sometimes two or three together, being small and gaping, of a blue colour and white intermixed, after which come small round seed, in small and somewhat long heads. The root is small and long, but of no use.

Place] It groweth generally throughout this land in divers places of the hedges and way sides, and other waste grounds.

Time] It flowereth in July, and the seed is ripe soon after.

Government and Virtues.] This is an herb of Venus, and excellent for the womb to strengthen and remedy all the cold griefs of it, as Plantain doth the hot. Vervain is hot and dry, opening obstructions, cleansing and healing. It helpeth the yellow jaundice, the dropsy and the gout; it killeth and expelleth worms in the belly, and causeth a good colour in the face and body, strengtheneth as well as correcteth the diseases of the stomach, liver, and spleen; helps the cough, wheezings, and shortness of breath, and all the defects of the reins and bladder, expelling the gravel and stone. It is held to be good against the biting of serpents, and other venomous beasts, against the plague, and both tertian and quartian agues. It consolidateth and healeth also all wounds, both inward and outward, stayeth bleedings, and used with some honey, healeth all old ulcers and fistulas in the legs or other parts of the body, as also those ulcers that happen in the mouth; or used with hog's grease, it helpeth the swellings and pains of the secret parts in man or woman, also for the piles or hæmorrhoids; applied with some oil of roses and vinegar unto the forehead and temples, it easeth the inveterate pains and ach of the head, and is good for those that are frantic. The leaves bruised, or the juice of them mixed with some vinegar, doth wonderfully cleanse the skin, and taketh away morphew, freckles, fistula, and other such like inflammations and deformities of the skin in any part of the body. The distilled water of the herb when it is in full strength, dropped into the eyes, cleanseth them from films, clouds, or mists, that darken the sight, and wonderfully strengthens the optic nerves: The said water is very powerful in all the diseases aforesaid, either inward or outward, whether they be old corroding sores, or green wounds.

The Vine.

THE leaves of the English Vine (I do not mean to send you to the Canaries for a medicine) being boiled, make a good lotion for sore mouths; being boiled with barley meal into a poultice, it cools inflammations of wounds; the droppings of the Vine, when it is cut in the Spring, which country people call Tears, being boiled in a syrup, with sugar, and taken inwardly, is excellent to stay womens longings after every thing they see, which is a disease many women with child are subject to. The decoction of Vine leaves in white wine doth the like; also the tears of the Vine, drink two or three spoonfuls at a time, breaks the stone in the bladder. This is a very good remedy, and it is discreetly done to kill a Vine to cure a man, but the salt of the leaves are held to do better. The ashes of the burnt branches will make teeth that are as black as a coal, to be as white as snow, if you but every morning rub them with it. It is a most gallant Tree of the Sun, very sympathetical with the body of man, and that is the reason spirit of wine is the greatest cordial among all vegetables.

Violets.

BOTH the tame and the wild are so well known, that they need no description.

They flower until the end of July, but are best in March and the beginning of April.

(Government and Virtues) They are a fine pleasing plant of Venus, of a mild nature, no way harmful. All the Violets are cold and moist while they are fresh and green, and are used to cool any heat, or distemperature of the body,

either

either inwardly or outwardly, as inflammations in the eyes, in the matrix or fundament, in imposthumes also, and hot swellings, to drink the decoction of the leaves and flowers made with water and wine, or to apply them poultice-wise to the grieved places. It likewise easeth pains in the head, caused through want of sleep; or any other pains arising of heat, being applied in the same manner, or with oil of roses. A dram weight of the dried leaves, or flowers of Violets, but the leaves more strongly, doth purge the body of choleric humours, and assuage the heat, being taken in a draught of wine or any other drink; the powder of the purple leaves of the flowers, only picked and dried and drank in water, is said to help the quinsy, and the falling sickness in children, especially in the beginning of the disease. The flowers of the white Violets ripen and dissolve swellings. The herb or flowers, while they are fresh, or the flowers when they are dry, are effectual in the pleurisy, and all diseases of the lungs, to lenify the sharpness of the rheum, and the hoarseness of the throat, the heat and sharpness of urine, and all the pains of the back or reins and bladder. It is good also for the liver and the jaundice, and all hot agues to cool the heat and quench the thirst, but the syrup of Violet is of most use, and of better effect, being taken in some convenient liquor, and if a little of the juice or syrup of lemons be put to it, or a few drops of the oil of vitriol, it is made thereby the more powerful to cool the heat and quench the thirst, and giveth to the drink a claret wine colour, and a fine tart relish, pleasing the taste. Violets taken or made up with honey, do more cleanse and cool, and with sugar contrarywise. The dried flowers of Violet are accounted amongst the cordial drinks, powders, and other medicines, especially where cooling cordials are necessary. The green leaves are used with other herbs to make plaisters and poultices for inflammations and swellings, and to ease all pains whatsoever arising of heat, and for the piles also, being fryed with yolks of eggs, and applied thereto.

Viper's Bugloss.

Descript. This hath many long rough leaves lying on the ground, from among which riseth up divers hard round stalks, very rough, as if they were set with prickles or hairs, whereon are set such like rough, hairy, or prickly sad green leaves, somewhat narrow; the middle rib for the most part being white. The flowers stand at the top of the stalk, branched forth in many long spiked leaves of flowers, bowing or turning like the turnsole, all opening for the most part on the one side, which are long and hollow, turning up the brims a little, of a purplish violet colour in them that are fully blown, but more reddish while they are in the bud, as also upon their decay and withering, but in some places of a paler purple colour, with a long pointel in the middle, feathered or parted at the top. After the flowers are fallen, the seeds growing to be ripe, are blackish, cornered and pointed somewhat like the head of a viper. The root is somewhat great and blackish, and woolly, when it groweth toward seed time, and perisheth in the Winter.

There is another sort little differing from the former only in this, that it beareth white flowers.

Place] The first groweth wild almost everywhere. That with white flowers about the castle walls in Lewes in Sussex.

Time] They flower in Summer, and their seed is ripe quickly after.

Government and Virtues] It is a most gallant herb of the Sun; it is a pity it is no more in use that it is. It is an especial remedy against the biting of the Viper, and all other venomous beasts, or serpents; as also against poison, or poisonous herbs. Dioscorides and others say, That whosoever shall take of the herb or root before they be bitten, shall not be hurt by the poison of any serpent. The root or seed is thought to be most effectual to comfort the heart, and expel sadness, or causeless melancholy; it tempers the blood, and allayeth hot fits of ague. The seed drank in wine, procureth abundance of milk in women breasts. The same also being taken, easeth the pain in the loins, back, and kidneys. The distilled water of the herb when it is in flower, or its chief strength, is excellent to be applied either inwardly or outwardly, for all the griefs aforesaid. There is a syrup made hereof very effectual for the comforting the heart, and expelling sadness and melancholy.

Wall-Flowers, or Winter-Gilliflowers.

THE garden kind are so well known, that they need no description.

Descript] The common single Wall Flowers, which grow wild abroad, have sundry small, long, narrow, dark green leaves, set without order upon small round, whitish woody stalks, which bear at the tops divers single yellow flowers one above another, every one bearing four leaves a piece, and of a very sweet scent, after which come long pods, containing a reddish seed. The roots are white, hard and thready.

Place] It groweth upon church walls, and old walls of many houses, and other stone-walls in divers places: The other sort in gardens only.

Time] All the single kinds do flower many times in the end of Autumn; and if the Winter be mild, all the Winter long, but especially in the months of February, March, and April, and until the heat of the Spring do spend them. But the double kinds continue not flowering in that manner all the year long, although they flower very early sometimes, and in some places very late.

Government and Virtues] The Moon rules them. Galen in his seventh book of simple medicines, saith, That the yellow Wall Flowers work more powerfully than any of the other kinds, and are therefore of more use in physic. It cleanseth the blood, and freeth the liver and reins from obstructions, provoketh womens courses, expelleth the secundine, and the dead child, helpeth the hardness and pains of the mother, and of the spleen also; stayeth inflammations and swellings, comforteth and strengtheneth any weak part, or out of joint, helpeth to cleanse the eyes from mists and films on them, and to cleanse the filthy ulcers in the mouth, or any other part, and is a singular remedy for the gout, and all aches and pains in the joints and sinews. A conserve made of the flowers, is used for a remedy both for the apoplexy and palsy.

The Walnut-Tree.

IT is so well known that it needeth no description.

Time] It flowereth not until the end of forth, and ... September.

Government and Virtues] It is also a plant of the Sun. Let the fruit of it be gathered accordingly, which you shall find

find to be of most virtues whilst they are green, before they have shells. The bark of the Tree doth bind and dry very much, and the leaves are much of the same temperature, but the leaves, when they are older, are heating and drying in the second degree, and harder of digestion than when they are fresh, which, by reason of their sweetness, are more pleasing, and better digesting in the stomach; and taken with sweet wine, they move the belly downwards, but being old, they grieve the stomach; and in hot bodies cause the choler to abound, and the head-ach, and are an enemy to those that have the cough; but are less hurtful to those that have a colder stomach, and are said to kill the broad worms in the belly or stomach. If they be taken with onions, salt and honey, they help the biting of a mad dog, or the venom, or infectious poison of any beast, &c. Caius Pompeius found in the treasury of Mithridates, king of Pontus, when he was overthrown, a scroll of his own hand writing, containing a medicine against any poison or infection, which is this: Take two dry walnuts, and as many good figs, and twenty leaves of rue, bruised and beaten together with two or three corns of salt, and twenty juniper berries, which take every morning fasting, preserves from danger of poison and infection that day it is taken. The juice of the other green husks boiled with honey is an excellent gargle for a sore mouth, or the heat and inflammations in the throat and stomach. The kernels when they grow old, are more oily, and therefore not fit to be eaten, but are then used to heal the wounds of the sinews, gangrenes and carbuncles. The said kernels being burned, are then very astringent and will stay lasks and womens courses, being taken in red wine, and stay the falling of the hair, and make it fair, being anointed with oil and wine. The green husks will do the like, being used in the same manner. The kernels beaten with rue and wine, being applied, helpeth the quinsey, and being applied with some honey, and applied to the ears, easeth the pains and inflammations of them. A piece of the green husk put into a hollow tooth, easeth the pain; and the kernel thereof, taken before they fall off, congealeth and drieth down them of in powder with wine, that is sour, being applied, helpeth those that are troubled with the involuntary passing of their urine. The oil that is pressed out of the kernels, is very profitable taken inwardly like oil of almonds,

to

to help the colic, and doth expel wind very effectually; an ounce or two thereof may be taken at any time. The young green nuts taken before they be half ripe, and preserved with sugar, are of good use for those that have weak stomachs, or defluctions thereon. The distilled water of the green husks, before they be half ripe, is of excellent use to cool the heat of agues, being drank an ounce or two at a time; as also to resist the infection of the plague, if some of the same be also applied to the sores thereof. The same also cooleth the heat of green wounds and old ulcers, and healeth them, being bathed therewith. The distilled water of the green husks being ripe when they are shelled from the nuts, and drank with a little vinegar, is good for the plague, so as before the taking thereof a vein be opened. The said water is very good against the quinsy, being gargled and bathed therewith, and wonderfully helpeth deafness, the noise, and other pains in the ears. The distilled water of the young green leaves in the end of May performeth a singular cure of foul running ulcers and sores, to be bathed with wet cloths or sponges applied to them every morning.

Wold, Weld, or Dyer's Weed.

THE common kind groweth bushing with many leaves, long, narrow and flat upon the ground, of a dark bluish green colour, somewhat like unto Woad, but nothing so large, a little crumpled, and as it were round pointed, which do so abide the first year, and the next Spring from among them rise up divers round stalks, two or three feet high, beset with many such like leaves thereon, but smaller, and shooting forth small branches, which with the fairs carry many small yellow flowers, in a long spiked head at the top of them, where afterwards come the seed, which is small and black, inclosed in heads that are divided at the top into four parts. The root is long, white, and thick, abiding the Winter. The whole herb changeth to be yellow, after it hath been in flower awhile.

Place] It groweth every where by the way sides, in moist grounds, as well as dry, in corners of fields and by lanes, and sometimes all over the field. In Sussex and Kent they call it green Weed.

Time]

Time] It floewereth about June.

Government and Virtues] Matthiolus saith, that the root hereof cureth cough phlegm, digesteth raw phlegm, thinneth gross humours, dissolveth hard tumours, and openeth obstructions. Some do highly commend it against the bitings of venomous creatures, to be taken inwardly and applied outwardly to the hurt place; as also for the plague or pestilence. The people in some counties of this land, do use to bruise the herb, and lay it to cuts or wounds in the hands or legs, to heal them.

Wheat.

ALL the several kinds hereof are so well known unto almost all people, that it is altogether needless to write a description thereof.

Government and Virtues] It is under Venus. Dioscorides saith, That to eat the corn of green Wheat is hurtful to the stomach, and breedeth worms. Pliny saith, That the corn of Wheat roasted upon an iron pan, and eaten, is a present remedy for those that are chilled with cold. The oil pressed from Wheat, between two thick plates of iron, or copper, heated, healeth all tetters and ringworms, being used warm: and hereby Galen saith, he hath known many to be cured. Matthiolus commendeth the same to be put into hollow ulcers to heal them up, and it is good for chops in the hands and feet, and to make rugged skins smooth. The green corns of Wheat being chewed, and applied to the place bitten by a mad dog, healeth it. Slices of Wheat bread soaked in red rose water, and applied to the eyes that are hot, red and inflamed, or blood-shotten, helpeth them. Hot bread applied for an hour at times, for three days together, perfectly healeth the kernel in the throat, commonly called the king's evil. The flour of Wheat mixed with the juice of henbane, stays the flux of humours to the joints, being laid thereon. The said meal boiled in vinegar, helpeth the shrinking of the sinews, saith Pliny; and mixed with vinegar, and boiled together, healeth all freckles, spots, and pimples in the face. Wheat flour, mixed with the yoke of an egg, honey and turpentine, doth draw, cleanse and heal any boil, plague sore, or foul ulcer. The bran of Wheat meal steeped in sharp vinegar, and then bound in a linen cloth, and rubbed on those

those places that have the scurf, morphew, scabs or leprosy, will take them away, the body being first well purged and prepared. The decoction of the bran of Wheat or barley, is of good use to bathe those places that are bursten by a rupture, and the said bran boiled in good vinegar, and applied to swollen breasts, helpeth them, and stayeth all inflammations. It helpeth also the biting of vipers (which I take to be no other than our English adder) and all other venomous creatures. The leaves of wheat meal, applied with salt, take away hardness of the skin, warts and hard knots in the flesh. Starch moistened in rose water, and laid to the cods, taketh away the itching. Wafers put in water, and drank, stayeth the lask and bloody flux, and are probably used both inwardly and outwardly for the ruptures in children. Boiled in water unto a thick jelly, and taken, it stayeth spitting of blood, and boiled with mint and butter, it helpeth the hoarsness of the throat.

The Willow-Tree.

THESE are so well known that they need no description. I shall therefore only shew you the virtues thereof.

Government and Virtues] The Moon owns it. Both the leaves, bark and the seed, are used to staunch bleeding of wounds, and at mouth and nose, spitting of blood and other fluxes of blood in man or woman, and to stay vomitings, and provocation thereunto, if the decoction of them in wine be drank. It helpeth also to stay thin, hot, sharp salt distillations from the head upon the lungs, causing a consumption. The leaves bruised with some pepper, and drank in wine, helpeth much the wind colic. The leaves bruised and boiled in wine, stayeth the heat of lust in man or woman and quite extinguisheth it, if it be long used. The seed is also of the same effect. Water that is gathered from the Willow, when it flowereth, the bark being slit, and a vessel fitting to receive it, is very good for redness and dimness of sight, or films that grow over the eyes, and stay the rheum that falls into them; to provoke urine, being stopped, if it be drank; to clear the face and skin from spots and discolourings. Galen saith, The flowers have an admirable faculty in drying up humours, being a medicine without any sharpness or corrosion, you may boil them in white wine, and drink as much

much as you will, so you drink not yourself drunk. The bark works the same effect if used in the same manner, and the tree hath always a bark upon it, though not always flowers; the burnt ashes of the bark being mixed with vinegar, taketh away warts, corns, and superfluous flesh, being applied to the place. The decoction of the leaves or bark in wine, takes away scurf and dandriff by washing the place with it. It is a fine cool tree, the boughs of which are very convenient to be placed in the chamber of one sick of a fever.

Woad.

Descript.] It hath divers large leaves, long, and somewhat broad withal, like those of the greater plantain, but larger, thicker, of a greenish colour somewhat blue withal. From among which leaves riseth up a lusty stalk, three or four feet high, with divers leaves set thereon, the higher the stalk riseth, the smaller are the leaves; at the top it spreadeth divers branches, at the end of which appear very pretty little yellow flowers, and after they pass away like other flowers of the field, come husks, long and somewhat flat withal, in form they resemble a tongue, in colour they are black, and they hang bobbing downwards. The seed contained within these husks (if it be a little chewed) give an azure colour. The root is white and long.

Place.] It is sowed in fields for the benefit of it, where those that sow it, cut it three times a year.

Time.] It flowers in June, but it is long after before the seed is ripe.

Government and Virtues.] It is a cold and dry plant of Saturn. Some people affirm the plant to be destructive to bees, and fluees them, which if it be, I cannot help it. I should rather think, unless bees be contrary to other creatures, it possesseth them with the contrary disease, the herb being exceeding dry and binding. However, if any bee be diseased thereby, the cure is, to set water by them, but set it in a vessel, that they cannot drown themselves, which may be remedied, if you put pieces of cork in it. The herb is so drying and binding, that it is not fit to be given inwardly. An ointment made thereof staunches bleeding. A plaister made thereof and applied to the region of the spleen which lies on the left side, takes away the hardness and pains thereof. The ointment is excellent
good

good in such ulcers as abound with moisture, and takes away the corroding and fretting humours: It cools inflammations, quencheth St Anthony's fire, and stayeth defluction of the blood to any part of the body.

Woodbine, or Honey-Suckles.

IT is a plant so common, that every one that hath eyes knows it, and he that hath none, cannot read a description, if I should write it.

Time.] They flower in June, and the fruit is ripe in August.

Government and Virtues.] Doctor Tradition, that grand introducer of errors, that hater of truth, that lover of folly, and that mortal foe to Dr Reason, hath taught the common people to use the leaves or flowers of this plant in mouth water, and by long continuance of time, hath so grounded it in the brains of the vulgar, that you cannot beat it out with a beetle: All mouth waters ought to be cooling and drying, but Honey Suckles are cleansing, consuming and digesting, and therefore no way fit for inflammations; thus Dr Reason. Again, if you please, we will leave Dr Reason awhile, and come to Dr Experience, a learned gentleman, and his brother: Take a leaf and chew it in your mouth, and you will quickly find it likelier to cause a sore mouth and throat than to cure it. Well then, if it be not good for this, What is it good for? It is good for something, for God and nature made nothing in vain. It is an herb of Mercury, and appropriated to the lungs; the celestial Crab claims dominion over it? neither is it a foe to the Lion, if the lungs be afflicted by Jupiter, this is your cure: It is fitting a conserve made of the flowers of it were kept in every gentlewoman's house: I know no better cure for an asthma than this; besides it takes away the evil of the spleen, provokes urine, procures speedy delivery of women in travail, helps cramps, convulsions, and palsies, and whatsoever griefs come of cold or stopping; if you please to make use of it as an ointment, it will clear your skin of morphew, freckles, and sun burning, or whatever else discolours it, and then the maids will love it. Authors say, The flowers are of more effect than the leaves, and that is true; but they say the seeds are least effectual of all. But Dr Reason told me, That there was a vital spirit in every seed to beget its like, and Dr Experience told me, That there was a greater heat in the seed than there was in any other part of the plant; and withal, that seat was the mother of action, and then judge if old Dr Tradition (who may well be honoured for his age, but not for his goodness) hath not so poisoned the world with errors before I was born, that it was never well in its wits since, and there is great fear it will die mad.

Wormwood.

THREE Wormwoods are familiar with us: one I shall not describe, another I shall describe, and the third be critical at, and I care not greatly if I begin with the last first.

Sea Wormwood hath gotten as many names as virtues, (and perhaps one more) Seriphian, Santonicon, Belenion, Narbinense, Hantonicon, Misneule, and a matter of twenty more which I shall not blot paper withal. A Papist got the toy by the end, and he called it Holy Wormwood, and in truth, I am of opinion, there giving so much holiness to herbs, is the reason there remains so little in themselves. The seed of this wormwood is that which usually women give their children for the worms. Of all wormwoods that grow here, this is the weakest, but doctors commend it, and apothecaries sell it, the one must keep his credit, and the other get money, and that is the key of the work. The herb is good for something, because God made nothing in vain. Will you give me leave to weigh things in the balance of reason; then thus: The seeds of the common Wormwood are far more prevalent than the seed of this to expel worms in children, or people of ripe age, of both, some are weak, some are strong. The Seriphian Wormwood is the weakest, and haply may prove to be fittest for the weak bodies, (for it is weak enough of all conscience.) Let such as are strong take the common Wormwood, for the others will do but little good. Again near the sea many people live, and Seriphian grows near them, and therefore is more fitting for their bodies, because nourished by the same air; and this I had from Dr Reason. In whose body Dr Reason dwells not, dwells Dr Madness, and he brings in his brethren, Dr Ignorance, Dr Folly, and Dr Sickness, and these together make way for death, and the latter end of that man is worse than the beginning. Pride was the cause of Adam's fall, pride begat a daughter, a daughter, I do not know the father of it, unless the devil, but she christened it, and called it Appetite, and sent her daughter to taste these Wormwoods, who finding this the least bitter, made the squeamish wench extol it to the skies, though the virtues of it never reached to the middle region of the air. Its due praise is this: It is weakest, therefore fittest for weak bodies, and fitter for those bodies that dwell near it, than those that live far from it; my reason is, the sea (those that live far from it, know when they come near it) casteth not such a smell as the land doth. The tender mercies of God being over all his works, hath by his eternal Providence planted Seriphian by the sea side, as a fit medicine for the bodies of those that live near it. Lastly, It is known to all that know any thing in the course of nature, that the liver delights in sweet things, if so it abhors bitter; then if your liver be weak, it is none of the wisest courses to plague it with an enemy. If the liver be weak, a consumption follows; would you know the reason? it is this, A man's flesh is repaired by blood, by a third concoction, which transmutes the blood into flesh, it is well I said (concoction) say I, if I had said (boiling) every cook would have understood me. The liver makes blood, and if it be weakened that it makes not enough, the flesh wasteth; and why must flesh always be renewed? Because the eternal God, when he made the creation, made one part of it in continual dependency upon another. And why did he so? Because himself only is permanent: to teach us, that we should not fix our affections upon what is transitory, but upon what endures for ever. The result of this is, if the liver be weak, and cannot make blood enough, (I would have said sanguify, if I had only written to scholars) the Seriphian, which is the weakest of Wormwoods, is better than the best. I have been critical enough, if not too much.

Place.] It grows familiarly in England, by the sea side.

Descript.] It starts up out of the earth, with many round, woody, hairy stalks from one root. Its height is four feet, or three at least. The leaves in longitude are long in latitude, narrow, in colour white in form hoary, in similitude like Southernwood, only broader and longer; in taste rather salt than bitter, because it grows so near the salt water. At the joints, with the leaves toward the tops it bears little yellow flowers; the root lies deep, and is woody.

Common

Common Wormwood I shall not describe, for every boy that can eat an egg knows it.

Roman Wormwood; and why Roman, seeing it grows familiarly in England? It may be so called, because it is good for a stinking breath, which the Romans cannot be very free from, maintaining so many bawdy-houses by authority of his Holiness.

Descript] The stalks are slender, and shorter than the common Wormwood by one foot at least, the leaves are more finely cut and divided than them, but something smaller, both leaves and stalks are ——— the flowers of a pale yellow colour; it is altogether like the common Wormwood, save only in bigness, for it is ——— ; in taste, for it is not bitter; in smell, for it is spicy.

Place] It groweth upon the tops of the mountains, (it seems it is aspiring) there 'tis natural ——— nursed up in gardens for the use of the apothecaries in London.

Time] All Wormwoods usually flower in August, a little sooner or later.

Government and Virtues] Will you give me leave to be critical a little? I must take leave. Wormwood is an herb of Mars, and if Pontanus say otherwise, he is beside the bridge; I prove it thus. What delights in martial places is a martial herb; but Wormwood delights in martial places, (so about forges and iron works you may gather a cart load of it) *ergo*, it is a martial herb. It is hot and dry in the first degree, viz. just as hot as your blood, and no hotter. It remedies the evils choler can inflict on the body of man by sympathy. It helps the evils Venus and the wanton boy produce, by antipathy: and it doth something else besides. It cleanseth the body of choler (who dares say Mars doth no good?) It provokes urine, helps surfeits, or swellings in the belly, it causeth appetite to meat, because Mars rules the attractive faculty in man: The sun never shone upon a better herb for the yellow jaundice than this. Why should men cry out so much upon Mars for an unfortunate? (or Saturn either?) Did God make creatures to do the creation a mischief? This herb testifies that Mars is willing to cure all diseases he causes; the truth is, Mars loves no cowards, nor Saturn fools, nor I neither. Take of the flowers of Wormwood, Rosemary, and Black Thorn, of each a like quantity, half that quantity of saffron; boil this in Rhenish vine, but put it not in saffron till it is almost boiled: This is the way to keep a man's body in health, appointed by Camerarius, in his book, intitled, *Hortus Medicus*, and it is a good one too. Besides all this, Wormwood provokes the terms. I would willingly teach astrologers, and make them physicians (if I knew how) for they are most fitting for the calling: if you will not believe me, ask Dr Hippocrates, and Dr Galen, a couple of gentlemen, that our College of Physicians keep to vapour with, not to follow. In this herb, I shall give the pattern of a ruler, the sons of art rough cast, yet as near the truth as the men of Benjamin could throw a stone: Whereby, my brethren, the astrologers may know by a penny how a shilling is coined. As for the College of Physicians, they are too stately to learn, and too proud to continue. They say a mouse is under the dominion of the Moon, and that is the reason they feed in the night; the house of the Moon is Cancer, rats are of the same nature with mice, but they are a little bigger; Mars receives his fall in Cancer, ergo, Wormwood being an herb of Mars, is a present remedy for the biting of rats and mice. Mushrooms (I cannot give them the title of Herbs, Fruits or Arbor) are under the dominion of Saturn, (and take one time with another, they do as much harm as good,) if any have poisoned himself by eating them, Wormwood, an herb of Mars, cures him, because Mars is exalted in Capricorn, the house of Saturn, and that it doth by sympathy, as it did the other by antipathy. Wheals, pushes, black and blue spots, coming either by bruises or beatings, Wormwood, an herb of Mars, helps; because Mars, (as bad as you love him, and as you hate him) will not break your head, but he will give you a plaster. If he do but teach you to know yourselves, his courtesy is greater than his discourtesy. The greatest antipathy between the planets, is between Mars and Venus; one is hot, the other cold; one diurnal, the other nocturnal; one dry, the other moist, their houses are opposite, one masculine, the other feminine, one public, the other private, one is valiant, the other effeminate, one loves the light, the other hates it; one loves the field, the other sheets; then the throat is under Venus, the quinsy lies in the throat, and is an inflammation there. Venus rules the throat (it being under Taurus her sign.) Mars eradicates all diseases in the throat by his herbs (of which

Worm-

wormwood is one) and sends them to Egypt on an errand never to return more, this done by antipathy. The eyes are under the Luminaries; the right-eye of a man, and the left-eye of a woman the Sun claims dominion over; the left eye of a man, and the right eye of a woman, are privileges of the Moon; Wormwood, an herb of Mars, cures both; what belongs to the Sun by sympathy, because he is exalted in his house, but what belongs to the Moon by antipathy, because he hath his fall in her's. Suppose a man be bitten or stung by a martial creature, imagine a wasp, a hornet, a scorpion, Wormwood, an herb of Mars, giveth you a present cure; then Mars, choleric as he is, hath learned that patience, to pass by your evil speeches of him, and tells you by my pen, that he gives you no affliction, but he gives you a cure; you need not run to Apollo, nor Esculapius, and if he was so choleric as you make him to be, he would have drawn his sword for anger, to see the ill conditions of those people that can spy his vices, and not his virtues. The eternal God, when he made Mars, made him for public good, and the sons of men shall know it in the latter end of the world. *E cœlum Mars solus habet* You say Mars is a destroyer; mix a little Wormwood, an herb of Mars, with your ink, neither rats nor mice touch the paper written with it, and then Mars is a preserver. Astrologers think Mars causeth scabs, and itch, and the virgins are angry with him, because wanton Venus told them he deforms their skins; but, quoth Mars, my only desire is, they should know themselves; my herb Wormwood, will restore them to the beauty they formerly had, and in that I will not come an inch behind my opposite, Venus; for which doth the greatest evil, he that takes away an innate beauty, and when he has done, knows how to restore it again? Or she that teaches a company of wanton lasses to paint their face? If Mars be in a Virgin, in the nativity, they say he causeth the colic (it is well God hath set somebody to pull down the pride of man.) He in the Virgin troubles none with the colic, but them that know not themselves (for who knows himself may easily know all the world.) Wormwood, an herb of Mars, is a present cure for it, and whether it be most like a Christian to love him for his good, or hate him for his evil, judge ye. I had almost forgotten, that charity thinks no evil. I was once in the Tower and viewed the wardrobe, and there was a great

many

many fine cloaths: (I can give them no other title, for I was never either linen or woollen-draper) yet as brave as they looked, my opinion was that the moths might consume them; moths are under the dominion of Mars; this herb Wormwood being laid among cloaths, will make a moth scorn to meddle with the cloaths, as much as a lion scorns to meddle with a mouse, or an eagle with a fly. You say Mars is angry, and it is true enough he is angry with many countrymen, for being such fools to be led by the noses by the college of physicians, as they lead bears to Paris garden. Melancholy men cannot endure to be wronged in point of good fame, and that doth sorely trouble old Saturn, because they call him the greatest unfortunate, in the body of man he rules the spleen, (and that makes covetous men so splenetic) the poor old man lies crying out of his left side. Father Saturn's angry, Mars comes to him; Come, brother, I confess thou art evil spoken of, and so am I: thou knowest I have my exaltation in thy house, I give him an herb of mine, Wormwood, to cure the poor man Saturn consented, but spoke little, and Mars cured him by sympathy When Mars was free from war, (or he loves to be fighting, and is the best friend a soldier hath) I say, when Mars was free from war, he called a council of war in his own brain, to know how he should do poor sinful man good, desiring to forget his abuses in being called an unfortunate. He musters up his own forces, and places them in battalia. Oh! quoth he, why do I hurt a poor silly man or woman? his angel answers him, It is because they have offended their God, (Look back to Adam!) Well, says Mars, though they speak evil of me, I will do good to them Death' cold, my herb shall heat them; they are full of ill humours (else they would never have spoken ill of me;) my herb shall cleanse them, and dry them, they are poor weak creatures, my herb shall strengthen them; they are dull witted, my herb shall fortify their apprehensions; and yet among astrologers all this does not deserve a good word. On the patience of Mars!

>*Felix qui potuit rerum cognoscere causas,*
>*Inque domus superum sea deæ cura facit.*
>
>Oh happy he that can the knowledge gain,
>To know th' eternal God made nought in vain.

To

To this I add,
I know the reason causeth such a dearth
Of knowledge; 'tis because men love the earth.

The other day Mars told me he met with Venus, and he asked her, What was the reason that she accused him for abusing women? He never gave them the pox. In the dispute they fell out, and in anger parted, and Mars told me that his brother Saturn told him, that an antivenerean medicine was the best against the pox. Once a month he meets with the Moon. Mars is quick enough of speech, and the Moon not much behind hand, (neither are most women) The Moon looks much after children, and children are much troubled with the worms; she desired a medicine of him, he bid her take his own herb, Wormwood. He had no sooner parted with the Moon but he met with Venus, and she was as drunk as a bitch: Alas! poor Venus, quoth he, What! thou a fortune, and be drunk? I'll give thee an antipathetical cure. Take my herb, Wormwood, and thou shalt never get a surfeit by drinking. A poor silly countryman hath got an ague, and cannot go about his business, he wishes he had it not, and so do I, but I will tell him a remedy, whereby he shall prevent it. Take the herb of Mars, Wormwood, and if misfortunes will do good, what will fortunes do? Some think the lungs are under Jupiter, and if the lungs, then the breath, and though sometimes a man gets a stinking breath, and yet Jupiter is a fortune, forsooth; up comes Mars to him: Come, brother Jupiter thou knowest I sent thee a couple of trines to thy house last night, the one from Aries, and the other from Scorpio, give me thy leave by sympathy to cure this poor man with drinking a draught of Wormwood beer every morning. The Moon came to me the other day, and she gave a man two terrible mischiefs, a dull brain and a weak sight; Mars laid by his sword and comes to her. Sister Moon, said he, this man hath angered thee, but I beseech thee take notice he is but a fool; prithee be patient, I will with my herb Wormwood, cure him of both infirmities by antipathy, for thou knowest thou and I cannot agree, with that the Moon began to quarrel, Mars (not delighting much in womens tongues) went away, and did it whether she would or no,

The English *Physician Enlarged.*

He that reads this, and understands what he reads, hath a jewel of more worth than a diamond, he that understands it not, is as little fit to give physic. There lies a key in these words which will unlock, (if it be turned by a wise hand) the cabinet of physic. I have delivered it as plain as I durst; it is not only upon Wormwood as I wrote, but upon all plants, trees and herbs, he that understands it not, is unfit (in my opinion) to give physic. This shall live when I am dead. And thus I leave it to the world, not caring a farthing whether they like or dislike it. The grave equals all men, and therefore shall equal me with all princes; until which time the eternal providence is over me. Then the ill tongue of a prating fellow, or of one that hath more tongue than wit, or more proud than honest, shall never trouble me. *Wisdom is justified of her children.* And so much for Wormwood.

Yarrow, called also Nose-bleed, Milfoil, and Thousand Leaf.

Descript.] It hath many long leaves spread upon the ground, finely cut, and divided into many small parts: its flowers are white, but not all of a whiteness, and fixed in knots, upon divers green stalks which rise from among the leaves.

Place.] It is frequent in all pastures.

Time.] It flowereth late, even in the later end of August.

Government and Virtues.] It is under the influence of Venus. An ointment of them cures wounds, and is most fit for such as have inflammations, it being an herb of Mars Venus, it stops the terms in women, being boiled in white wine, and the decoction drunk, as also the Bloody Flux, the ointment of it is not only good for green wounds, but also for ulcers and fistulas, especially such as abound with moisture. It stays the shedding of hair, the head being bathed with the decoction of it, inwardly taken it helps the retentive faculty of the stomach, it helps the running of the reins in men, and the whites in women, and helps such as cannot hold their water, and the leaves chewed in the mouth easeth the tooth-ach, and these virtues being put together, shew that the herb is drying and binding. Achilles is supposed to be the first that left the virtues of this herb to posterity, having learned them of his master Chiron, the centaur: and certainly, a very profitable herb it is in cramps, and therefore called Militaris.

DIRECTIONS

DIRECTIONS.

HAVING in divers places of this treatise promised you the way of making syrups, conserves, oils, ointments, &c. of herbs, roots, flowers, &c. whereby you may have them ready for your use at such times when otherwise they cannot be had, I come now to perform what I promised, and you shall find me rather better than worse than my word.

That this may be done methodically, I shall divide my directions into two grand sections, and each section into several chapters, and then you shall see it look with such a countenance as this is.

SECT. I.

Of gathering, drying, and keeping Simples, and their Juices.

Chap. 1. Of Leaves, of Herbs, &c. | Chap. 4. Of Roots.
Chap. 2. Of Flowers. | Chap. 5. Of Barks.
Chap. 3. Of Seeds. | Chap. 6. Of Juices.

SECT. II.

Of making and keeping Compounds.

Chap. 1. Of distilled Waters | Chap. 10. Of Ointments.
Chap. 2. Of Syrups. | Chap. 11. Of Plaisters.
Chap. 3. Of Juleps. | Chap. 12. Of Poultices.
Chap. 4. Of Decoctions. | Chap. 13. Of Troches.
Chap. 5. Of Oils. | Chap. 14. Of Pills.
Chap. 6. Of Electuaries. | Chap. 15. The way of fitting
Chap. 7. Of Conserves. | Medicines to Compound
Chap. 8. Of Preserves. | Diseases.
Chap. 9. Of Lohochs. | Of all these in order.

SECT.

SECT. I.

The way of gathering, and preserving Simples and their Juices.

CHAP. I.

Of Leaves, of Herbs, or Trees.

OF leaves, choose only such as are green and full of juice, pick them carefully, and cast away such as are any ways declining, for they will putrify the rest: So shall one handful be worth ten of those you buy in Cheapside.

2. Note in what places they most delight to grow in, and gather them there; for Betony that grows in the shade is far better than that which grows in the Sun, because it delights in the shade; so also such herbs as delight to grow near the water, let such be gathered as grow near the water, though hapily you may find some of them upon dry ground: the treatise will inform you where every herb delights to grow.

3. The leaves of such herbs as run up to seed are not so good when they are in flower as before, (some few excepted, the leaves of which are seldom or never used) in such cases, if through ignorance they were not known, or through negligence forgotten, you had better take the top and the flowers, than the leaf.

4. Dry them well in the sun, and not in the shade, as the saying of physicians is; for if the sun draws away the virtues of the herb, it must needs do the like by hay, by the same rule, which the experience of every country farmer will explode for a notable piece of nonsense.

5. Such as are artists in astrology, (and indeed none else are fit to make physicians) such I advise; let the planet that governs the herb be angular, and the stronger the better, if they can, in herbs of Saturn, let Saturn be in the ascendant; in the herbs of Mars, let Mars be in the mid-heaven, for in those houses they delight; let the Moon apply to them by good aspect, and let her not be in the houses of her enemies; if you cannot well stay till she apply to them, let her apply

to a planet of the same triplicity; if you cannot wait that time neither, let her be with a fixed star of their nature.

6. Having well dried them, put them up in brown paper, sewing the paper up like a sack, and press them not too hard together, and keep them in a dry place near the fire.

7. As for the duration of dried herbs, a just time cannot be given; let authors prate their pleasure, for,

First, Such as grow upon dry grounds will better keep, than such as grow on moist.

Secondly, Such herbs as are full of juice, will not keep so long as such as are drier.

Thirdly, Such herbs as are well dried, will keep longer than such as are slack dried.

Yet this I say, by this you may know when they are corrupted, viz. by their loss of colour, or smell or both, and if they be corrupted, reason will tell you that they must needs corrupt the bodies of those people that take them.

8. Gather all leaves in the hour of that planet that governs them.

CHAP. II. *Of Flowers.*

THE flower, which is the beauty of the plant, and of none of the least use in physic, groweth yearly, and is to be gathered when it is in its prime.

2. As for the time of gathering them, let the planetary hour, and the planet they come of, be observed, as we shewed you in the foregoing chapter; as for the time of the day, let it be when the Sun shines upon them, that so they may be dry, for if you gather either flowers or herbs when they are wet or dewy, they will not keep; and this I forgot before.

3. Dry them well in the sun, and keep them in papers near the fire, as I shewed you in the foregoing chapter.

4. So long as they retain the colour and smell, they are good; either of them being gone, so is their virtue also.

CHAP. III. *Of Seeds.*

1. THE seed is that part of the plant which is endowed with a vital faculty to bring forth its like, and it contains potentially the whole plant in it.

2. As for place, let them be gathered from the place where the thing ought to grow.

3. Let them be full ripe when they are gathered; and for-

get

get not the celestial harmony before mentioned, for I have found by experience that their virtues are twice as great at such times as others: *There is an appointed time for every thing under the Sun.*

4. When you have gathered them, dry them a little, and but a little in the Sun before you lay them up.

5. You need not be so careful of keeping them so near the fire, as the other before mentioned, because they are fuller of spirit, and therefore not so subject to corrupt.

6. As for the time of their duration, 'tis palpable they will keep a good many years; yet this I say, they are in best till two years, and this I make appear by a good argument. They will grow the soonest then next year they be set, therefore then they are in their prime, and it is an easy matter to discern them early.

CHAP. IV. *Of Roots.*

1. Of Roots, chuse such as are neither rotten nor worm-eaten, but proper in their taste, colour and smell; such as exceed neither in softness nor hardness.

2. Give me leave to be a little critical against the vulgar received opinion, which is, that the sap falls down into the root in the Autumn, and rises again in the Spring, as men go to bed at night and rise in the morning; and this idle talk or untruth is so grounded in the heads, not only of the vulgar, but also of the learned, that a man cannot drive it out by reason. I pray let such fashion-ers answer me to this argument. If the sap falls into the roots in the fall of the leaf, and lies there all the Winter, then must the root grow only in the Winter. Experience witnesseth, but the root grows not at all in the Winter, as the same experience teacheth, but only in the Summer, *ergo*,

If you set an apple-kernel in the Spring, you shall find the root to grow to a pretty bigness in that Summer, and be not a whit bigger next Spring. What doth the sap do in the root all that while, pick straws? It is as rotten as a rotten post.

The truth is, when the Sun declines from the tropic of Cancer, the sap begins to congeal both in root and branch; when he toucheth the tropic of Capricorn, and ascends to us-ward, it begins to wax thin again, and by degrees as it congealed. But to proceed,

P 3

3 The drier time you gather the roots in, the better they are; for they have the less excrementitious moisture in them.

4 Such roots as are soft, your best way is to dry in the Sun, or else hang them in the chimney corner, upon a string; as for such as are hard, you may dry them any where.

5. Such roots as are great, will keep longer than such as are small, yet most of them will keep a year.

6 Such roots as are soft, it is your best way to keep them always near the fire, and to take this general rule for it, if in Winter time you find any of your roots, herbs or flowers begin to be moist, as many times you shall, especially in the Winter time (for it is your best way to look to them once a month) dry them by a very gentle fire; or if you can with convenience keep them near the fire, you may save yourself the labour.

7. It is in vain to dry roots as may commonly be had, as Parsley, Fennel, Plantain, &c. but gather them only for present need.

CHAP. V. *Of Barks.*

BARKS, which physicians use in medicines, are of these sorts. Of fruits, of roots, of boughs.

2 The barks of fruits are to be taken when the fruit is full ripe, as Oranges, Lemons, &c. but because I have nothing to do with exotics here, I pass them without any more words.

3. The barks of trees are best gathered in the Spring, if it be of great trees, as oaks or the like; because then they come easier off, and so you may dry them if you please; but indeed the best way is to gather all barks only for present use.

4. As for the barks of roots, it is this, and thus to be gotten. Take the roots of such herbs as have a pith in them, as Parsley, Fennel, &c. slit them in the middle, and when you have taken out the pith (which you may easily and soon do) that which remains is called (though something improperly) the bark, and indeed is only to be used.

CHAP. VI. *Of Juices.*

1. JUICES are to be pressed out of herbs when they are young and tender, and also out of some stalks, and tender tops of herbs and plants, and also out of some flowers.

2. Having gathered the herb you would preserve the juice of, when it is very dry (for otherwise the juice will not

be

be worth a button) bruise it very well in a stone mortar with a wooden pestle, then having put it into a canvas bag, the herb I mean not the mortar, for that will give but little juice, press it hard in a press: then take the juice and clarify it.

3. The manner of clarifying it is this: put it into a pipkin or skillet, or some such thing, and set it over the fire, and when the scum ariseth, take it off; let it stand over the fire till no more scum arise, when you have your juice clarified, cast away the scum as a thing of no use.

4. When you have thus clarified it, you have two ways to preserve it all the year.

First, when it is cold put it into a glass, and put so much oil on it as will cover it to the thickness of two fingers, the oil will swim at the top, and so keep the air from coming to putrify it, when you intend to use it, do no more but so pour out into a porringer a little more than you intend to use, and if any oil come out with it (as if the glass be not full, it is an hundred to one if there do) you may easily scum it off with a spoon, and put the juice you use not into the glass again, it will quickly sink under the oil. This is the first way.

Secondly, The second way is a little more difficult, and the juice of fruits is usually preserved this way. When you have clarified the juice as before, boil it over the fire till (being cold) it be of the thickness of honey. This is most commonly used for diseases of the mouth, and is called Roba and Saba. And thus much for the first section, the second follows.

SECT. II.

The way of making and keeping all necessary Compounds.

CHAP. I.

Of Distilled Waters.

HITHERTO we have spoke of medicines which consist in their own nature, which authors vulgarly call Simples, though something improperly, for indeed and in truth, nothing

thing is simple but pure elements; all things else are compounded of them. We come now to treat of the artificial medicines, in the front of which (because we must begin somewhere) we shall place distilled waters; in which consider,

1. Waters are distilled out of herbs, flowers, fruits, and roots.

2. We treat not of strong waters, but of cold, as being to act Galen's part, and not Paracelsus.

3. The herbs ought to be distilled when they are in the greatest vigour, and so ought the flowers also.

4. The vulgar way of distillations, which people use, because they know no better, is in a pewter still; and although distilled waters are the weakest of artificial medicines, and good for little, unless for mixtures of other medicines, though this may be distilled, they are weaker by many degrees than they would be, were they distilled in sand. If I thought it not impossible to teach you the way of distilling in sand by writing, I would attempt it.

5. When you have distilled your water, put it into a glass, and having bound the top of it over with a paper, pricked full of holes, so that the excrementitious and fiery vapours may exhale, which indeed are they that cause that settling in distilled waters called the Mother, which corrupts waters, and might this way be prevented, cover it close, and keep it for your use.

6. Stopping distilled waters with a cork makes them musty, and so will a paper also, if it do but touch the water, your best way then is to stop them with a bladder, being first put in water, and bound over the top of the glass.

Such cold waters as are distilled in a pewter still (if well kept) will endure a year; such as are distilled in sand, as they are twice as strong, so they endure twice as long.

CHAP. II. *Of Syrups.*

1. A SYRUP is a medicine of a liquid form, composed of infusion, decoction and juice. And, 1. For the more grateful taste. 2. For the better keeping of it, with a certain quantity of honey or sugar, hereafter mentioned, boiled to the thickness of new honey.

2. You see at the first view, That this aphorism divides itself into three branches, which deserve severally to be treated of, viz.

a. Syrups

1 Syrups made by infusion.
2 Syrups made by decoction.
3 Syrups made by juice.

Of each of these, (for your instruction sake, kind countrymen and women) I speak a word, or two, or three apart.

First, Syrups made by infusion are usually made of flowers, and of such flowers as soon lose their colour and strength by boiling, as Roses, Violets, Peach Flowers, &c. My translation of the *London Dispensatory* will instruct you in the rest. They are thus made. Having picked your flowers clean, to every pound of them add three pounds or three pints, which you will (for it is all one) of spring water, made boiling hot by the fire, first put your flowers into a pewter pot, with a cover, and pour the water to them, then shutting the pot, let it stand by the fire, to keep hot twelve hours, and strain it out. (in such syrups as purge) as damask roses, peach flowers, &c. the usual and indeed the best way, is to repeat this infusion, adding fresh flowers to the same liquor divers times, that so it may be the stronger) having strained it out, put the infusion into a pewter bason or an earthen one well glazed, and to every pint of it add two pound of sugar, which being only melted over the fire, without boiling, and scummed, will produce you the syrup you desire.

Secondly, Syrups made by decoction are usually made of compounds, yet may any simple herb be thus converted into syrup. Take the herb, root, or flowers you would make into a syrup, and bruise it a little, then boil it in a convenient quantity of spring water, the more water you boil it in the weaker it will be, a handful of the herb or root, &c. is a convenient quantity for a pint of water, boil it till half the water be consumed, then let it stand till it be almost cold, and strain it (being almost cold) through a woollen cloth, letting it run out a leisure, without pressing; to every pint of this decoction add one pound of sugar, and boil it over the fire till it come to a syrup, which you may know, if you now and then cool a little of it in a spoon, scum it all the while it boils, and when it is sufficiently boiled, whilst it is hot, strain it again through a woollen cloth, but press it not. Thus you have the syrup perfect.

Thirdly, Syrup made of juices, are usually made of such herbs as are full of juice, and indeed they are better made into a syrup this way than any other, the operation is thus:

P 5

Having beaten the herb in a stone mortar, with a wooden pestle, press out the juice, and clarify it, as you are taught before in the juices; then let the juice boil away till a quarter of it (or near upon) be consumed; to a pint of this add a pound of sugar, and boil it to a syrup, always scumming it, and when it is boiled enough, strain it through a woollen cloth, as we taught you before, and keep it for your use.

3. If you make syrup of roots that are any thing hard, as Parsley, Fennel, and Grass roots, &c. when you have bruised them, lay them in steep some time in that water which you intend to boil them in, hot, so will the virtue the better come out.

4. Keep your syrups either in glasses or stone pots, and stop them not with cork nor bladder, unless you would have the glass break, and the syrup lost; and as many opinions as there are in this nation, I suppose there are but few or none of this, only bind paper about the mouth.

5 All syrups, if well made, continue an year with some advantage; yet of all, such as are made by infusion keep the least while.

CHAP. III. *Of Juleps.*

1. JULEPS were first invented, as I suppose, in Arabia; and my reason is, because the word julep is an Arabic word.

2. It signifies only a pleasant potion, as is vulgarly used by such as are sick, and want help, or such as are in health, and want no money to quench thirst.

3 Now a day it is commonly used,
   1 *To prepare the body for purgation.*
   2. *To open obstructions and the pores.*
   3 *To digest tough humours.*
   4 *To qualify hot distempers, &c*

4 It is thus made (I mean simple juleps, for I have nothing to say to compound. here, all compounds have as many simple ideas, as men have crotchets in their brain) I say simple juleps are thus made. Take a pint of such distilled water, as conduces to the cure of your distemper, which this treatise will plentifully furnish you withal, to which add two ounces of syrup, conducing to the same effect, (I shall give you rules for it in the last chapter) mix them together, and drink a draught of it at your pleasure.

I

If you love tart things, add ten drops of oil of vitriol to your pint, and shake it together, and it will have a fine grateful taste.

5. All juleps are made for present use, and therefore it is in vain to speak of their duration.

CHAP. IV. *Of Decoctions.*

1. ALL the difference between decoctions and syrups made by decoction, is this; syrups are made to keep, decoctions only for present use; for you can hardly keep a decoction a week at any time; if the weather be hot, not half so long.

2. Decoctions are made of leaves, roots, flowers, seeds, fruits or barks, conducing to the cure of the disease you make them for; in the same manner they are made as we shewed you in syrups.

3. Decoctions made with wine last longer than such as are made with water; and if you take your decoction to cleanse the passages of the urine, or open obstructions, your best way is to make it with white wine instead of water, because this is penetrating.

4. Decoctions are of most use in such diseases as lie in the passages of the body; as the stomach, bowels, kidneys, passages of urine and bladder, because decoctions pass quicker to those places than any other form of medicines.

5. If you will sweeten your decoction with sugar, or any syrup fit for the occasion you take it for, which is better, you may and no harm do.

6. If in a decoction, you boil both roots, herbs, flowers, and seed together, let the roots boil a good while first, because they retain their virtue longest; then the next in order by the same rule, viz. 1. Barks. 2. The herbs. 3. The seeds. 4. The flowers. 5. The spices, if you put any in, because their virtues come soonest out.

7. Such things as by boiling cause sliminess to a decoction, as Figs, Quince-seed, Linseed, &c. your best way is, after you have bruised them, to tie them up in a linen rag, as you tie up a calf's brains, and so boil them.

8. Keep all decoctions in a glass close stopped, and in the cooler place you keep them, the longer they will last e'er they be sour.

Lastly, The usual dose to be given at one time, is usually two,

two, three, four, or five ounces, according to the age and strength of the patient, the season of the year, the strength of the medicine, and the quality of the disease.

CHAP. V. *Of Oils.*

OIL olive, which is commonly known by the name of sallad oil, I suppose, because it is usually eaten with sallads by them that love it, if it be pressed out of ripe olives, according to Galen, is temperate, and exceeds in no one quality.

2. Of oils, some are simple, and some are compound.

3. Simple oils are such as are made of fruits or seeds by expression, as oil of sweet and bitter almonds, linseed and rape-seed oil, &c. of which see in my *Dispensatory*.

4. Compound oils are made of oil of olives, and other simples, imagine herbs, flowers, roots, &c.

5. The way of making them is this: having bruised the herb or flower, you would make your oil of, put them into an earthen pot, and to two or three handfuls of them pour a pint of oil, cover the pot with a paper, set it in the sun about a fortnight or less, according as the sun is in hotness, then having warmed it very well by the fire press out the herbs, &c. very hard in a press, and add as many more herbs to the same oil; bruise the herbs (I mean not the oil) in like manner, set them in the sun as before, the oftener you repeat it the stronger your oil will be, at last, when you conceive it strong enough, boil both herbs and oil together till the juice be consumed, which you may know by its leaving its bubbling, and the herbs will be crisp, then strain it while it is hot, and keep it in a stone or glass vessel for your use.

6. As for chymical oils, I have nothing to say in this treatise.

7. The general use of these oils, is for pains in the limbs, roughness of the skin, the itch, &c. as also for ointments and plaisters.

8. If you have occasion to use it for wounds or ulcers, in two ounces of oil dissolve half an ounce of turpentine, the heat of the fire will quickly do it, for oil itself is offensive to wounds, and the turpentine qualifies it.

CHAP.

CHAP. VI. *Of Electuaries.*

PHYSICIANS make more a quoil than needs, by half, about electuaries. I shall prescribe but one general way of making them up; as for the ingredients you may vary them as you please, and according as you find occasion by the last chapter.

1. That you may make electuaries when you need them, it is requisite that you keep always herbs, roots, seeds, flowers, &c. ready dried in your house, that so you may be in a readiness to beat them into powder when you need them.

2. Your better way is to keep them whole than beaten; for being beaten, they are the more subject to lose their strength, because the air soon penetrates them.

3. If they be not dry enough to beat into powder when you need them, dry them by a gentle fire till they be so.

4. Having beaten them, sift them through a fine tiffany searce, that so there may be no great pieces found in your electuary.

5. To one ounce of your powder add three ounces of clarified honey; this quantity I hold to be sufficient, I confess authors differ about it. If you would make more or less electuary, vary your proportion accordingly.

6. Mix them well together in a mortar, and take this for a truth, you cannot mix them too much.

7. The way to clarify honey, is to set it over the fire in a convenient vessel, till the scum rise, and when the scum is taken off, it is clarified.

8. The usual dose of cordial electuaries, is from half a dram to two drams, of purging electuaries, from half an ounce to an ounce.

9. The manner of keeping them is in a pot.

10. The time of taking them is either in a morning fasting, and fasting an hour after them, or at night going to bed, three or four hours after supper.

CHAP. VII. *Of Conserves*

THE way of making conserves is twofold, one of herbs and flowers, and the other of fruits.

2. Conserves of herbs and flowers are thus made: If you
make

make your conserves of herbs, as of Scurvy-grass, Wormwood, Rue, and the like, take only the leaves and tender tops (for you may beat your heart out before you can beat the stalks small) and having beaten them, weigh them, and to every pound of them add three pound of sugar, beat them well together in a mortar, you cannot beat them too much.

3. Conserve of fruits, as of Barberries, Sloes, and the like, is thus made. First scald the fruit, then rub the pulp through a thick hair sieve made for the purpose, called a pulping sieve: you may do it for a need with the back of a spoon; then take this pulp thus drawn, and add to it its weight of sugar, and no more; put it in a pewter vessel, and over a charcoal fire; stir it up and down till the sugar be melted, and your conserve is made.

4. Thus have you the way of making conserves; the way of keeping them is in earthen pots.

5. The dose is usually the quantity of a nutmeg at a time, morning and evening, or (unless they are purging) when you please.

6. Of conserves, some keep many years, as conserves of Roses; others but a year, as conserves of Borage, Bugloss, Cowslips, and the like.

7. Have a care of the working of some conserves presently after they are made, look to them once a day, and stir them about; conserves of Borage, Bugloss, Wormwood, have gotten an excellent faculty at that sport.

8. You may know when your conserves are almost spoiled by this, you shall find a hard crust at top with little holes in it, as though worms had been eating there.

CHAP. VIII. *Of Preserves.*

OF Preserves are sundry sorts, and the operations of all being somewhat different, we will handle them all apart. These are preserved with sugar,

    1 *Flowers.*
    2. *Fruit.*
    3 *Roots.*
    4 *Barks.*

1 Flowers are but very seldom preserved; I never saw any that I remember, save only Cowslip flowers, and that was a great fashion in *Sussex* when I was a boy: It is thus done;

done: First, take a flat glass, we call them jat-glasses, strew in a laying of fine sugar, on that a laying of flowers, on that another laying of sugar, on that another laying of flowers, so do till your glass be full; then tie it over with a paper, and in a little time you shall have very excellent and pleasant preserves.

There is another way of preserving flowers, namely, with vinegar and salt, as they pickle Capers and Broom buds, but because I have little skill in it myself, I cannot teach you.

2. Fruits, as Quinces, and the like, are preserved two ways.

First, boil them well in water, and then pulp them through a sieve, as we shewed you before, then with the like quantity of sugar, boil the water they were boiled in into a syrup, viz. A pound of sugar to a pint of liquor; to every pound of this syrup, add four ounces of the pulp; then boil it with a very gentle fire to their right consistence, which you may easily know, if you drop a drop of it upon a trencher; if it be enough, it will not stick to your fingers when it is cold.

Secondly, another way to preserve fruits is this; first, pare off the rind, then cut them in halves, and take out the core; then boil them in water till they are soft; if you know when beef is boiled enough, you may easily know when they are; then boil the water with its like weight of sugar into a syrup; put the syrup into a pot, and put the boiled fruit, as whole as you left it when you cut it into it, and let it remain till you have occasion to use it.

3. Roots are thus preserved; first, scrape them very clean and cleanse them from the pith, if you have any, for some roots have not, as Eringo and the like, boil them in water till they be soft, as we shewed you before in the fruits, then boil the water you boiled the root in, into a syrup, as we shewed you before, then keep the root whole in the syrup till you use them.

4. As for Barks, we have but few come to our hands to be done, and those, of those few that I can remember, are Oranges, Lemons, Citrons, and the outer Bark of Walnuts which grow without side the shell, for the shells themselves would make but scurvy preserves; these be they I can remember, if there be any more, put them into the number.

The way of preserving these is not all one in authors, for
some

some are bitter, some are hot: such as are bitter, say authors, must be soaked in warm water, oftentimes changing till their bitter taste be fled. But I like not this way, and my reason is this: Because I doubt when their bitterness is gone, so is their virtue also. I shall then prescribe one common way, namely, the same with the former, viz. First boil them whole till they be soft, then make a syrup with sugar and the liquor you boiled them in, and keep the Barks in the syrup.

5. They are kept in glasses, or in glazed pots.

6. The preserved flowers will keep a year, if you can forbear eating them, the roots and bark much longer.

7. This art was plainly and first invented for delicacy, yet came afterwards to be of excellent use in physic. For,

First, hereby medicines are made pleasant for sick and queasy stomachs, which else would loath them.

Secondly, hereby they are preserved from decaying a long time.

CHAP. IX. *Of Lohochs.*

1. THAT which the *Arabians* call *Lohochs* and the *Greeks Elegma*, the *Latins* call *Linctus*, and in plain *English* signifies nothing else, but a thing to be licked up.

2. Their first invention was to prevent and remedy afflictions of the breast and lungs, to cleanse the lungs of phlegm, and make it fit to be cast out.

3. They are in body thicker than a syrup, and not so thick as an electuary.

4. The manner of taking them, is often to take a little with a liquorish stick, and let it go down at leisure.

5. They are easily thus made: make a decoction of pectoral herbs, and the treatise will furnish you with enough, and when you have strained it, with twice its weight of honey or sugar, boil it to a *Lohoch*, if you are molested with tough phlegm, honey is better than sugar, and if you add a little vinegar to it, you will do well, if not I hold sugar to be better than honey.

6. It is kept in pots, and may be kept a year and longer.

7. It is excellent for roughness of the wind pipe, inflammations of the lungs, ulcers in the lungs, difficulty of breath, asthmas, coughs, and distillations of humours.

CHAP.

CHAP. X. *Of Ointments.*

1. VARIOUS are the ways of making ointments, which authors have left to posterity, which I shall omit, and quote one which is easiest to be made, and therefore most beneficial to people that are ignorant in physic, for whose sake I write this. It is thus done.

Bruise those herbs, flowers, or roots, you will make an ointment of, and to two handfuls of your bruised herbs add a pound of hog's grease dried, or cleansed from the skins, beat them very well together in a stone mortar with a wooden pestle, then put it in a stone pot, (the herb and grease I mean, not the mortar) cover it with a paper, and let it either in the sun, or some other warm place, three, four, or five days, that it may melt, then take it out and boil it a little; then whilst it is hot, strain it out, pressing it out very hard in a press; to this grease add as many more herbs bruised as before, let them stand in like manner as long; then boil them as you did the former; if you think your ointment be not strong enough, you may do it the third and fourth time; yet this I tell you, the fuller of juice the herbs are, the sooner will your ointments be strong. The last time you boil it, boil it so long till your herbs be crisp, and the juice consumed, then strain it, pressing it hard in a press, and to every pound of ointment add two ounces of turpentine, and as much wax, because grease is offensive to wounds, as well as oil.

2. Ointments are vulgarly known to be kept in pots, and will last above a year, some above two years.

CHAP. XI. *Of Plaisters.*

1. THE *Greeks* made their plaisters of divers simples, and put metals into most of them if not all, for having reduced their metal into powder, they mixed them with that fatty substance whereof the rest of the plaister consisted, whilst it was yet hot, continually stirring it up and down, lest it should sink to the bottom, so they continually stirred it till it was finished, then they made it up in rolls, which when they needed for use, they could melt by fire again.

2. The

2. The *Arabians* made up theirs with oil and fat, which needeth not so long boiling.

3. The *Greeks* emplaisters consisted of these ingredients, metals, stones, divers sorts of earth, feces, juices, liquors, seeds, roots, herbs, excrements of creatures, wax, rosin, gems.

CHAP. XII. *Of Poultices.*

1. POULTICES are those kind of things which the *Latins* call *Cataplasmata*, and our learned fellows, that if they can read *English*, that's all, call them *Cataplasms*, because it is a crabbed word few understand; it is indeed a very fine kind of medicine to ripen sores.

2. They are made of herbs and roots, fitted for the disease and members afflicted, being chopped small, and boiled in water almost to a jelly; then by adding a little Barley-meal, or meal of Lupins, and a little oil, or rough sweet suet, which I hold to be better, spread upon a cloth and applied to the grieved place.

3. Their use is to ease pains, to break sores, to cool inflammations, to dissolve hardness, to ease the spleen, to concoct humours, and dissipate swellings.

4. I beseech you take this caution along with you; use no poultices (if you can help it) that are of an healing nature, before you have first cleansed the body, because they are subject to draw the humours to them from every part of the body.

CHAP. XIII. *Of Troches.*

1. THE *Latins* call them *Placentula*, or little cakes, (and you might have seen what the *Greeks* call them too, had not the last edition of my *English Dispensatory* been so hellishly printed, that's all the kingdom gets by one stationer printing another's copies. viz. to plague the country with false prints, and disgrace the author) the *Greeks* τροχισκοι, κυκλισκοι, and αρτισκοι, they are usually little round flat cakes, or you may make them square if you will.

2. Their first invention was, that powders being so kept might resist the intromission of air, and so endure pure the longer.

3. Besides, they are the easier carried in the pockets of such

such as travel; as many a man (for example) is forced to travel whose stomach is too cold, or at least not so hot as it should be, which is most proper, for the stomach is never cold till a man be dead; in such a case, it is better to carry troches of Wormwood, or Galangal, in a paper in his pocket, and more convenient by h.r, than to lug a gallipot along with him.

4. They are made thus. At night when you go to bed, take two drams of fine gum-tragacanth; put it into a gallipot, and put half a quarter of a pint of any distilled water, fitting for the purpose you would make your troches for, to it, to cover it, and the next morning you shall find it in such a jelly as the physicians call Mucilage. with this you may (with a little pains taking) make a powder into paste, and that paste into cakes called troches.

5. Having made them, dry them in the shade, and keep them in a pot for your use.

CHAP. XIV. *Of Pills.*

1. THEY are called *Pilulæ*, because they resemble little balls; the *Greeks* call them *Catapotia*.

2. It is the opinion of modern physicians, that this way of making medicines, was invented only to deceive the palate, that so by swallowing them down whole, the bitterness of the medicine might not be perceived, or at least it might not be unsufferable, and indeed most of their pills, though not all, are very bitter.

3. I am of a clean contrary opinion to this; I rather think they were done up in this hard form, that so they might be the longer in digesting; and my opinion is grounded upon reason too, not upon fancy or hear say. The first invention of pills was to purge the head; now as I told you before, such infirmities as lie near the passages, were best removed by decoctions, because they pass to the grieved part soonest; so here, if the infirmity lies in the head, or any other remote part, the best way is to use pills, because they are longer in digestion, and therefore the better able to call the offending humour to them.

4. If I should tell you here a long tale of medicines working by sympathy and antipathy, you would not understand a word of it; they that are set to make physicians may find it in the treatise. All modern physicians know not what belongs to a sympathetical cure, no more than a cuckow what belongs

belongs to flats and sharps in music; but ollow the vulgar road, and call it a hidden quality, because it is hidden from the eyes of dunces, and indeed none but astrologers can give a reason for it; and physic without reason, is like a pudding without fat.

5. The way to make pills is very easy, for with the help of a pestle and mortar, and a little diligence, you may make any powder into pills, either with syrup, or the jelly I told you before.

CHAP ult. *The way of mixing Medicines, according to the cause of the Disease, and Part of the Body afflicted.*

THIS being indeed the key of the work, I shall be somewhat the more diligent in it. I shall deliver myself thus

1. To the Vulgar.
2. To such as study Astrology; or such as study Physic astrologically

First, To the vulgar. Kind souls, I am sorry it hath been your hard mishap to have been so long trained in such Egyptian darkness, even darkness which to your sorrow may be felt. The vulgar road of physic is not my practice, and I am therefore the more unfit to give you advice, and I have now published a little book which will fully instruct you not only in the knowledge of your own bodies, but also in fit medicines to remedy each part of it when afflicted; in the mean season take these few rules to stay your stomachs.

1 With the disease, regard the cause and the part of the body afflicted, for example, suppose a woman be subject to miscarry through wind, thus do

1. Look abortion in the table of diseases, and you shall be directed by that, how many herbs prevent miscarriage.
2. Look wind in the same table, and you shall see how many of those herbs expel wind

These are the herbs medicinal for your grief.

2 In all diseases strengthen the part of the body afflicted.
3. In mixt diseases there lies some difficulty, for sometimes two parts of the body are afflicted with contrary humours, as sometimes the liver is afflicted with choler and

water,

water, as when a man hath both the dropsy and the yellow jaundice; and this is usually mortal.

In the former, suppose the brain be too cold and moist, and the liver be too hot and dry; thus do.

1. Keep your head outwardly warm.
2. Accustom yourself to smell of hot herbs.
3. Take a pill that heats the head at night going to bed.
4. In the morning take a decoction that cools the liver, for that quickly passeth the stomach, and is at the liver immediately.

You must not think (courteous people) that I can spend time to give you examples of all diseases; these are enough to let you see so much light as you without art are able to receive; if I should set you to look at the sun, I should dazzle your eyes and make you blind.

Secondly, To such as study astrology, (who are the only men I know that are fit to study physic, physic without astrology being like a lamp without oil) you are the men I exceedingly respect, and such documents as my brain can give you at present (being absent from my study) I shall give you.

1. Fortify the body with herbs of the nature of the Lord of the Ascendant, it is no matter whether he be a fortune or infortune in this case.
2. Let your medicine be something antipathetical to the Lord of the sixth.
3. Let your medicine be something of the nature of the sign ascending.
4. If the Lord of the tenth be strong, make use of his medicines.
5. If this cannot well be, make use of the medicines of the light of time.
6. Be sure always to fortify the grieved part of the body by sympathetical remedies.
7. Regard the heart, keep that upon the wheels, because the sun is the fountain of life, and therefore those universal remedies, *Aurum Potabile*, and the philosopher's stone, cure all diseases by fortifying the heart.

The TABLE of Diseases.

A
ABORTION 50 263 292
After birth 25 97 300
Agues 14 134 284
Aposthumes 78 126 221
St Anthony's fire 33 165
Almonds in the ears 41 237
Asthma 317
Apoplexy 169 89 194

B
Blindness 175 109
Blows 181 203
Belly-ach 63 202
Bloody urine 5 38
Barrenness 18 206
Belching 56
Biting of mad dogs 35 157
Bruises inward 5
Brains 126
Bleeding 5 153 301
Bloody flux 5 122 159
Black jaundice 281 291
Breast 89 128 305
Burning 33 221
Bruises 30 79 206
Boils 26 81 263
Bones broken 48 114 275
Bowels 68 249
Back 91 309
Bladder 59 173

C
Conception helpeth 67 264
Carbuncles 272 311
Consumption of the lungs 184
Catarrhs 236 287
Cancers 5 79 125
Cankers 41 64 113 205
Child-birth 35 120
Chincough 300
Cholic 5 110 202 274
Cough 5 48 157 265 300
Choler 10 170 248

Cold 35 229 314
Chilblains 123 165
Convulsion 2 48 143 296
Cramp 22 116 186
Costiveness 78
Curdled milk 30 142

D
Drowsiness 254
Difficulty of making water 22
Difficulty of breathing 58 97
Defluxions of blood 316
Dead child 48 118 223
Deafness 66 184 283
Distillations 47 51
Dropsy 10 35 146 199 291
Dimness of sight 8 223
Dreams 170 190 238
Defluxions of rheum 236 253
Deformity 121 287
Dysury 30 89 142

E
Expel the dead birth 264
Eyes pained and watering 8
Expel wind 161 300
Ears 72 166 272
Epidemical diseases 12 41
Eyes 4 30 307 308

F
Films in the eyes 119
Flux of blood 279 315
Falling sickness 79 152 264
Flegm 9 121 303
Fevers 27 103 315
Flux 14 56 161 211
Freckles 48 113 317
French pox 14 149 291
Frenzy 159 307

G
Gout in the hands 9
Green wounds 229 275
Gout 13 107 300 311
Gravel 107 237 307

Gout

The TABLE of Diseases.

Groin 202

H
Hip gout 79
Hectic fever 47
Head-ach 108 277
Heart 56 309
Hemorrhoids 121 202
Hoarseness 79 264
Humours 126
Hiccough 102 190
Heat of urine 173

I
Inflammations 108 149
——— in the breasts 11
——— in wounds 204
Iliac passion 272
Imposthumes 126 190
Itch 79 237 251
Indigestion 68 249

K
Kibes 149
Knots and kernels in the flesh 79 85 100
King's evil 17 257
Kidneys 92 309

L
Lasks 201 249
Loins pained 309
Leprosy 121 250 314
Lethargy 169 237
Liver 90 157 301
Lice 52 155 291
Loathing of meat 104 187
Loose teeth 238 293
Lungs 12 122 317
Lust provokes 77 190 211

M
Milk amends 119 309
Member disjointed 147 233
Marks 175 223 267
Mad dogs biting 73 190
Measles 48 286 301

Melancholy 25 198 309
Memory 20 163 264
Mother 16 103 272
Milk in Nurses 45 234
Morphew 48 104 237
Miscarriage 187
Mushrooms 25 119

N
Nocturnal pollutions 111 10
Navels of children 238 290
Nipples 126
Nerves 28 211
Noise in the ears 8 155
Nose 160
Noli me tangere 128

O
Obstructions of the liver 20 114
——— of the reins 202
——— of the spleen 21 214
Open the spleen and the liver 12

P
Pain in the bowels 290
——— in the stomach 27 285
Preserve health 318
Plague sores 241
Pin and web 147 172
Passion of the heart 112 253
Pestilential fevers 173 229
Pains in the ears and sides 78 184
Palsy 79 163 264 317
Piles 86 187 232
Pissing of blood 92 158
Plague 8 24 286
Pestilence 13 56 254 307
Pleurisy 126 237
Poison 12 103 190 281
Phythisic 173 255
Pushes 126 250
Pimples 103 249 293

P 4 pus

The TABLE of Diseases.

Polypus 97 233
Privities 175

Q
Quartian agues 114 233
Quinsy 43 155
Quotidian agues 113

R
Raw humours 90 102
Retention of meat 249
Rheum 90 167
Red face 77 158
Reins 173 249
Rickets 108 296
Ringworms 48 147
Ruptures 41 79 100 301

S
Sore breast 124 238
Scabby head 181 301
Sore gums 237
Sore mouth and throat 267 276 308
Skin 97 301
Scabs 45 79 100 257
Sours 17 24
Sciatica 126 237 293
Scurf 121 181 315
Shortness of breath 97 253
Small pox 186 301
Spleen 17 190 237
Spitting of blood 104 291
Surfeits 2 6
Stitches 52 264
Stranguary 178 190
Swellings of the cods 108 260
Stone 81 251
Swooning 45 223

Teeth clean 10
Testicles 93 205

Tough phlegm 2 2
Tertian agues 210 289
Tetters 157 249 314
Tooth-ach 22 79 282
Trembling 91 169

U
Urine provokes 20 22
Ulcers in the privities 9 293 307
——— in the nose 260
Venereal sores 272
Vertigo 20 109
Veneri 31 210
Vomiting 56 190 249

W
Womens courses stop or provoke 78 79 272 273
Womens breasts 250
Whites stop 52 205
Wheals 234 21
Wheesing 1 237 307
Wind cholic 68 271
Watching 109 217
Worts 53 12 22
Weariness 2 237
Wen 121 303
Witchcraft 28 154
Women in easy delivery 86 225
Whitlow 8 206
Wind 52 122
Warts 9 264 311
Womb 16 123 307
Wound 25 161 301
Wry neck 114 203
Weakness 91

Y
Yellow jaundice 79 157 254

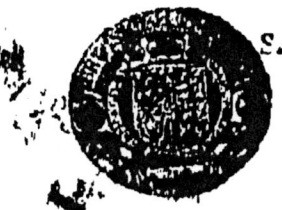

The TABLE of Diseases

... 97 233
Privities 175

Q
Quartian agues 114 233
... 153
Quotidian ... 133

R
Raw humours 90 102
Retention of meat 249
Return 90 167
Red faces 77 158
Reins 173 249
Rickets 108 296
Ringworms 48 147
Ruptures 41 79 100 307

S
Sore breast 124 138
Scabby head 181 301
Swoln gums 263
Sore mouth and throat 264
... 276 307
... 97 307
Scabs 46 79 100 347
Scars 17 2 4
Sciatica 126 237 293
Scurf 124 181 315
Shortness of breath 97 233
Small pox 186 301
Spleen 17 190 237
Spitting of blood 104 291
Surfeits ... 256
Stitches 52 261
... 173 190
Swellings of the cods 108 260
Stone 66 251
Swooning 46 223

T
Teeth clean 10
... 93 205

Tough phlegm 3 21
Tertian agues ... 289
Tetters 137 249 314
Tooth-ach 22 79 ...
Trembling 91 169

U
Urine provokes 20 2 2
Ulcers in the privities 9 293 307
——— in the nose 260
Venereal sores 272
Vertigo 28 169
Venery 31 210
Vomiting 56 190 249

W
Womens courses stop or provoke 78 79 2 2 273
Womens breasts ... 250
Whites stop 52 205
Wheals 234 2 1
Waceful... 15 237 307
Wind cholic 68 271
Watching 149 217
Worts 53 12 202
Weariness 32 237
Wens 121 303
Witchcraft 28 154
Womens speedy delivery 86 225
Whitloes 8 206
Wind 52 122
Worms 9 264 311
Womb 16 120 307
Wounds 35 161 301
Wry neck 114 203
Wrinkles 91

Y
Yellow jaundice 79 157 254

CPSIA information can be obtained at www.ICGtesting.com
Printed in the USA
LVOW121927031011

248894LV00013B/113/P